ASSESSING

GENETIC RISKS

IMPLICATIONS FOR HEALTH AND SOCIAL POLICY

Lori B. Andrews, Jane E. Fullarton,
Neil A. Holtzman, and Arno G. Motulsky, *Editors*

Committee on Assessing Genetic Risks
Division of Health Sciences Policy
Institute of Medicine

NATIONAL ACADEMY PRESS
Washington, D.C.   1994

NATIONAL ACADEMY PRESS • 2101 Constitution Ave., N.W. • Washington, D.C. 20418

NOTICE: The project that is the subject of this report was approved by the Governing Board of the National Research Council, whose members are drawn from the councils of the National Academy of Sciences, the National Academy of Engineering, and the Institute of Medicine. The members of the committee responsible for the report were chosen for their special competencies and with regard for appropriate balance.

This report has been reviewed by a group other than the authors according to procedures approved by a Report Review Committee consisting of members of the National Academy of Sciences, the National Academy of Engineering, and the Institute of Medicine.

The Institute of Medicine was chartered in 1970 by the National Academy of Sciences to enlist distinguished members of the appropriate professions in the examination of policy matters pertaining to the health of the public. In this, the Institute acts under both the Academy's 1863 congressional charter responsibility to be an adviser to the federal government and its own initiative in identifying issues of medical care, research, and education. Dr. Kenneth I. Shine is president of the Institute of Medicine.

This project was funded by the National Center for Human Genome Research of the National Institutes of Health (Contract No. NO1-HG-0-001) and by the Health Effects Research Program of the Department of Energy (Contract No. DE-FG05-91ER61115; DOE's support does not constitute an endorsement of the views expressed in the report). The Lucille B. Markey Charitable Trust provided supplemental funding of the study. Additional support for this project was provided by independent Institute of Medicine funds.

Library of Congress Cataloging-in-Publication Data

Assessing genetic risks : implications for health and social policy /
    Lori B. Andrews . . . [et al.] editors.
         p. cm.
    Includes bibliographical references and index.
    ISBN 0-309-04798-6
    1. Medical genetics—Social aspects. 2. Human chromosome
abnormalities—Diagnosis—Social aspects. 3. Medical policy—United
States. I. Andrews, Lori B., 1952- .
    [DNLM: 1. Hereditary Diseases—genetics. 2. Hereditary Diseases—
epidemiology. 3. Risk Factors. 4. Health Policy—United States.
QZ 50 A846 1994]
RB155.A76 1994
616'.042—dc20
DNLM/DLC
for Library of Congress   93-47973
                                        CIP

Printed in the United States of America.

The serpent has been a symbol of long life, healing, and knowledge among almost all cultures and religions since the beginning of recorded history. The image adopted as a logotype by the Institute of Medicine is based on a relief carving from ancient Greece, now held by the Staalichemuseen in Berlin.

COMMITTEE ON ASSESSING GENETIC RISKS

ARNO G. MOTULSKY (Chair),*+ Professor of Medicine and Genetics, Department of Medicine, Division of Medical Genetics, University of Washington, Seattle, Washington

LORI B. ANDREWS, Fellow, American Bar Foundation, Chicago, Illinois

BARBARA BOWLES BIESECKER, Genetic Counselor, University of Michigan Medical Center, Department of Internal Medicine, Ann Arbor, Michigan

JAMES F. CHILDRESS, Chairman, Department of Religious Studies, Edwin B. Kyle Professor of Religious Studies, University of Virginia, Charlottesville, Virginia

BARTON CHILDS,* Emeritus Professor of Pediatrics, The Johns Hopkins University School of Medicine, Baltimore, Maryland

FRANCIS S. COLLINS,*‡ Associate Investigator, Howard Hughes Medical Institute, and Professor, University of Michigan Medical Center, Ann Arbor, Michigan

P. MICHAEL CONNEALLY, Distinguished Professor of Medical and Molecular Genetics and Neurology, Indiana University School of Medicine, Indianapolis, Indiana

HELEN R. DONIS-KELLER, Director, Division of Human Molecular Genetics, Professor of Surgery and Genetics, Department of Surgery, Washington University School of Medicine, St. Louis, Missouri

NORMAN C. FOST, Professor of Pediatrics, University of Wisconsin School of Medicine, Department of Pediatrics, Madison, Wisconsin

NEIL A. HOLTZMAN, Professor of Pediatrics, Health Policy, and Management and Epidemiology, The Johns Hopkins University Hospital, Baltimore, Maryland

MICHAEL M. KABACK, Professor of Pediatrics and Reproductive Medicine, University of California-San Diego, San Diego, California

MARY-CLAIRE KING, Professor of Genetics and Epidemiology, Department of Molecular and Cell Biology, School of Public Health, University of California at Berkeley, Berkeley, California

PATRICIA A. KING,* Professor of Law, Georgetown University Law Center, Washington, D.C.

ALEXANDER LEAF,* Jackson Professor of Clinical Medicine, Emeritus, Harvard University Medical School and Distinguished Physician, Veterans Affairs Medical Center, Brockton/West Roxbury, Massachusetts

PETER LIBASSI, Dean, Barney School of Business and Public Administration, University of Hartford, West Hartford, Connecticut; formerly Senior Vice President, Travelers, Hartford, Connecticut

ROBERT F. MURRAY, Jr.,* Professor of Pediatrics, Medicine, Oncology, and Genetics, Howard University College of Medicine, Washington, D.C.

GERALD D. ROSENTHAL,*§ Resident Consultant, Egyptian Junior Medical Doctors Association, c/o Pathfinder International, Watertown, Massachusetts

MARK A. ROTHSTEIN, Law Foundation Professor of Law, and Director, Health Law and Policy Institute, University of Houston Law Center, Houston, Texas

CLAUDIA T. WEICKER, Hartford, Connecticut

NANCY SABIN WEXLER, Professor of Clinical Neuropsychology, Departments of Neurology and Psychiatry, College of Physicians and Surgeons, Columbia University, New York, New York; President, Hereditary Disease Foundation, Santa Monica, California

Liaison Panel to the Committee on Assessing Genetic Risks

FRANK FUJIMURA, Scientific Director of Molecular Biology, Nichols Institute Reference Laboratories, San Juan Capistrano, California

PHILIP R. REILLY, Executive Director, Shriver Center for Mental Retardation, Waltham, Massachusetts

Staff

JANE EVALYN FULLARTON, Study Director
C. ELAINE LAWSON, Research Associate
RUTH ELLEN BULGER, Director, Division of Health Sciences Policy
MARY JANE BALL, Project Assistant
NANCY DIENER, Financial Assistant
PHILOMENA MAMMEN, Administrative Assistant

---

*Member, Institute of Medicine
+Member, National Academy of Sciences
‡Resigned from the committee April 1993.
§Resigned after first meeting of the committee.

Preface

The last decade has seen remarkable growth in the understanding of genetics as applied to medicine. In addition, the technology for the detection of genetic diseases has developed rapidly, and testing for genetic diseases with DNA techniques has become increasingly possible. The last few years have also seen the initiation of the Human Genome Project, the aim of which is mapping and ultimately sequencing all human genes—giving special attention to genes that cause or may predispose to disease. As part of this ambitious project, and for the first time in the history of science, a special effort is being made as part of a large research project to explore its broader social implications. Three to five percent of the funding available for the Human Genome Project has been set aside to study the many social, ethical, and legal implications that will result from better understanding of human heredity and its impact on disease. Since assessment of genetic risks by genetic testing is expanding rapidly, the Institute of Medicine (IOM) of the National Academy of Sciences undertook this study to assess the current status and future implications of such testing. This study deals with some of the scientific aspects of genetic risk assessment as well as the many societal problems that have already arisen and are likely to be posed by future developments. The study was supported jointly by the National Center for Human Genome Research at the National Institutes of Health and by the Department of Energy, Health Effects Program of the Life Science Research Office. Supplemental funding was provided by the Markey Charitable Trust, a private foundation, and these funds were matched by the Institute of Medicine.

A multidisciplinary Committee on Assessing Genetic Risks was constituted and held a series of workshops and meetings (including a public meeting) on the many phases of genetic testing and its impact on patients, providers, and laboratories. Based on the information gleaned from the many expert participants in these workshops, the public, the appropriate scientific and policy literature, and extensive discussions at committee meetings, the report was written. As part of its process, the committee had the benefit of a Liaison Panel whose members had industrial relationships. This panel worked with the committee during the information gathering activities; once recommendations and report writing began, the liaison members no longer participated.

The rapidly changing nature of the science and practice of genetic testing has led the committee to approach its recommendations by providing general principles that we hope will be useful today and for the next few years. We tried, whenever possible, to avoid technical complexities without sacrificing scientific accuracy to make our conclusions available to as large an audience as possible.

Our committee hopes that this report will be widely read, not only by various health professionals interested in genetics and medicine, but by a broad audience who makes and influences public policy, such as federal and state legislators, other officials and their staff, members of genetic support groups, and the public. Health professionals, an interested public, and policy makers will need to be well informed to move forward with thoughtful and judicious decision making in this area. These recommendations must be based on solid facts and, at the same time, recognize and respect the multifaceted aspects of our pluralistic society. These recommendations are the result of carefully considered judgment, based on a careful review of the state of the art of genetic testing today and our vision of the future. Since currently no single voice has the authority to make policy recommendations in the field of genetic risk assessment and testing, it is hoped the findings of this broadly based multidisciplinary IOM committee will serve as a set of recommendations on which future decisions can be based.

We addressed the need for better professional training of health professionals and of human and medical geneticists. Many genetic tests will be ordered and interpreted by primary care health practitioners, and not only by geneticists or genetic counselors. A good understanding of genetics will therefore be required for all health care professionals. A movement of genetic testing from academic institutions to commercial laboratories is taking place already and will increase as larger volumes of genetic tests are being ordered. The regulation of laboratories sufficiently expert to carry out genetic testing as well as quality control of testing takes on great importance and we have developed a series of recommendations on these important matters.

Various health care providers and medical geneticists already have considerable experience with newborn screening, with prenatal diagnosis, with carrier testing in high-risk populations, and with testing for a variety of genetic diseases. However, the development of genetic tests for diseases that manifest in middle and late life is just beginning to be explored. It is in this area that much new ground needs to be covered. While interpretation of tests for single gene disorders of late onset, including familial cancer, is not easy, the complexities of testing and interpretations for the gene constellations that predispose to many common diseases such as coronary heart disease, diabetes mellitus, hypertension, and others raise new problems. These dilemmas will become particularly thorny if testing for the yet undiscovered genes predisposing to common psychiatric diseases such as schizophrenia and manic depressive disorders becomes a reality.

Testing of DNA from various body tissues for the early mutational events that predispose to a variety of common cancers is on the horizon. This area of genetic testing promises to revolutionize early cancer detection and poses many problems of health monitoring.

Many issues raised by genetic testing do not have a single or unambiguous solution, and different well-informed and well-meaning observers may disagree with each other. Public health oriented policy makers, many physicians, and a significant proportion of the public might consider the reduction of genetic disease as a principal goal of work in this area. Our committee stressed the importance of autonomous decision making by individuals and by the family even if the development of a genetic disease might be the outcome. We believe that in a society such as ours, autonomy far outweighs any public health considerations. In practice, most informed couples do, in fact, select various courses of actions that lead to a lower frequency of genetic disease.

There is a strong and continuing tradition of nondirective genetic counseling in medical genetics, and we were emphatic in stressing nondirectiveness. However, impressed by medical advances that can lead to prevention and treatment of some genetic diseases, many of us feel that there is an obligation under such circumstances to provide appropriate medical advice with guidance to select a specific preventive or therapeutic course of action after a full discussion of all consequences (including possible insurance repercussions and employment discrimination). At the same time, all committee members strongly uphold the principle of nondirective counseling for *reproductive* decisions.

Arno G. Motulsky, M.D., Sc.D.
Chair

ADDITIONAL VIEWS OF THE CHAIRMAN*

Our report may strike some observers as emphasizing the problematic aspects of genetic testing. All members of the Committee on Assessing Genetic Risks are excited about the great promise and potential of genetic testing for the prevention and treatment of genetic diseases. Since the positive aspects of genetic testing are clear, this perspective required less explication. Our report, therefore, covers in

*The opinions expressed are my own and do not represent the consensus of a majority of the committee.

some detail the difficulties raised by genetic testing and screening, and suggests some solutions and guidelines.

Our emphasis on genetic education may be considered somewhat utopian when an increasing proportion of the population is illiterate and dropout rates in high schools are rising. Nevertheless, we feel that an understanding of genetics will be most important in the future, not only for an appreciation of the role of genetics in health and disease, but also for making decisions on issues such as the use of foods developed with DNA technologies. Even though we may not be able to educate everyone, much more intensive coverage of genetics in the schools at all levels, as well as responsible reporting in the media, is something to which all of us strongly subscribe.

The recommendations regarding newborn screening represent somewhat ideal scenarios that may require some modification in practice. For example, even though full genetic education and counseling would be ideal prior to newborn screening, such a practice may not be currently realistic. For every single affected infant, there will be many thousands of unaffected children. Pretest education and counseling in such a situation cannot, by necessity, be as comprehensive as in scenarios where the pretest probability for a child to be affected is high. However, once a child is found to be affected, equally intensive counseling and appropriate follow-up are indicated in both situations.

The majority of our committee was persuaded that voluntary participation in neonatal screening was the best way to ensure that children would be screened and parental autonomy maintained. Everyone agreed that testing should always be offered for phenylketonuria (PKU) and hypothyroidism since early treatment is highly successful. Some committee members feel that mandatory screening for these two conditions would be a simpler solution.

The common, medically innocuous sickle cell trait will frequently be detected in African-American children as a side product of newborn testing for sickle cell anemia. Once this knowledge—with its significant reproductive implications for the parents—is available, such information is difficult to withhold and in my opinion should be given to the mother with appropriate genetic counseling.

There is agreement that information regarding carrier status of a medically innocuous genetic trait should not be used to discriminate against a child being considered for adoption. However, once a disease has been diagnosed or if there is a high risk of a medically significant condition, I believe strongly that prospective adoptive parents should be provided this information.

Arno G. Motulsky, M.D., Sc.D.
Chair

Acknowledgments

In addition to the work of the committee and staff, the successful completion of a study such as this requires assistance from many people. The committee wishes to express its sincere gratitude to those who participated in and prepared papers for the workshops and public forum (see Appendix A and Volume 2). The committee also wishes to thank those who prepared background papers: David A. Micklos, Director of the DNA Learning Center at the Cold Spring Harbor Laboratory, for his paper on issues in public education (Volume 2); Ann C. M. Smith for her background paper on professional personnel issues prepared in collaboration with Jane Fullarton and C. Elaine Lawson of the committee staff; and Kathi E. Hanna who contributed background papers on genetic testing and genetic counseling, as well as material on personnel issues.

We owe special recognition and thanks to Jane Fullarton, study director, who helped to organize the committee, guided us through the study process, organized the workshops that were essential to the committee's deliberations, edited Volume 2 of the committee report, and assumed substantial responsibility for the preparation of this report. C. Elaine Lawson, research associate, also contributed to this report by collecting and cataloging references, by drafting charts and tables throughout the report, by preparing the data base on public education in genetics, and especially by developing the public education chapter. We also thank Linda Clark and Mary Jane Ball, project assistants, who helped with meeting planning and logistics and prepared briefing books, and especially Mary Jane Ball for her work on the papers in Volume 2. Thanks to Nancy Diener, financial assistant for her help throughout the project. For their editorial assistance, the committee thanks Michael Edington and Betsy Turvene, Institute of Medicine (IOM) editors, and Florence Poillon and Paul Phelps for their consultant editing on the report. Many thanks to Ruth Ellen Bulger, director of the Division of Health Sciences Policy, IOM, who provided policy advice and guidance throughout the course of this study.

This study took place during a period of transition at the Institute of Medicine. Samuel Thier was president of the IOM at the initiation of the study. Stuart Bondurant served as acting president during the transition to the presidency of Kenneth Shine, who assumed his full responsibilities in July 1992. The committee appreciates the leadership provided by them during the course of the study, as well as the oversight provided by Enriqueta Bond, IOM executive officer.

Finally, support for this study was provided jointly by the National Center for Human Genome Research of the National Institutes of Health (NIH) and the Health Effects Research Program of the Department of Energy (DOE). Our special thanks go to Eric Juengst, NIH project officer, and Daniel Drell, DOE project officer, for their support during the study and for their approval of the change in study scope that made the current state-of-the-art assessment of genetic testing possible. We also wish to thank Robert Glaser and Nancy Weber of the Markey Charitable Trust for their supplemental funding of the study, and the Institute of Medicine for matching the Markey Trust funding.

Contents

This report includes a number of recommendations that the committee hopes will achieve the goal of acquiring and using genetic information in health care in a manner that respects the autonomy of individuals.

Genetic testing may raise complex or novel questions about the right to access information, and these questions may have legal ramifications. This report should not be interpreted as creating a set of legal guidelines. Relevant laws and regulations will vary from state to state. Clinicians or other persons who have questions about the appropriate management of genetic information may on occasion wish to consider seeking legal counsel.

Assessing
Genetic Risks

Executive Summary

Approximately 3 percent of all children are born with a severe disorder that is presumed to be genetic in origin, and several thousand definite or suspected single-gene diseases have been described. Most of these diseases manifest themselves early in life, although some inherited diseases—and many others that have a genetic component—have their onset much later in life (e.g., diabetes mellitus or mental illness). Then there are many disorders in which both genetic and environmental factors play major roles (e.g., coronary heart disease, hypertension). These "complex" disorders are more common than single-gene diseases and thus, in the aggregate, constitute a greater public health burden. Many disease genes can be detected in individuals before symptoms occur, but for many common diseases with some genetic basis, such as heart disease and cancer, the detection of genetic alterations might only indicate susceptibility, not the certainty of disease.

PROMISE AND PROBLEMS IN GENETIC TESTING

The ability to diagnose genetic disease has developed rapidly over the past 20 years, and the Human Genome Project, with its ambitious goal of mapping and sequencing the entire genome, will bring a further explosion in our knowledge of the structure and function of human genes. The ultimate goals of these scientific advances are the treatment, cure, and eventual prevention of genetic disorders, but effective interventions lag behind the ability to detect disease or increased susceptibility to disease. Thus, many genetic services today consist of diagnosis and counseling; effective treatment is rare. Nevertheless, as more genes are identified, there is growing pressure to broaden existing screening programs, and otherwise increase both the number of available genetic tests and the volume of genetic information they generate.

The rapidly changing science and practice of genetic testing raise a number of scientific, ethical, legal, and social issues. The national investment in the Human Genome Project will greatly increase the capacity to detect genes leading to disease susceptibility. It will also greatly increase the availability of genetic testing over the next 5 to 10 years, identifying the genetic basis for diseases—even some newly discovered to be genetic—and increasing the number of tests for detecting them. The emergence of the biotechnology industry increases the likelihood that these findings will be rapidly translated into widely available test kits and diagnostic products. Entrepreneurial pressure may also lead to the development of commercial and academic "genetic testing services" that would not be regulated under current Food and Drug Administration (FDA) procedures. Problems of laboratory quality control would be heightened by the introduction of "multiplex" tests that detect the presence of numerous genetic markers—for disease, carrier status, and susceptibility alike—at the same time. And the potential for generating all of this genetic information about individuals raises serious questions of informed consent, confidentiality, and discrimination. Over the next five to ten years, there will be an increasing number of personal and public policy decisions related to genetic testing; well-trained health professionals and an interested and informed public will both be key to that decision making.

As genetic screening becomes more widespread, these issues threaten to outrun current ethical and regulatory standards, as well as the training of health professionals. There will be a need for greater numbers of genetics specialists, but genetic testing is no longer just for specialists. Increasingly, primary care providers will be called upon to administer tests, counsel patients, and protect their privacy. Government officials and the broader public will also be called upon to participate in setting public policy for genetic testing and in making difficult decisions, public and private, based on the results of genetic tests. Consequently, there must be a significant increase in genetics education, both in the medical curriculum and for all Americans. Finally, there will be a need for centralized oversight to ensure that new genetic tests are accurate and effective, that they are performed and interpreted with close to "zero-error" tolerance, and that the results of genetic testing are not used to discriminate against individuals in employment or health insurance.

COMMITTEE ON ASSESSING GENETIC RISKS

This study of the scientific, ethical, legal, and social issues implicit in the field of genetic diagnosis, testing, and screening was supported jointly by the National Center for Human Genome Research at the National Institutes of Health and the Department of Energy's Health Effects and Life Sciences Research Office. Supplemental funding was also provided by the Markey Charitable Trust and the Institute of Medicine. The Committee on Assessing Genetic Risks hopes that this report will be widely read, not only by various health professionals interested in genetics and preventive medicine, but by a wide-ranging audience who makes and influences public policy in the United States, including members of genetic support groups and the public.

The establishment of the Ethical, Legal, and Social Implications (ELSI) Program in the Human Genome Project (HGP) and the set-aside of the first 3 to 5 percent of the HGP research budget for the study of ethical, legal, and social issues is unique in the history of science. This support gives us the opportunity to "worry in advance" about the implications and impacts of the mapping and sequencing of the human genome, including several thousand human disease genes, *before* wide-scale genetic diagnosis, testing, and screening come into practice, rather than *after* the problems have presented themselves in full relief.

The committee took its starting point from the wise advice of the 1975 National Academy of Sciences study *Genetic Screening: Programs, Principles, and Research*:

> Screening programs for genetic diseases and characteristics . . . have multiplied rapidly in the past decade, and many have been begun without prior testing and evaluation and not always for reasons of health alone. Changes in disease patterns and a new emphasis on preventive medicine, as well as recent and rapid advances in genetics, indicate that screening for genetic characteristics will become more common in the future. These conditions, together with the mistakes already made, suggested the need for a review of current screening practices that would identify the problems and difficulties and give some procedural guidance, in order to minimize the shortcomings and maximize the effectiveness of future genetic screening programs.

These words, written almost 20 years ago, remain just as valid today for genetic testing and diagnosis. The committee reaffirms the sentiments expressed in the 1975 report and hopes to update and broaden their application for the 1990s and beyond.

As a result, the committee has posed its recommendations in terms of general principles that we hope will be useful today—and for some years into the future—for the evaluation of expanded genetic diagnosis, testing, and screening. Although these recommendations reflect what is known today, and what experts foresee for the next few years, the committee had no crystal ball and, therefore, tried to develop criteria and to suggest processes for assessing when new tests are ready for pilot introduction and for widespread application in the population.

The committee's fundamental ethical principles include *voluntariness, informed consent, and confidentiality,* which in turn derive from respect for autonomy, equity, and privacy. Other committee principles described in the report include the necessity of (1) *high-quality tests (of high specificity and sensitivity) performed with the highest level of proficiency and interpreted correctly*; and (2) *conveying information to clients—both before and after testing—in an easily understood manner through genetic education and counseling that is relevant to the needs and concerns of the client.* These principles are the absolute foundation of genetic testing.

It is the view of the committee that, *until benefits and risks have been defined, genetic testing and screening programs remain a form of human investigation.* Therefore, routine use of tests should be preceded by pilot studies that demonstrate their safety and effectiveness. Standard safeguards should be applied in conducting these pilot studies, and independent review of the pilot studies should be conducted to determine whether the test should be offered clinically. Publicly supported population-based screening programs are justified only for disorders of significant severity, impact, frequency, and distribution, and when there is consensus that the available interventions warrant the expenditure of funds. **Informed consent should be an essential element of all screening. These principles and procedures described above should apply to genetic testing regardless of the setting, whether in primary medical practice, public programs, or any other settings.**

GENETIC TESTING AND ASSESSMENT

Genetic tests include the many different laboratory assays used to diagnose or predict a genetic condition or the susceptibility to genetic disease. *Genetic testing* denotes the use of specific assays to determine the genetic status of individuals already suspected to be at high risk for a particular inherited condition because of family history or clinical symptoms; *genetic screening* involves the use of various genetic tests to evaluate populations or groups of individuals independent of a family history of a disorder. However, these terms are commonly used interchangeably, and the committee has generally used the term *genetic testing* unless a specific aspect of genetic screening alone is being discussed. *Genetic counseling* refers to the communication process by which individuals and their family members are given information about the nature, recurrence risk, burden, risks and benefits of tests, and meaning of test results, including reproductive options of a genetic condition, as well as counseling and support concerning the implications of such genetic information.

Newborn Screening

At the present time, there are 10 genetic conditions for which some states screen newborns, although the scope of such screening varies by state (see Table 1). It is also possible to extract DNA from the newborn blood "spots" that are used for these tests. There is increasing pressure to test old blood samples for a wide variety of disorders, as well as to do DNA testing on newborns for a wide

TABLE 1 Genetic Disorders for Which Newborns Were Screened in the United States in 1990

Disorder	No. of States That Provided Screening[a]
Phenylketonuria	52
Congenital hypothyroidism[b]	52
Hemoglobinopathy	42[c]
Galactosemia	38
Maple syrup urine disorder	22
Homocysteinuria	21
Biotinidase deficiency	14
Adrenal hyperplasia	8
Tyrosinemia	5
Cystic fibrosis	3[d]

[a]Includes District of Columbia, Puerto Rico, and U.S. Virgin Islands.
[b]Only a proportion of cases have a genetic etiology.
[c]Utah's hemoglobinopathy pilot study (6-1-90 through 3-31-91) has been discontinued.
[d]Wisconsin's cystic fibrosis screening program is for research purposes only.

SOURCE: Council of Regional Networks for Genetic Services, 1992.

variety of disorders in the future. **As basic principles to govern newborn screening, the committee recommends that such screening take place only when (1) there is a clear indication of benefit to the newborn, (2) a system is in place to confirm the diagnosis, and (3) treatment and follow-up are available for affected newborns.** In addition, the committee does not believe that newborns should be screened using multiplex testing for many disorders at one time unless all of the disorders meet the principles described by the committee in this report (see Chapters 2 and 8).

To determine clear benefit to the newborn, well-designed and peer-reviewed pilot studies are required to demonstrate the safety and effectiveness of the proposed screening program. In pilot studies for new population-based newborn screening programs, parents should be informed of the investigational nature of the test and have the opportunity to consent to the participation of their infant. **Since some existing programs may not have been subject to careful evaluation, the committee recommends that ongoing programs be reviewed periodically, preferably by an independent body that is authorized to add, eliminate, or modify existing programs** (see Chapters 1, 3, and 9). The need for ongoing review and revision also suggests that detailed statutory requirements for specific tests may be unduly inflexible; state statutes should provide guidance for standards—not prescriptions. **The committee recommends that states with newborn screening programs for treatable disorders also have programs** available to ensure that necessary treatment and follow-up services are provided to affected children identified through newborn screening without regard to ability to pay. Informed consent should also be an integral part of newborn screening, including disclosure of the benefits and risks of the tests and treatments. **Finally, mandatory screening has not been shown to be essential to achieve maximum public health benefits; however, it is appropriate to mandate the** *offering* **of established tests (e.g., phenylketonuria, hypothyroidism) where early diagnosis leads to improved treatable outcomes.** (See Chapter 8.)

Newborns should not be screened for the purpose of determining the carrier status of the newborn or its parents for autosomal recessive disorders. Instead, couples in high-risk populations who are considering reproduction should be offered carrier screening for themselves (see below). When carrier status may be incidentally determined in newborn screening (e.g., in sickle cell screening), parents should be informed in advance about the benefits and limitations of genetic information, and that this information is not relevant to the health of their child. If they ask for the results of the incidentally determined carrier status for their own reproductive planning, it should be communicated to them in the context of genetic counseling, and they should be informed that misattributed paternity could be revealed. **Newborn screening programs should include provision for counseling of parents who are informed that the child is affected with a genetic disorder.**

The committee recognizes the complexities of identifying information about misattributed paternity. **On balance, the committee recommends that information on misattributed paternity be communicated to the mother, but not be volunteered to the woman's partner.** There may be special circumstances that warrant such disclosure, but these situations present difficult counseling challenges (see Chapters 4 and 8).

Stored newborn blood spots should be made available for additional research only if identifiers have been removed. As with other research involving human subjects, research proposals for the subsequent use of newborn blood spots should be reviewed by an appropriate institutional review board. If identifiable information is to be disclosed, informed consent of the infant's parent or guardian should be obtained prior to use of the specimen (see Chapters 2 and 8 for further discussion). Although DNA typing will provide new tools for newborn screening, in general, the committee recommends that these tools be employed only (1) when genetic heterogeneity of conditions to be detected is small; (2) when the sensitivity of detecting disease-causing mutations is high; (3) when costs are reasonable; and (4) when the benefits to newborns of early detection are clear.

Carrier Identification

Carrier testing is usually provided for purposes of reproductive planning. **The committee recommends that couples in high-risk populations who are** considering reproduction be offered carrier screening before pregnancy if possible. Standard safeguards such as institutional review and demonstrated safety and effectiveness should be applied in initiating any carrier detection program. First, the test should be accurate, sensitive, and specific. In the future, such screening will be done increasingly as part of routine medical care; the same principles should apply regardless of the setting. Carrier testing and screening should also be voluntary, with high standards of informed consent and attention to telling individuals or couples, in easily understood terms, the medical and social choices available to them should they be found at risk for disease in their off-spring, including termination of the pregnancy. Research is needed to develop innovative methods for providing carrier testing in young adults before pregnancy and to evaluate these methods through pilot studies. The committee had reservations about carrier screening programs in the high school setting in the United States and about carrier screening of persons younger than age 18.

With improving technology, carrier status for many different rare autosomal and X-linked recessive disorders will be detectable by multiplex technology (see Chapters 1 and 8). Obtaining appropriate informed consent before testing for each of these disorders will be a challenge (see Chapter 4). **Multiplexed tests should, therefore, be grouped into categories of tests (and disorders) that raise similar issues and implications for informed consent and for genetic education and counseling** (see Chapters 1, 4, and 8). If carrier status is detected, individuals should be informed of their carrier status to allow testing and counseling to be offered to their partners. Usually, the partner will be found not to be a carrier; however, if both partners are carriers, they should be referred for genetic counseling to help them understand available reproductive options, including the possibility of abortion of an affected fetus identified through prenatal diagnosis.

Prenatal Diagnosis

Anyone considering prenatal diagnosis must be fully informed about the risks and benefits of both the testing procedure and the possible outcomes, as well as alternative options that might be available. Disclosure should include full information concerning the spectrum of severity of the genetic disorders for which prenatal diagnosis is being offered (e.g., cystic fibrosis or fragile X). Furthermore, invasive prenatal diagnosis is only justified if the diagnostic procedures are accurate, sensitive, and specific for the disorder(s) for which prenatal diagnosis is being offered. **Standards of care for prenatal screening and diagnosis should also include education and counseling before and after the test, either directly or by referral, and ongoing counseling should also be available following termination of pregnancies.**

The committee believes that *offering* prenatal diagnosis is an appropriate standard of care in circumstances associated with increased risk of carrying a fetus with a diagnosable genetic disorder, including the increased risks associated with advanced maternal age. However, the committee was concerned about the use of prenatal diagnosis for identification of trivial characteristics or conditions. **It was the consensus of this committee that prenatal diagnosis should only be offered for the diagnosis of genetic disorders and birth defects.** A family history of a diagnosable genetic disorder warrants the offering of prenatal diagnosis, regardless of maternal age, as does determination of carrier status in both parents of an autosomal recessive disorder for which prenatal diagnosis is available. Prenatal diagnostic services for detection of genetic disease for which there is a family history should be reimbursed by insurers (see Chapters 2 and 7). Ability to pay should not restrict appropriate access to prenatal diagnosis or termination of pregnancy of an affected fetus.

The committee felt strongly that the use of fetal diagnosis for determination of fetal sex and the subsequent use of abortion for the purpose of preferential selection of the sex of the fetus represents a misuse of genetic services that is inappropriate and should be discouraged by health professionals. More broadly, reproductive genetic services should not be used to pursue eugenic goals, but should be aimed at increasing individual control over reproductive options. As a consequence, additional research is needed on the impact of prenatal diagnosis, particularly its immediate and long-term impact on women, and on the design and evaluation of genetic counseling techniques for prenatal diagnosis for the future.

Testing for Late-Onset Disorders

Science is moving closer to defining the genetics of such adult disorders as Alzheimer disease, a variety of cancers, heart disease, and arthritis, to name a few (see Chapter 2). A combination of genetic and environmental factors plays a predominant role in most people afflicted with these disorders, but we do not yet understand why some people with a certain gene(s) develop a disease and others do not. Although further work may eventually elucidate the gene(s) involved, there may be long delays until the time when effective interventions are available for many disorders. Furthermore, not all affected individuals will have an identifiable genetic basis to their disorder. Thus, the complexities involved in determining and establishing susceptibility, sorting out potential environmental influences, and devising a strategy for counseling and treatment will pose tremendous challenges in the future.

Many of these diseases do not manifest clinically until adulthood and may become apparent only in middle age or later. *Predictive* or *presymptomatic* testing and screening can provide clues about genetic susceptibility or predisposition to genetic disorders. For monogenic disorders of late onset, such as Huntington disease, tests will usually be highly predictive. Many common diseases usually have multifactorial—or complex—causation, including both multiple genetic factors and environmental effects; for these disorders, prediction will be less certain.

Many common diseases of adulthood, including coronary artery disease, some cancers, diabetes, high blood pressure, rheumatoid arthritis, and some psychiatric diseases, fall into this category. However, in rare forms of these common diseases, single genes may play the decisive role; screening for disease-causing alleles of these genes will be of much greater predictive value.

The committee therefore recommends caution in the use and interpretation of presymptomatic or predictive tests. The nature of these predictions will usually be probabilistic (i.e., with a certain degree of likelihood of occurrence) and not deterministic (i.e., not definite, settled, or without doubt). The dangers of stigmatization and discrimination are areas of concern, as is the potential for harm due to inappropriate preventive or therapeutic measures. Since environmental factors are often essential for the manifestation of complex diseases, the detection of those at high risk will identify certain individuals who will most benefit from certain interventions (e.g., dietary measures in coronary heart disease). Identification of some persons at high risk for certain cancers suggests that more frequent monitoring may identify the earliest manifestations of cancer when treatability is greatest (e.g., colon cancer); research is needed on the psychosocial implications of such testing in both adults and children.

Further research and the unfolding of the Human Genome Project are likely to reveal the underlying genes mediating predisposition to numerous common diseases, and genetic susceptibility testing will be increasingly possible. Certain environmental factors may interact with only one set of genes and not with another. There may also be interaction between the various genes involved, so that the effects of multiple gene action cannot be predicted by separate analyses of each of the single genes. In such cases, definitive prediction will rarely, if ever, be possible. When dealing with genetic testing for some non-Mendelian diseases, it will be impossible to group individuals into two distinct categories—those at no (or very low) risk and those at high risk. Extensive counseling and education will be essential in any testing for genetic susceptibility. The benefits of the various presymptomatic interventions must be weighed against the potential anxiety, stigmatization, and other possible harms to individuals who are informed that they are at increased risk of developing future disease.

Population screening for predisposition to late-onset monogenic diseases should only be considered for treatable or preventable conditions of relatively high frequency. Under such guidelines, population screening should only be offered after appropriate, reliable, sensitive, and specific tests become available. Such tests do not yet exist. The committee recommends that the predictive value of genetic tests be thoroughly validated in prospective studies of sufficient size and statistical power before their widespread application. Since there will be a considerable time lag before the appearance of confirmatory symptoms, these studies will require support for long periods of time (see Chapter 3).

In the case of predictive tests for mental disorders, results must be handled with stringent attention to confidentiality to protect an already vulnera-

ble population. If no effective treatment is available, testing may not be appropriate since more harm than good could result from improper use of test results. On the other hand, future research might result in psychological or drug treatments that could prevent the onset of these diseases. Carefully designed pilot studies should be conducted to determine the effectiveness of such interventions and to measure the desirability and psychosocial impact of such testing. Interpretation and communication of predictive test results in psychiatry will be particularly difficult. To prepare for the issues associated with genetic testing for psychiatric diseases in the future, psychiatrists and other mental health professionals will need more training in genetics and genetic counseling; such training should include the ethical, legal, and social issues in genetic testing.

Because of their wide applicability, it is likely there will be strong commercial interests in the introduction of genetic tests for common, high-profile complex disorders. **Strict guidelines for efficacy therefore will be necessary to prevent premature introduction of this technology.**

Testing of Children or Minors

Children should generally be tested only for genetic disorders for which there exists an effective curative or preventive treatment that must be instituted early in life to achieve maximum benefit. Childhood testing is not appropriate for carrier status, untreatable childhood diseases, and late-onset diseases that cannot be prevented or forestalled by early treatment. In general, the committee believes that testing of minors should be discouraged unless delaying such testing would reduce benefits of available treatment or monitoring. It is essential that the individual seeking testing understand the potential abuse of such information in society, including in employment or insurance practice, and that the provider should ensure that confidentiality is respected (see Chapter 8 for discussion of disclosure to relatives).

Because only certain types of genetic testing are appropriate for children, multiplex testing that includes tests specifically directed to obtaining information about carrier status, untreatable childhood diseases, or late-onset diseases should not be included in the multiplex tests offered to children. **Research should be undertaken to determine the appropriate age for testing and screening for genetic disorders, both to maximize the benefits of therapeutic intervention and to avoid the possibility of generating genetic information about a child when there is no likely benefit and there is possibility of harm to the child.**

LABORATORY ISSUES IN GENETIC TESTING

The committee's review of laboratory issues in genetic testing included a workshop with the nation's experts in laboratory quality assurance in genetic testing and meetings with federal officials responsible for implementing federal regulations under the Clinical Laboratory Improvement Amendments of 1988 (CLIA88) and the medical devices legislation under which the Food and Drug Administration regulates genetic testing products such as test kits, probes, and reagents. **The committee found that although adequate legislative authority exists to oversee the quality of genetic testing, this authority is not in fact being implemented for genetic testing.** For example, existing CLIA88 regulations could ensure the quality of genetic laboratory testing, but these regulations are not being applied to genetic testing at all. Similarly, FDA has authority to regulate genetic testing kits and associated genetic test reagents and DNA probes, but such tests are rarely being submitted to FDA for approval.

The safety and effectiveness of genetic tests should be established before they are used routinely and, even when that comes to pass, great care should be taken in performing the tests and interpreting the results. The committee is concerned that the regulatory burden not impede further development of tests or the offering of genetic testing services by laboratories; nevertheless, the committee believes that the nature of genetic tests and their interpretation, and the magnitude of the personal and clinical decisions that may be made based on those results—including the abortion of affected fetuses—warrant a standard with close to "zero" chance of error for such tests. Consequently, laboratories and personnel performing these tests should participate in proficiency testing programs, including review of the interpretation provided by the laboratory to referring physicians. Laboratories with any error should be placed on probation, and proficiency testing repeated, preferably using blinded methods. Unless the laboratory can attain this standard, its certification to perform this test should be removed.

Existing quality assurance in genetic testing is voluntary and has improved laboratory quality in its participants, but the committee finds that current laboratory quality control programs are inadequate to address the special issues posed by genetic testing primarily because these programs lack essential enforcement authority. As genetic testing expands, these voluntary programs should and will be replaced by the requirements of CLIA88. **In the interim, the committee believes that the impact of voluntary programs could be strengthened by publishing the names of laboratories that have satisfied proficiency and other requirements.** This is now done by the National Tay-Sachs Disease and Allied Disorders Association, Inc., which publishes results of the quality assessment conducted by the International Tay-Sachs Disease Quality Control Reference Standards and Data Collection Center. Before publication, any laboratory not satisfying these requirements should be given ample opportunity to rectify its deficiencies.

Genetics laboratories should provide reports in an easily understandable form for referring physicians who are not genetics specialists. The evaluation of the quality of these reports should be an important component of the proficiency testing process. These reports, including interpretation of the results, should also be reviewed by the Health Care Financing Administration (HCFA) as part of its inspection of laboratories performing genetic tests under CLIA88. The committee also recommends that laboratories performing genetic tests maintain a data base of qualified genetic counselors, genetic centers, and support groups (see Chapters 3, 4, and 6).

Genetic Tests for Rare Disorders

Genetic tests for rare disorders pose special problems in laboratory quality assurance because individual laboratories throughout the country are unlikely to perform enough of these tests to maintain proficiency. **Therefore, the committee recommends that tests for rare diseases be centralized in a few laboratories, to which specimens could be referred from other institutions.** The committee strongly urges the genetics community under the leadership of its professional societies to designate a small number of laboratories to serve as centralized facilities for rarely performed tests. An external proficiency testing program should be established for these central laboratories, and the genetics community should also study the possibility of setting a minimum volume for a specific genetic test that a laboratory must perform annually in order to obtain certification for that test and to ensure the quality of test performance. With its informatics and data base capabilities, the Special Information Services Program of the National Library of Medicine might also maintain a data base of centralized laboratories performing tests for rare disorders, as well as genetic counseling centers and support groups, which should be available to laboratories, providers, and consumers at no charge.

CLIA88

The committee recommends that most genetic tests be classified as "high complexity" under CLIA88, primarily to ensure the highest level of federal oversight of laboratories performing genetic tests. The committee recommends that HCFA create a new specialty of clinical genetics, incorporating the existing subspecialty of clinical cytogenetics, and the new subspecialties of biochemical genetics and molecular genetics as well. Maternal serum alpha-fetoprotein (MSAFP) testing and other methods of prenatal testing for birth defects should be incorporated into one of these three subspecialties. **The Centers for Disease Control and Prevention (CDC) should expand its proficiency testing programs for newborn screening.** HCFA should also give high priority to setting specific requirements for frequently performed prenatal tests and incorporating these standards in its training programs for current and new laboratory inspectors. All laboratories performing genetic screening, including state laboratories, should be required to participate in proficiency testing.

Laboratories using investigational devices for genetic tests (see below) are still covered under CLIA88 as long as test results are reported and used in clinical decision making and counseling, and these laboratories should also be subject to external quality assessment. **Laboratories in academic health centers and elsewhere that conduct research, but that also perform genetic tests as a service (providing the results to referring laboratories or physicians, or directly to patients), fall under the purview of CLIA88 and should be subject to the same criteria, standards, and regulation as commercial genetic testing laboratories.**

Genetic Tests and the FDA

The committee is concerned that tests for newborns and other types of screening may be offered to the public before their safety, effectiveness, and clinical utility have been adequately assessed. **To remedy this, the manufacturer or user of a device for a new screening test (including state laboratories or health departments) should comply with the FDA's regulations for Investigational Device Exemptions (IDE).** For example, the investigational or "pilot" phase of screening should be conducted under a protocol approved by an institutional review board (IRB), and the pilot phase should be evaluated by an entity independent of the organization conducting the pilot study.

Compliance with FDA requirements is essential to ensuring safe and effective use of genetic tests, just as compliance with CLIA88 is essential for any laboratory performing genetic tests for clinical purposes. **All genetic tests should either be designated as investigational devices—subject to IRB approval and FDA regulation—or be submitted to the FDA for full premarket approval.** An Advisory Panel on Genetic Test Devices to the FDA should be established to ensure appropriate expert review for genetic testing products. Genetic diagnostic devices should be classified for full premarket approval by FDA (Class III), and the FDA should develop guidance to manufacturers for preparing premarket applications for genetic test devices (see Chapter 3).

DNA probes and other reagents that are essential to the performance of genetic tests are medical devices under current FDA law and regulation. **Consequently, whenever probes and reagents are used for clinical purposes, they must either be labeled "for investigational use only" (and must comply with FDA requirements for investigational use) or have FDA approval for marketing.** When genetic test devices are used investigationally for clinical purposes, manufacturers—including commercial or academically based laboratories preparing their own devices—should apply for FDA approval of an IDE, including an IRB-approved protocol and periodic reports on the results of their investigations.

Many institutional review boards lack experience in the review of investigational genetic testing protocols. The National Institutes of Health (NIH) Office for Protection from Research Risks has recently issued initial guidance for research involving genetics in its IRB *Guidebook*. **The NIH Office for Protection from Research Risks (OPRR) and the National Center for Human Genome Research (NCHGR) ELSI Program should continue to coordinate efforts to assist IRBs in coping with this responsibility.** Other federal agencies and professional groups should also consider developing guidelines to help IRBs cope with this added responsibility, such as the informed consent guidelines for research involving genetic testing developed by the Alliance of Genetic Support Groups and the American Society of Human Genetics (ASHG) (see Chapter 4).

The committee recognizes that, for very rare diseases and diseases with a long lead time between the time of the test and the appearance of disease, it will be difficult for FDA applicants to provide adequate data on safety and effectiveness for subjects of the type in whom the test would be applied (e.g., presymptomatic individuals). It may also be impossible to assess the sensitivity and specificity of prenatal tests by independent tests or histopathological examination of aborted fetuses. **For rare diseases, the FDA could grant the applicant "provisional premarket approval," a designation under which the test could be made more widely available while making the manufacturer responsible for obtaining additional postmarket data until sufficient data are available to warrant full "premarket" approval.** This process may require new legislation, but the committee believes that provisional premarket approval, with the sponsor responsible for periodic postmarket study, adequately covers the development of tests for rare conditions, which is the intent of the "humanitarian device exemption" (contained in the Safe Medical Device Amendments of 1990). And since manufacturers may be unwilling to go through premarket approval of tests for rare diseases, Congress should also consider the need for legislation in the spirit of the Orphan Drug Act that would give manufacturers an incentive to develop diagnostic medical devices for genetic tests of limited marketability.

GENETIC COUNSELING

Genetic counseling and education must be an integral part of genetic testing. Anyone who is offering (or referring for) genetic testing must provide (or refer for) appropriate genetic counseling and education prior to testing. To ensure that adequate genetic counseling is provided to all those seeking genetics services, a cadre of individuals trained in medical genetics and counseling must be available. Primary care practitioners and allied health professionals must have a minimal basic understanding of medical genetics and counseling (see Chapters 4 and 6). Efforts must also be made to ensure that the public is sufficiently educated to be informed consumers of genetics services (see Chapter 5).

Basic Tenets of Genetic Counseling

The committee believes that certain basic tenets apply, regardless of who is conducting the counseling and where it is being done. These include respect for the autonomy and privacy of the individual, the need for informed consent and confidentiality, and sensitivity to the counselor's tendency toward directiveness and paternalism (see Chapters 1, 4, and 8). The standard of care should be to support the client in making voluntary informed decisions and to provide sensitive and empathic support for the emotional suffering caused by the genetic problem. **The goal of reducing the incidence of genetic conditions is not acceptable, since this aim is explicitly eugenic; professionals should not present any reproductive decisions as "correct" or advantageous for a person or society.** Research is needed to test alternative methods for providing genetic counseling (e.g., interactive video and computer methods with referral to a counselor for answers to questions), and to evaluate the costs and effectiveness of such changes.

One key to effective genetics services is the concept of the *teachable moment*, that is, the point(s) at which an individual, couple, or family, is best able to comprehend the information being given them. Unfortunately, the genetic counselor may not have the opportunity to counsel clients at more advantageous teachable moments—after some of the early shock and denial that often accompany genetic diagnosis have abated—because of restrictions on insurance reimbursement (see Chapter 7) and administrative impediments such as scheduling counseling on the day of testing. Studies are therefore needed on alternative approaches to genetic counseling, including the effects of differing levels of intensity of counseling and education both before testing—to help those at risk to decide whether or not they want to be tested—and after testing—to deal with the consequences of having the information (see below).

Physicians need to balance their desire to provide medical advice with respect for the patient's right to make an informed decision that may be different from the one recommended by the physician. This is especially crucial in genetic testing, since genetic information carries more personal, family, and social risks and burdens than many other kinds of medical information. In particular, decisions about whether to reproduce or to abort an affected fetus are individual choices that should be left to each couple. Similarly, a decision about whether to test for the presence of genes or gene complexes that predict the likely development of future disease that cannot be treated should be an individual decision. And when treatment becomes possible, some of these decisions may still be painful, costly, and uncertain, and still require genetic counseling. **Nondirectiveness should always remain the standard of care for reproductive planning and decisions, and full informed consent before genetic testing will continue to be essential.**

Since genetics education and counseling are likely to be provided increasingly by primary care practitioners, these practitioners will need training to help them perform these functions appropriately and to know when to refer patients to specialized genetics personnel. Innovative educational devices to support genetics education and counseling should be designed and evaluated (e.g., video, interactive computer systems, and on-line data bases) in primary care settings. **Finally, the genetic counselor, as the messenger of potentially devastating or discriminatory information, must honor the patient's desire for confidentiality except under rare special circumstances where breach of**

confidentiality is necessary to avert serious harm (discussed in Chapters 4 and 8). These special circumstances may involve the potential effects of genetic information on other family members or the potential harm to others if the information is not disclosed. Should a counselor anticipate a professional or personal need to disclose genetic information to a party other than the patient with whom he or she is consulting, then the potential for that disclosure should be addressed before any genetic testing services are rendered.

Tailoring Counseling to the Client

Research on the best ways to provide essential genetics education and counseling—by a variety of providers in a variety of settings—must precede efforts to streamline genetic counseling (see Chapters 6 and 9). The committee believes that understanding and recall of numerical risks of recurrence are too limited as measures of the success of or need for counseling. Beyond mere comprehension of numerical risk, genetic counseling is intended to assist individuals in evaluating the implications of genetic testing and genetic information, and in determining their own acceptable risk. **Since risk perceptions vary among individuals and among counselees and counselors, there is no one right way to present or interpret risk information; however, information must be balanced, and the process must be tailored to the client.**

Ethnic and cultural sensitivity is particularly important—genetic counseling should be tailored to the cultural perspective of the client, with special attention to differing cultures between client and health care professional. Research is needed to determine how best to provide genetic counseling in ways that are sensitive and appropriate to a variety of cultures and languages. Training in culturally appropriate language and delivery of genetic services should be included in the training of genetics and other health professionals who are likely to provide genetic testing and counseling in the future. It is also vital to destigmatize language describing genetic disorders and disabilities, and to present information about these conditions as fairly as possible. As one step in this process, genetic counseling and other genetics training programs should actively seek to increase the number of minority practitioners prepared to provide a variety of genetic counseling roles in a variety of settings (see Chapters 4 and 6).

PUBLIC EDUCATION

Much of the responsibility for preparing individuals to deal effectively with the ramifications of genetics must fall to the public education system. This includes both formal education, which takes place in the schools, and informal education, which takes place outside of school (see Chapter 5). Data from large-scale testing programs suggest that a clinic or a doctor's office is not the best context for a first exposure to genetic testing information, and that public education campaigns and counseling, generally, have a greater impact on individuals with some previous exposure to genetic concepts. Decisions about genetic testing and its potential personal impact ultimately must be tied to preexisting knowledge and value systems; without such knowledge, individuals are more likely to make uninformed decisions or to cede all decisions about genetic testing to their health care professionals.

What do we want people to know, value, and do about genetic information? For example, people should know that DNA is the information molecule; they should value the variation and diversity that are expressed from that molecule, but they also need to appreciate the nature of the interaction among genes, the individual, and the environment. Perhaps the most important contribution of new knowledge about genetics is its ability to document a major biological basis for human variation. The old argument about nature versus nurture is outdated: as discussed throughout the report, both nature (biology) and nurture (environment) are important to health, and broad public understanding of the role of genetics (and its limits) is essential to avoid genetic reductionism and a "new eugenics."

Genetics education should also focus on concepts of genetic variability, diversity, and kinship. Such a focus will help to avoid simplistic explanations such as dichotomizing of genetic risks of complex diseases with genetic determinants as either categorically good news—that an individual has essentially zero risk for a particular disease—or categorically bad news—that he or she is virtually certain to develop it. Many disorders are of variable and often unpredictable severity, and much genetic risk assessment is of an inherently probabilistic nature. **Genetic testing is not an end in itself but rather a method for gaining information and insight to help people make personal and family health decisions.** The basic task is to educate the public so that each individual is capable of making an informed decision about seeking or using genetic testing and considering personal courses of action. In addition, the public and policy makers must be educated to help them develop appropriate public policy regarding genetic testing and screening. Genetic counseling will ultimately be made more effective by a better-educated public. This approach to public education about genetics will not be a simple or a small task.

The Human Genome Project's Ethical, Legal, and Social Implications Program should coordinate a public education initiative in genetics and expand its support for such efforts. Key policy and research strategies to be considered are (1) ensuring that appropriate educational messages about genetic tests and their implications reach the public; (2) incorporating principles, concepts, and skills training that support informed decision making about genetic testing into all levels of schooling—kindergarten through college; (3) enhancing consumers' knowledge and ability to make informed decisions in either seeking or accepting genetic tests; (4) establishing systems for designing, implementing, and maintaining community-based genetics education among population groups at higher risk of particular genetic disorders (e.g., increased risk related to race or ethnicity); and (5) enlisting the mass media to help decrease consumer confusion and increase the knowledge and skills that will equip consumers to make the most appropriate decisions for themselves (see Chapter 5).

The National Science Foundation, the Department of Energy, the National Institutes of Health, and other organizations should expand their investment in public education related to the human genome. These efforts should (1) expand programs that support model educational initiatives for precollege science and undergraduate molecular biology; (2) collaborate with the Ethical, Legal, and Social Implications component of the Human Genome Project to encourage such programs to focus on the health, social, legal, and ethical issues raised by genetic testing and screening; and (3) require evaluation of educational interventions.

Broad public participation will be required to develop educational approaches that respect the widely varying personal and cultural perspectives on issues of genetics, and are tolerant and respectful of individuals with genetic disorders of all kinds. Particular effort will be needed to include the perspectives of women, minorities, and persons with disabilities, who may feel especially affected by developing genetic technologies. There is much to be learned from those who are particularly affected by genetic testing technologies, and from those affected by genetic disorders, including persons with disabilities and their families and support groups. The committee believes that genetics professionals and qualified educators must work with public representatives to identify the essential components of genetic literacy.

A "Consumer's Guide to Genetic Testing" should be developed (also see Chapters 1, 5, and 9) to provide information on genetic services, various genetic tests, and the implications of the tests so as to aid in providing balanced, reliable, readily understandable, and available sources of needed information. Innovative computer and interactive computer systems should also be developed to provide patients/clients with the latest information on genetic disorders and on genetic diagnosis, testing, and screening. If designed and used appropriately, such computer resources could assist genetics specialists and primary care practitioners by presenting patients with basic, self-paced genetics education and even presenting possible options for consideration of patients. The ELSI Program should therefore coordinate with the National Library of Medicine in developing innovative methods of providing information to the public similar to the on-line AIDS bibliography. More research is needed to determine which tasks in genetics education and counseling can be appropriately accomplished by using such techniques and to evaluate these techniques in various settings and populations.

PROFESSIONAL EDUCATION

The committee sees no prospect, in the foreseeable future, of having enough highly specialized genetics personnel to handle all genetic testing, including essential genetics education and genetic counseling. Therefore, policy discussion should focus not only on training more genetic counselors and other genetic specialists, but on better educating the obstetrics, pediatrics, and family practice communities about the nature of genetic testing, diagnosis, and counseling.

Some progress has been made in increasing physicians' knowledge of genetic testing and their ability to take good family histories, particularly in specialties that involve more genetic tests (e.g., pediatrics and obstetrics; see Chapter 6). More recent graduates also know more than older physicians. Nevertheless, the committee is very concerned that relatively little progress has been made—certainly not enough to prepare physicians-in-training for the increasing requirements for genetic testing, education, and counseling projected for the future. **The committee strongly recommends that medical education begin to incorporate a genetic point of view throughout its curriculum, but especially in the critical clinical years, and that medical board examinations should include more questions on genetics.** More research is needed on knowledge of genetics and skills needed for genetics education and genetic counseling among all of these professional groups so that proper reforms can be implemented.

The biggest potential contribution of genetics to medical education may be its ability to document a major biological basis for human variation. Conventional teaching in medical school often disregards differences in etiology, presentation, response to therapy, personal preferences, and prognosis of people who may be "lumped" together under a single disease label. A true revolution will come much more from introducing a new way of learning about disease and health, of emphasizing the importance of individual differences, some but not all of which are genetically determined. Historically, the discovery of germs as causative agents in disease led to a reductionist germ theory that explained everything in terms of germs; the committee is concerned that the explosion of genetics knowledge may replace the reductionist germ theory with a *reductionist gene theory*—to the detriment of medical progress.

Genetics professionals and all others offering or referring for genetic testing should be trained in the ethical, legal, and social issues surrounding genetic diagnosis, testing, and screening. Laboratory personnel should be a special focus of such training about the complexities of genetic testing to adequately interpret tests, including a knowledge of test limitations and social issues surrounding genetic testing. **Of particular importance is training to deal with the sensitivities of genetics education and counseling, including the need for nondirectiveness, in counseling about reproductive options and about disorders for which no treatment exists.** Expanded undergraduate and graduate training of nurses in genetics, genetics education, and genetic counseling is also needed, along with the training of social workers in the special requirements of genetics education and counseling. With proper training, the integration of other health professionals such as nurses, nurse practitioners, social workers, psychologists, and primary care physicians, into the existing genetics services network will supplement the time and skills of traditional genetic counseling (see Chapter 4).

The accelerating developments of new knowledge in genetic testing will also require expanded formal continuing education programs in clinical genetics, including those geared to the genetic counselor, primary care practitioner, and social worker (see Chapter 5). The Ethical, Legal, and Social Implications Program should coordinate with professional genetics organizations and the National Library of Medicine to develop genetics education and dissemination programs for interested health professionals. Genetics specialists should develop and provide continuing education and training for other professionals, as well as take a leadership role in genetics education for the public. Other health care professionals should also participate in programs intended to increase public awareness and education about genetics.

More minorities should be recruited for training programs in all aspects of clinical genetics. This will be especially important in providing culturally sensitive and appropriate genetic testing, education, and counseling services in the future (see above), when so-called minority groups will comprise a majority of the population of the United States (see Chapters 4 and 6).

FINANCING OF GENETIC TESTING SERVICES

The cost and financing of genetic testing and counseling have had a profound effect on access to these services in the United States. No matter what aspect of genetics is discussed, it is almost impossible to keep the discussion from turning to issues related to financing, in particular the role of health insurance in genetic testing and counseling (see Chapter 7). The United States is the only developed country in the world without a social insurance or statutory system to cover basic expenses for medical services for most of its population. This creates problems of access and equity, especially for those low-income or high-risk individuals who are self-employed, work part-time, or are employed by small businesses and who may not be able to afford or obtain health insurance. Over 37 million people are without health insurance coverage in the United States.

Even for those who have health insurance, coverage for most preventive, screening, and counseling services may be excluded. These limitations of health care coverage in the United States particularly affect genetic services, which have an important counseling component. Insurance reimbursement or other financing of genetic testing is not generally available now in the United States. The committee also heard testimony that individuals whose insurance does cover some or all genetic services may be reluctant or unwilling to file claims for such services. They may fear that the genetic information they sought might be used to evaluate and deny their future applications for health or life insurance coverage, or lead to higher premiums or limited coverage. And, because so much coverage in the United States is employment based, people may also worry that their employer will have access to the information and use it (overtly or covertly) to discriminate against them (see Chapters 7 and 8).

In order to develop appropriate financing for genetic testing and counseling services, private and public health plans, and geneticists and consumers, should work together to develop guidelines for the reimbursement of genetic services. Such guidelines should address the issue of how each new genetic test should be assessed for its sensitivity and specificity in light of the availability of effective treatment, the consequences of the test, the evaluation of pilot study results, and when new tests are appropriate for use in routine clinical practice (see Chapters 1 and 7).

In addition, the insurance concept of what is considered *medically necessary* (and therefore reimbursable) should be expanded to include the *offering* of *appropriate genetic testing* and related education and counseling, making these genetic services reimbursable under health insurance plans. Medical appropriateness can often be established by a family history of the disorder. In pregnancy, medical necessity should be considered established for cytogenetic testing in pregnancies in women of advanced maternal age or considered at high risk based on other methods of assessing risk. The committee also recommends that newborn screening and MSAFP screening in pregnant women of any age be considered within the insurance definition of medically appropriate and be reimbursable under health insurance plans (see Chapter 7).

SOCIAL, LEGAL, AND ETHICAL ISSUES IN GENETIC TESTING

The committee recommends that vigorous protection be given to *autonomy, privacy, confidentiality, and equity.* These principles should be breached only in rare instances and only when the following conditions are met: (1) the action must be aimed at an important goal—such as the protection of others from serious harm—that outweighs the value of autonomy, privacy, confidentiality, or equity in the particular instance; (2) it must have a high probability of realizing that goal; (3) there must be no acceptable alternatives that can also realize the goal without breaching those principles; and (4) the degree of infringement of the principle must be the minimum necessary to realize the goal.

Voluntariness

Voluntariness should be the cornerstone of any genetic testing program. The committee found no justification for a state-sponsored *mandatory* public health program involving genetic testing of adults or for unconsented-to genetic testing of patients in the clinical setting. There is evidence that voluntary screening programs achieve a higher level of efficacy in screening, and there is no evidence that mandating newborn screening is necessary or sufficient to ensure that the vast majority of newborns are screened. Mandatory *offering* of newborn screening is appropriate for disorders with treatments of demonstrated efficacy where very early intervention is essential to improve health outcomes (e.g., phenylketonuria and congenital hypothyroidism). One benefit of voluntariness and informing parents about newborn screening is that of quality assurance: parents can check to see if the sample was actually drawn. In addition, since people will be facing the possibility of undergoing many more genetic tests in their lifetimes, the disclosure of information to parents about newborn screening prior to the event can be an important tool for education about genetics.

Informed Consent

Obtaining informed consent should be the method of ensuring that genetic testing is voluntary. By *informed consent* the committee means a *process* of education and the opportunity to have questions answered—not merely the signing of a form. The patient or client should be given information about the risks, benefits, efficacy, and alternatives to the testing; information about the severity, potential variability, and treatability of the disorder being tested for; information about the subsequent decisions that will be likely if the test is positive (such as a decision about abortion); and information about any potential conflicts of interest of the person or institution offering the test (see Chapters 1, 3, and 8). **Research should therefore also be undertaken to determine what patients *want* to know in order to make a decision about whether or not to undergo a genetic test.** People often have less interest in the label for the disorder and its mechanisms of action than in how certainly the test predicts the disorder, what effects the disorder has on physical and mental functioning, and how intrusive, difficult, or effective any existing treatment protocol would be. Research is also necessary to determine the advantages and disadvantages of various means of conveying that information (e.g., through specialized genetic counselors, primary care providers, single disorder counselors, brochures, videos, audiotapes, computer programs).

Confidentiality

All forms of genetic information should be considered confidential and should not be disclosed without the individual's consent (except as required by state law, or in rare instances discussed in Chapters 4 and 8). This includes genetic information that is obtained through specific genetic testing of a person, as well as genetic information about that person that is obtained in other ways (e.g., physical examination, past treatment, or a relative's genetic status). The confidentiality of genetic information should be protected no matter who obtains or maintains that information. This includes genetic information collected or maintained by health care professionals, health care institutions, researchers, employers, insurance companies, laboratory personnel, and law enforcement officials. To the extent that current statutes do not ensure such confidentiality, they should be amended.

Codes of ethics for professionals providing genetic services should contain specific provisions to protect autonomy, privacy, and confidentiality. The committee endorses the 1991 National Society of Genetic Counselors (NSGC) statement of guiding principles on confidentiality of test results:

> The NSGC support individual confidentiality regarding results of genetic testing. It is the right and responsibility of the individual to determine who shall have access to medical information, particularly results of testing for genetic conditions.

Confidentiality should be breached and relatives informed about genetic risks *only* when (1) attempts to elicit voluntary disclosure fail, (2) there is a high probability of irreversible harm that the disclosure will prevent, and (3) there is no other reasonable way to avert the harm. When disclosure is to be attempted over the patient's refusal, the burden should be on the person who wishes to disclose to justify to the patient, to an ethics committee, and perhaps in court that the disclosure was necessary and met the committee's test. Thus, the committee has determined that the disadvantages of informing relatives over the patient's refusal generally outweigh the advantages, except in the rare instances described above (see Chapters 4 and 8). **The committee recommends that health care providers not reveal genetic information about a patient's carrier status to the patient's spouse without the patient's permission, and that information on misattributed paternity should be given to the mother, but not be volunteered to her partner.**

As a matter of general principle, the committee believes strongly that patients should disclose to relatives genetic information relevant to ensuring the health of those relatives. Patients should be encouraged and aided in sharing appropriate genetic information with spouses and relatives. To facilitate the disclosure of relevant genetic information to family members, accurate and balanced materials should be developed to assist individuals in informing their families, and in providing access to further information, as well as access to testing if relatives should choose to be tested. Under those rare circumstances where unauthorized disclosure of genetic information is deemed warranted, the genetic counselor should first try to obtain the permission of the person to release the information.

The committee also endorses the principles on the protection of DNA data and DNA data banking developed in 1990 by the ASHG Ad Hoc Committee on Identification by DNA Analysis. In short, patients' consent should be obtained before their names are provided to a genetic disease registry, and their consent should also be obtained before information is redisclosed. **Each entity that receives or maintains genetic information or samples should have procedures in place to protect confidentiality.** Information or samples should be kept free of identifiers and instead use encoding to link the information or sample to the individual's name. Finally, any entity that releases genetic information about an individual to someone other than that individual should ensure that the recipient of the genetic information has procedures in place to protect the confidentiality of the information.

Genetic Discrimination in Health Insurance

Legislation should be adopted to prevent medical risks, including genetic risks, from being taken into account in decisions on whether to issue or how to price health care insurance. Because health insurance differs significantly from other types of insurance in that it regulates access to health care—an important social good—risk-based health insurance should be eliminated. Access to health care should be available to every American without regard to the individual's present health status or condition; in particular, the committee recommends that insurability decisions not be based on genetic status (see Chapters 7 and 8).

Some of the committee's concerns about genetic discrimination in health insurance would be obviated by current proposals for national health insurance reform that would eliminate most, if not all, aspects of medical underwriting. **The committee recommends that insurance reform preclude the use of genetic information in establishing eligibility for health insurance.** As health insurance reform proposals are developed, those concerned with genetic disorders will need to assess whether th. y adequately protect genetic information and persons with genetic disorders from health insurance discrimination and discrimination in the provision of medical services (see Chapters 7 and 8).

Genetic Discrimination in Employment

Legislation should be adopted that forbids employers to collect genetic information on prospective or current employees unless it is clearly job related. Sometimes employers will have employees submit to medical exams to see if they are capable of performing particular job tasks. If an individual consents to the release of genetic information to an employer or potential employer, the releasing entity should not release specific information, but instead answer only yes or no regarding whether the individual was fit to perform the job at issue.

The committee urges the Equal Employment Opportunity Commission to recognize that the language of the Americans with Disabilities Act (ADA) provides protection for presymptomatic people with genetic risks for late-onset disorders, unaffected carriers of disorders that might affect their children, and individuals with genetic profiles indicating the possibility of increased risk of a multifactorial disorder. State legislatures should adopt laws to protect people from genetic discrimination in employment. In addition, ADA should be amended (and similar state statutes adopted) to limit the type of medical testing employers can request and to ensure that the medical information they can collect is job related.

RESEARCH AND POLICY AGENDA

In its efforts to complete a comprehensive overview of issues in genetic testing and screening, the Committee on Assessing Genetic Risks identified significant gaps in data, research, and policy analysis that impede informed policy making for the future. Surprisingly few data exist on the extent of genetic testing and screening today, for example, and no system is in place to gather data or to assess practices in relation to the committee's principles and recommendations for the future. The committee's review of the key data, research, and policy needs in genetic testing and screening has generated recommendations addressed to the Ethical, Legal, and Social Implications Program of the Human Genome Project, and several recommendations are addressed to other relevant agencies, including other components of the National Institutes of Health, the Agency for Health Care Policy and Research (AHCPR), the Centers for Disease Control and Prevention, the Food and Drug Administration, the Public Health Service (PHS), the Health Care Financing Administration, the Department of Health and Human Services (DHHS), the Department of Energy (DOE), the National Science Foundation (NSF), and a broad range of private organizations.

Policy Oversight

The committee strongly believes that effective oversight will be essential as genetic testing develops to ensure that genetic tests are validated and used appropriately, with respect for the potential harms such testing may pose. **For effective overall and continuing policy oversight, the majority of the committee recommends the creation of a broadly representative National Advisory Committee and Working Group on Genetic Testing to oversee professional practices and determine when new genetic tests are ready for wide-scale use in medical practice** (see Chapters 1 and 9).

Although the American Society of Human Genetics, National Society of Genetic Counselors, American Academy of Pediatrics, American College of Obstetricians and Gynecologists, and other professional organizations have developed policy statements on key policy issues in genetic testing, genetic testing has moved beyond the domain of genetics specialists alone. There is also a need for broad public involvement in the development of public policy concerning genetic testing and screening. As discussed throughout this report, genetic testing has broad health and social implications of both immediate and future concern to individuals and families with genetic disorders, genetic support groups, and the public at large. Increased public education will be required to equip the public to make informed personal and policy decisions in genetic testing (see Chapter 5). The proposed National Advisory Committee on Genetic Testing and its Working Group are intended to provide the essential broadly based scientific and public oversight for genetic testing and screening.

The committee also sees a need for broadly representative advisory bodies at the state level (see Chapters 1 and 9). These advisory bodies should be guided by the principles outlined in this report. They should guide state health departments and legislatures on such issues as when tests should be added to state-run screening programs and how to ensure that the offering, testing, and associated education and counseling are conducted in accord with the principles outlined in this report. **State statutes affecting genetic testing should not be unduly prescriptive or restrictive, and should provide latitude to such advisory bodies to modify state-run genetic testing programs.**

Research Policy

Much of current genetic testing grew out of the context of research studies, and some genetic testing is still being done in research settings. Research initiatives involving genetic testing are being supported and developed not only within the Human Genome Project, but also within the research programs of various components of the National Institutes of Health (including the National Institute of General Medical Sciences, National Cancer Institute, National Heart, Lung, and Blood Institute, National Institute of Child Health and Human Development, National Institute of Diabetes and Digestive and Kidney Diseases) and the Human Genome Program of the Department of Energy. **In developing and approving research protocols, the committee recommends that the NIH and the DOE consider the recommendations of this committee within the context of their research programs, including study of the psychosocial issues and implications of genetic testing and the potential for harm from the use and misuse of genetic information.** This is especially significant where there is no treatment available for the disorders, as will often be the case in the near future. In developing requests for proposals and requests for applications and in reviewing research, demonstration projects, pilot studies, clinical trials, and family studies in genetics, funding agencies should pay particular attention to psychosocial issues and should assess the availability of appropriate genetic counseling and follow-up services as elements of study design.

Need for Additional Standards

The committee identified several areas for which additional standards were needed concerning who should be tested, for what disorders, and at what age. **While existing standards may have been adequate for the past, new standards must be developed in response to rapid developments in genetic testing methods that are now experimental. In particular, additional standards are needed for prenatal diagnosis, predispositional testing, and multiplex testing** (see Chapter 9). Research and policy analysis is needed in prenatal genetic diagnosis to address problems such as the complexities of identifying fetal cells in maternal blood, maternal serum alpha-fetoprotein screening, notions of "perfectibility," use of prenatal diagnosis and selective abortion to choose the sex of the fetus, the special impact of prenatal diagnosis on women, and carrier detection in pregnancy rather than prior to conception (see Chapters 2 and 9). Reproductive genetic decisions raise some of the most deeply personal and troubling issues in genetic testing. Professional groups need to work together and develop innovative methods for involving the public in the development of standards for the use of these technologies (see Chapters 2, 3, 4, and 9).

Standards are also needed for genetic testing for predisposition to late-onset disorders. There is an important "window of opportunity" for considering these issues now, before predispositional genetic testing becomes widespread. Tests for predisposition to common disorders will be of great commercial interest, and could have substantial potential for harm to individuals and families in terms of insurability and employability, as well as substantial benefit from the potential of early preventive and therapeutic interventions. Strict guidelines for efficacy will be necessary to prevent premature introduction of this technology (see Chapters 1, 2, and 9). **The committee believes that population screening for late-onset diseases should be considered only for treatable or preventable conditions of relatively high frequency and only after appropriate, reliable, sensitive, and specific tests become available; and such tests should be voluntary.** In general, because of the significant medical and psychosocial consequences of predictive testing, the committee believes that testing of minors should be discouraged. Instead, **research should be undertaken to determine the appropriate age for testing and screening for genetic disorders in minors in order to maximize the benefits of therapeutic intervention.**

Multiplex testing—multiple genetic tests on a single blood or other tissue sample—represents one of the most likely innovations in genetic testing. **Consequently, the committee also recommends the development of standards for multiplex genetic testing.** Innovative methods are needed to group tests by related types of disorders that raise similar issues (including the availability of effective treatment and how soon treatment needs to be instituted), as a basis for appropriate education, informed consent, and genetic counseling. This will allow potential screenees (or parents) to choose which, if any, group of tests they feel is appropriate for them. Tests for untreatable disorders should not be multiplexed with tests for disorders that can be cured or prevented by treatment or by avoidance of particular environmental stimuli. Multiplex testing is also an area in which more research is needed to develop ways to ensure that patient autonomy is recognized (see Chapters 1, 2, 3, 4, and 8).

Policy Research Needs

The committee identified significant data and policy research needs related to genetic testing (see Chapter 9). In addition to its other recommendations, the committee identified several areas in which policy research is needed, including

- **pilot studies of new tests before wide-scale introduction;**
- **cost-effectiveness analysis of genetic testing;**
- **critical deficiencies in data on genetic services;**
- **research on population distribution and heterogeneity of traits involved in genetic or genetically influenced disease; and**
- **assessment of what has been learned thus far from ELSI research and policy studies.**

1

Setting the Stage

The prospect of identifying all of our genes raises the hope of understanding and finding ways to alleviate the diseases that afflict humankind. Some diseases are caused by mutations of a single gene; identifying the gene often may be helpful in learning its normal function, and understanding function can greatly accelerate development of therapies to prevent manifestations of these diseases, or even arrest or reverse their course. Conventional therapies, such as drugs or special diets, can compensate for the genetic aberration. Other therapies, based on identification and cloning of the normal gene, can supply the product of the normal gene. Gene therapy might substitute or add a normal gene for the defective one, inactivate a defective gene, or even repair it.

Most single-gene diseases are rare, but some of these rare diseases have more common analogues. Learning more about the basic defect in rare, single-gene forms of hyperlipidemic heart disease, Alzheimer disease, and some cancers, may teach us more about the nature of the defect in the common forms, and might also help us design effective treatments.

Knowing which genes cause or contribute to the occurrence of disease also permits scientists to develop tests to detect people who will suffer the disease, *before they experience symptoms*, so they can benefit from early intervention (if it is available). Tests for many single-gene disorders already exist, and some of them are described in this report. Tests for detecting genetic predispositions to more common, complex disorders are under development. And even when treatments have not yet been developed, genetic tests can nevertheless help people decide about conceiving or bearing children. In addition to the benefits to be derived from genetic testing, a number of concerns have been raised about the use of genetic testing. One such concern is that those who are poor or live in rural areas will not have access to testing. The development and widespread use of genetic tests before safe and effective treatments are available have raised fears about the uses of genetic testing—that genetic tests will be imposed while other approaches to alleviating human suffering are neglected. Their use also raises issues about discrimination and privacy—that people found to possess certain genetic characteristics will lose opportunities for employment, insurance, and education. Finally, genetic testing raises worries about inequities and intolerance—that not everyone will share equitably in the benefits of genetic testing, that some will be stigmatized, and that the beauty of human diversity will be denigrated due to a narrowed definition of what is acceptable.

This is not the first time the National Academy of Sciences (NAS) has addressed issues related to genetic testing. Since *Genetic Screening: Programs, Principles and Research* was published by the academy in 1975 (NAS, 1975), the technology underlying genetic testing has been revolutionized, greatly expanding the number of diseases for which genetic testing will be possible. This has brought new urgency to many of the issues raised in the 1975 report and raised some additional issues as well. In this chapter, we briefly review the technological changes and their implications for assessing genetic risks. We revisit the first NAS report, and consider its applicability today.

RECOMBINANT DNA TECHNOLOGY, GENE MAPPING, AND IDENTIFICATION OF DISEASE-RELATED GENES

During the 1970s, researchers discovered that human DNA (as well as DNA from other organisms) could be cut reproducibly into small segments, each of which could then be rapidly reproduced (cloned) by inserting it into a microorganism. Cloned segments can then be prepared in sufficient quantity to serve as "probes" to find the longer piece of human DNA from which the segment has been cut. Further advances facilitate determination of the chromosome on which the segment of DNA resides.

The availability of DNA probes made it possible to search for individual variation in DNA. Different kinds of DNA variation have been found. Probes can detect such DNA sequence variation among individuals (polymorphisms), and the inheritance of chromosome segments containing polymorphisms can be easily traced from parents to offspring (Botstein et al., 1980). Using DNA sequence variations as "markers," researchers began constructing maps defining their order and spacing along chromosomes (e.g., Donis-Keller et al., 1987). An important application of this genetic mapping technology was the localization at specific chromosomal sites of genes responsible for inherited disorders.

If, for instance, within a large family the relatives who had a genetic disease were found to have one form of a polymorphism significantly more often than blood relatives who did not have the disease, the disease-causing gene (still unidentified) was probably "linked" to that polymorphism. Different families might have polymorphisms on the same chromosome and very close to the marker, or might have different forms of the same polymorphism, but if each of them had an inherited disease that originated from the same gene, they would be "linked" to that same marker. Since the chromosome location of the marker was known (or could be easily determined), the chromosome location of the disease gene was immediately evident. Then the search for the gene itself could begin. There can be a very long gap between gene localization—finding the general location of the gene on the chromosome—and gene identification and isolation. The Huntington disease gene was the first autosomal gene to be localized using new DNA marker techniques (Gusella et al., 1983). Ten years later, it was found (Huntington's Disease Research Collaborative Group, 1993). Many marker genes including those responsible for cystic fibrosis (CF) (Rommens et al., 1989; Collins, 1992), neurofibromatosis (Collins et al., 1989), and a form of colon cancer (Fearon and Vogelstein, 1990) have been isolated using this approach.

The international effort to map the human genome is accelerating the development of new markers and the construction of detailed linkage maps of the human genome. Disease-causing genes are also being discovered at an accelerating pace (NIH-CEPH Collaborative Mapping Group, 1992; Weissenbach et al., 1992). New technological innovation in mapping and sequencing will lead to the cloning of disease-causing genes and the discovery of alterations in those genes (mutations) that lead to the occurrence of specific disease. As of July 15, 1992, 3,836 polymorphic markers had been localized on specific regions of chromosomes, and 611 disease-related genes had been mapped (Donis-Keller et al., 1987, 1992; see Figure 1-1).

As a result of these discoveries, it is still a very difficult but technically more straightforward matter to localize and identify disease-causing genes for single-gene diseases—those that follow the rules of inheritance established by Gregor Mendel in 1865—provided that families in which the disease occurs are willing to participate in linkage studies and are of sufficient size to study. As the Human Genome Project progresses, genes will be found by means other than their association with a specific disease in such families. Theoretically, there could be as many diseases as there are genes (50,000 to 100,000 human genes by current estimates), although some genes are so essential to embryonic and fetal development that defects in them will result in spontaneous abortion rather than postnatal disease. It is possible that some functioning genes are so nonessential that defects in them will not result in any impairment. As is the case with most single-gene diseases, many of those waiting to be discovered will be rare. There is considerable conservation of gene sequences across species. This allows scientists to find homologous genes in mice, fruit flies, or primates, and to create artificial manifestations in the DNA to mimic the mutation in the human gene. Animal models carrying the actual human gene will permit the study of the normal and abnormal function of the gene in the development of new therapies.

32

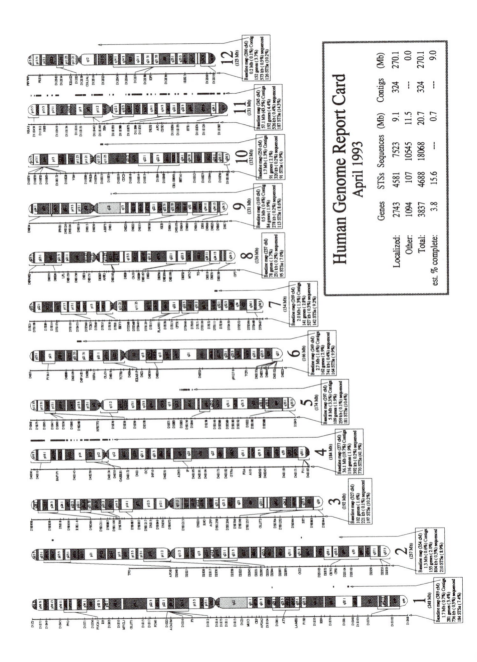

Human Genome Report Card
April 1993

	Genes	STSs	Sequences	(Mb)	Contigs	(Mb)
Localized:	2743	4581	7523	9.1	324	270.1
Other:	1094	107	10545	11.5	---	0.0
Total:	3837	4688	18068	20.7	324	270.1
est. % complete:	3.8	15.6	---	0.7	---	9.0

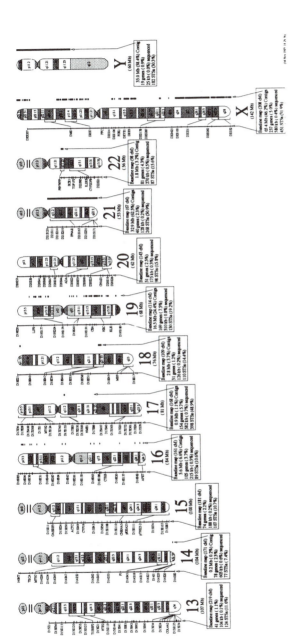

FIGURE 1-1 Simplified gene map. SOURCE: National Center for Human Genome Research, National Institutes of Health, 1993.

When diseases that are suspected to be gene-influenced do not follow usual Mendelian patterns of inheritance, more than one gene, or a variety of environmental factors to which susceptible individuals are exposed, play a role. This is the case for many common diseases, including several birth defects, some forms of heart disease, hypertension, cancer, diabetes, mental illness, and infectious disorders. Evidence supporting the promise of linkage mapping for common diseases has been found in families in which the disease is inherited as a single-gene dominant disorder. For example, two different genes, each by itself responsible for Alzheimer disease have been mapped (Goate et al., 1991; Schellenberg et al., 1992). In another case, a gene thought to be responsible for only a rare form of colon cancer was later found to be implicated in the more common sporadic form of the disease (Fearon and Vogelstein, 1990). Success of the linkage approach in complex disorders has been tempered, however, by several failures. Earlier reports of linkage in manic-depressive illness in the Old-Order Amish could not be confirmed when new individuals in the family became ill (Egeland and Kidd, 1989); reports of linkage on the X chromosome previously reported for manic depression were recently retracted (Baron et al., 1992).

For disorders with complex etiologies, such as coronary artery disease, identification of a genetic defect in a rare, single-gene form may provide invaluable clues to causation and approaches to therapy in general. This has been demonstrated for familial hypercholesterolemia (Goldstein and Brown, 1989). It is possible, however, that mutations in the gene that is involved in the rare, single-gene forms of other common, complex disorders will not play a role in the complex forms. Moreover, it will be very difficult to use linkage studies to establish the role of genes that are neither necessary nor sufficient to cause the disease (Greenberg, 1993).

Implications of Recombinant DNA Technology for Genetic Testing

Prior to the discovery of recombinant DNA techniques, the determination of a person's risk of harboring genes that could lead to disease in that person, or in her or his offspring, was limited to those diseases for which a clinical diagnosis could be made or for which tests were available to detect an altered gene product (an enzyme or other protein) or a metabolite that accumulated in a readily accessible tissue such as blood, urine, skin (by biopsy), mucosa of the mouth, or hair. In the late 1960s, it proved possible to detect some altered gene products in cells obtained from the amniotic fluid by midtrimester amniocentesis, thus making prenatal diagnosis possible (Fuchs, 1966; Steele and Breg, 1966; Jacobson and Barter, 1967; Hahneman and Mohr, 1968; Nadler, 1968). However, effective treatment was not available for most prenatally diagnosable disorders. In the absence of effective treatment, prenatal diagnosis had to be done at a gestational age at which the mother had the option of aborting the affected fetus safely and legally. The number of diseases that could be diagnosed prenatally increased markedly when it became possible to localize a disease-related gene by linkage studies and then identify the gene. Based on the same techniques that made localization and identification possible, tests could be developed whose purpose was to show whether mutations capable of causing a specific disease, or conferring susceptibility to its occurrence, were present or absent. Since all of a person's genes are present in all nucleated cells from the moment of conception, the requirements of having an accessible tissue or an active gene (resulting in the appearance of a gene product) were eliminated. For any disease-related gene that has been localized, linkage studies can be done in families in which the disease has already occurred to determine whether other relatives are likely to be affected. For any disease for which the disease-causing gene and, within it, disease-causing mutations have been identified, direct tests for the presence of those mutations can be done on anyone: having a family history is not a prerequisite; entire populations can be screened for the presence of specific mutations.

The development of genetic tests to assess individual risks of diseases followed quickly on the heels of the discovery of disease-related genes and mutations. For most diseases, testing has been confined to families in which the disease has already occurred, even when direct tests for mutations have been developed. This has greatly increased the opportunity for people in these families to learn their risks of disease or of having children with the disease. In the case of sickle cell anemia and thalassemia (autosomal recessive disorders for which carrier screening was possible by "gene product" techniques), direct tests of mutation have permitted safe and reliable prenatal diagnosis. As the Human Genome Project and other research lead to the discovery of more disease-related genes, the scope of testing will expand further. Tests for genetic predispositions to multifactorial disorders will also be possible, and eventually technologies will be available to simultaneously test for hundreds of different disease-causing mutations, either in the same or in different genes.

Other Recent Advances and Their Implications for Genetic Testing

A number of other techniques have been developed recently that also expand the opportunities for genetic testing. The most far-reaching is the polymerase chain reaction (PCR), a technique that permits the rapid amplification (reproduction) of predetermined segments of DNA. By starting with the DNA from as little as one cell, a sufficient amount of material can be replicated within hours to allow the amplified segment to be detected easily. This has greatly simplified genetic testing.

New techniques have also been developed for prenatal diagnosis. *Chorionic villus sampling* permits prenatal diagnosis as early as 9 weeks of gestation, compared to amniocentesis, which until recently was seldom performed before 16 weeks. *Earlier amniocentesis* is currently being investigated.

Very recently, successful prenatal diagnosis has been reported before the embryo is implanted in the uterus. The technique, known as *preimplantation diagnosis*, involves removing cells at the blastocyst stage and using PCR to amplify the segments of DNA (one from each parent) containing the part of the disease-related gene that contains the disease-causing mutation of interest. If the disease-causing mutation is absent, the embryo(s) is then implanted in the woman's uterus (Simpson and Carson, 1992). Prefertilization determination of whether an ovum contains a specific disease-causing mutation has also been accomplished by *polar body analysis* (Verlinsky and Pergament, 1984; Verlinsky and Kuliev, 1992). If the ovum does not contain such a mutation, in vitro fertilization is carried out, and the resulting embryo is implanted in the woman's uterus; this technique also involves the use of PCR. These techniques are still considered experimental and are discussed further in Chapter 2.

Recombinant DNA technology has also added new techniques for detecting changes in the number of chromosomes present in a fetus's cells (aneuploidy). The technique involves fluorescent in situ hybridization (FISH) of chromosome-specific probes with cells obtained prenatally (Klinger, 1992). It is far less time-consuming and labor-intensive than the earlier technique of karyotyping, which nevertheless is capable of detecting a much wider range of disorders than FISH.

Empiric observations have revealed that when a woman is carrying a fetus with an extra chromosome (i.e., trisomy), she is likely to have altered concentrations of alpha-fetoprotein (AFP), chorionic gonadotropin, and estradiol in her blood (so-called *triple-marker* testing for increased risk of abnormalities in the fetus) (Haddow et al., 1992). This has permitted the development of maternal blood tests for these substances as initial screens of pregnant women for increased risk of such fetal abnormalities. Confirmatory tests are necessary for actual diagnosis.

New techniques for prenatal diagnosis are also being evaluated involving fetal cells that are usually present in and can be isolated from the maternal circulation in the first trimester of pregnancy. These techniques are still highly experimental (Bianchi et al., 1991; Elias et al., 1992). Although this technique is noninvasive of the fetus, the scientific, ethical, legal, and social issues associated with other forms of prenatal diagnosis are still present (see Chapters 2 and 4).

Many of the techniques discussed thus far involve gene changes (mutations) that are—with rare exceptions (i.e., *mosaicism*)—usually present in all cells of the body, having occurred as *germline mutations* and inherited from one or both parents. On the other hand, there is now evidence that as cells become cancerous they undergo a number of nongermline, noninherited, *somatic cell mutations* in different genes (Fearon and Vogelstein, 1990). Preliminary work suggests that the presence of these somatic cell mutations may be detected (via PCR) by analysis of fluids in which mutated cells might be shed (e.g., fecal matter in the case of colon cancer), which would serve as an early warning of the development of malignancy (Sidransky et al., 1992).

Advances in ultrasound have resulted in its use to detect structural changes in the fetus, some of which may be associated with genetic or chromosomal abnormalities. Although not a genetic test in itself, ultrasonography is used as an adjunct to help detect structural abnormalities. In some countries, ultrasonography is performed on every pregnant woman, and its use is increasingly common in the United States as well. It may be the most frequently used prenatal diagnostic test. The general consensus is that ultrasound should not be used *routinely* in every pregnancy (NIH, 1984; ACOG, 1988), but that consensus may not reflect actual obstetrical practice today. Recent reviews in the literature have identified some factors affecting reliability in identification of fetal anomalies through ultrasound (Filly et al., 1987; Goldstein et al., 1989); others have reported variability in quality by center and practitioner and error rates of more than 10 percent (Levi et al., 1991; Lancet, 1992). The committee heard testimony that raised its concern about the reliability of interpretation of prenatal ultrasound images and about the consequences of decisions based on such interpretation (see Chapter 2).

Limitations of Genetic Testing

Genetic tests are seldom perfect predictors of clinical risk. No biochemical screening test is sensitive enough to detect all cases, and even current DNA methods cannot detect all possible mutations that cause a specific disease. For example, more than 300 mutations in the CF transmembrane regulator gene have been found that cause CF; most of them are extremely rare. Current technology permits the simultaneous detection of approximately 20 of the most common ones, accounting for about 85 to 90 percent of mutations in whites but a much smaller proportion of mutations in nonwhites (Cutting et al., 1992). Moreover, the frequency of the different mutations for CF can vary within subpopulations; what applies to a northern European population does not necessarily apply to Italian or Jewish populations. The 0.4 to 0.6 percent of normal individuals who carry undetectable mutations will not know—even after testing—that they are at risk, if they mate with another carrier, of having a child with CF. Similar *allelic diversity* occurs in many other disorders. Thus it becomes important to distinguish between *analytic sensitivity*, the ability of a test to detect the various mutations it was designed to detect, and *clinical sensitivity*, the ability of the test to detect all patients who will get, or who have, the disease.

A way could be found around the less-than-perfect sensitivity of current DNA tests in the presence of allelic diversity. The multiple mutations that result in a specific disease all impair the normal expression of the gene. Consequently, a test that measures normal gene expression could tell, indirectly, whether any mutation capable of altering expression is present. Tests of altered gene product antedated DNA-based tests, but they could only be performed when evidence of gene expression could be found in readily accessible tissues. Recent work indicates that minute amounts of mRNA for proteins that are detectable only in specialized tissues are present in accessible tissues such as white blood cells and cultured chorionic villus cells (Chelly et al., 1989; Sarkar and Commer, 1989). The protein could be translated from the mRNA and its structure and function assayed.

Even when a test can detect a mutation capable of causing a single-gene disease, the test may not be able to predict with certainty whether disease symptoms will appear or when they will appear. In such cases of *incomplete penetrance*, the specific mutation may be a *necessary but not a sufficient condition* for the disease to become manifest; other conditions must be present as well. These may be mutations at other gene loci or environmental factors; some or all of these other factors may be unknown. As a result, genetic test information on predispositions to a disorder has a potential for falsely labeling persons as being at risk for the disorder.

Many factors may modify the severity of single-gene diseases: the disease can have *variable expressivity*. The degree of severity (or extent of expressivity) cannot usually be predicted by a genetic test, even a test for a specific mutation; however, some specific mutations tend to be associated with specific levels of severity of the disorder.

Aside from problems that arise as a result of allelic diversity, incomplete penetrance, and variable expressivity, tests for genes implicated in single-gene disorders have other limitations. The accuracy of linkage tests will be impaired when an incorrect diagnosis is made in a relative or when the social father is not, in fact, the biological father. Linkage studies often have some uncertainty attached to them because the DNA marker linked to a disease gene can be separated by recombination. Such recombination events become more frequent as the physical distance between the marker and the disease gene increases. Tests will also be imperfect predictors if the laboratories performing them do not do so correctly and accurately.

Problems of penetrance and expressivity become even greater in testing for complex disorders in which multiple factors, of which the gene being tested is only one, contribute to the causation of the disease. In some of these disorders, a gene at a different locus (or genes at more than one locus) than the one being tested could contribute to causation. This is a form of *genetic heterogeneity*.

For some disorders, treatments of proven effectiveness will be available, but these treatments could be harmful to people who do not have the genetic disease (such as those in which a test was falsely positive). For many diseases, however, no definitive therapy will be possible when testing becomes available, although identification of the underlying genetic defect is likely to accelerate the discovery of future treatments. The duration of the lag period between testing and treatment capabilities will vary from disease to disease. For some disorders, the lag time will be so long that (1) individuals confronted with having to decide whether to be tested will not have any prospect of effective treatment to benefit them, and (2) they could not postpone having children long enough to see whether a treatment to benefit a prenatally diagnosed fetus will be discovered. Under such circumstances, nonmedical benefits and harms, as well as ethical considerations, dominate the decision about whether testing should be undertaken, both for individuals and for society.

Because of the imperfect nature of genetic tests and the implications of both true positive and false positive test results, as well as false negative results, the understanding of those who offer tests and of the recipients themselves is crucial to appropriate use of genetic testing. It was these issues that prompted the first NAS report on genetic screening.

LESSONS FROM THE PAST

From 1972 to 1975, a committee convened by the National Research Council (NRC) considered problems related to genetic testing. At that time, the most frequent use of genetic tests was in screening programs. That committee defined genetic screening "as a search in a population for persons possessing certain genotypes that (1) are already associated with disease or predispose to disease, (2) may lead to disease in their descendants, or (3) produce other variations not known to be associated with disease" (NAS, 1975, p. 9). A report on screening had been published by Wilson and Jungner (1968), but genetic aspects were not emphasized in that report. Thus, the NAS committee set out to gather ideas and information with the intention of producing a review of current practices and recommendations for the future. That NAS report focused on two disorders for which screening programs had recently been developed: the testing of newborns for phenylketonuria (PKU), which started in the late 1950s; and screening for sickle cell anemia and carriers, which started in 1971. The 1975 committee quickly perceived that much of the genetic testing then being done was undertaken prematurely and was haphazard or ill-informed. The Tay-Sachs carrier screening program, which started in the Jewish community in Baltimore in 1971, suggested that screening could be organized rationally (Kaback and Zeiger, 1972). The report also considered screening for Tay-Sachs disease and thalassemia. A brief description of early screening programs follows.

Phenylketonuria

Screening for PKU began with the testing of infants' urine for a metabolite of phenylalanine, an amino acid that accumulated in PKU. Within a few years it became apparent that as many as half of infants with PKU were missed by the urine test (Medical Research Council, 1968). It was replaced by a test for phenylalanine in the blood. This test could be performed on a spot of blood obtained from a heel prick before the infant left the hospital nursery. After a short field trial, this test was made mandatory by most states. Some state laws gave parents a right to refuse testing, primarily on religious grounds. In most states, however, screening was done without informing the parents about the test or their right to refuse.

Mandatory screening was based on the belief that restricting the phenylalanine in the diet of infants with PKU would prevent the mental retardation that was almost invariably associated with the disorder. Scientists had proven that the low-phenylalanine diet promptly lowered serum phenylalanine levels in infants with PKU. However, at the time mass screening began, there was no conclusive evidence that the diet prevented mental retardation. Because of the claims of benefit, it was impossible to mount a randomized controlled trial to determine the effectiveness of the diet. (In retrospect, 14 children detected by screening, and meeting rigorous criteria for PKU, would have been needed in a two-year trial to demonstrate the effectiveness of the diet; Holtzman, 1977.) Only after 10 years did a collaborative trial (in which all infants were treated with the special diet, but to varying degrees) provide convincing evidence of an association between early institution of the low-phenylalanine diet and maintenance of good dietary control on the one hand, and intellectual performance on the other (Committee on Genetics, 1982; N. Holtzman et al., 1986).

In the meantime, it also became apparent that not all infants with elevated phenylalanine had classical PKU. Some infants had variant forms of PKU that resulted in seizures, retardation, and death even with dietary restriction of phenylalanine; fortunately, these variants are very rare (Scriver et al., 1989). In other infants, the elevation of phenylalanine was transient or, if it persisted, was mild and not associated with mental retardation. A few infants who did not actually have PKU died or suffered irreversible damage when they were started—without proper monitoring—on the low-phenylalanine diet, resulting in depletion of their supply of phenylalanine, an essential amino acid (Holtzman, 1970).

A 1970 survey of health department and PKU clinics indicated that 5 to 10 percent of infants with PKU were being missed by screening and were being diagnosed because of mental retardation. Although it is not altogether clear what accounts for some infants being missed, two factors contribute significantly: (1) the inherent lack of sensitivity of the screening test, particularly when it is performed the first day after birth, and (2) human errors in the performance of the test, which include errors in specimen collection, laboratory procedure, or followup, such as failure to notify parents or the infant's physician (C. Holtzman et al., 1986). The current practice to reduce the length of stay of newborns in order to reduce hospital costs may well contribute to an increasing rate of false negatives with the PKU screening test.

Thus, screening for PKU had been undertaken widely before either the validity of the test, the quality of the laboratories performing it, or the efficacy or safety of the treatment had been firmly established. As a result, some infants suffered irreparable harm; however, many more infants benefited from early PKU detection and appropriate therapy.

Sickle Cell Anemia and Trait

A more serious set of errors was made in the establishment of sickle cell screening programs in the African-American community in the early 1970s. Some of these screening programs were established without adequate consultation and education of the affected communities. A test then in common use failed to distinguish individuals with the disease from those who were only carriers. No treatment for sickle cell anemia as effective as the low-phenylalanine diet for PKU was available or on the horizon. The only benefit of early detection for infants with the disease was to ensure that children would receive medical care promptly when they became sick, yet improved access to medical care was not usually part of the programs. Nor was prenatal diagnosis available at that time; the only way parents could avoid having affected children was not to have children at all or to avoid mating with another carrier.

Since 8 percent of African-Americans are carriers of the sickle cell trait, many carriers were detected in screening programs. However, knowledge of having the sickle cell trait had no medical benefit since carriers are healthy. Detection of the trait was appropriate only for reproductive purposes since there is a 1 in 4 risk of having an infant with sickle cell anemia if both parents carry the trait. However, confusion about the significance of carrying the common sickle cell trait (about 1 in 12 African-Americans) and the rare sickle cell anemia (with a frequency of about 1 in 600) often led to stigmatization and discrimination.

In the early 1970s, seven states passed mandatory laws requiring sickle cell screening, while ten others had voluntary laws. Some laws called for newborn screening. Others erroneously regarded sickle cell anemia as an infectious disease and called for screening before a child could enter school. Others required it as a condition of obtaining a marriage license. In at least one state law, as well as in the National Sickle Cell Anemia Control Act of 1972, it was evident that legislators had confused the frequency of the trait (about 1 in 12 African-Americans) with the frequency of the disease of about 1 in 600 (Reilly, 1977). The national act required programs supported with federal funds to be voluntary, not mandatory. Nevertheless, even in the late 1970s, some screening in at least one state was done without informed consent (Farfel and Holtzman, 1984).

The experiences in the sickle cell screening programs of the early 1970s reinforce the need for education before screening and for counseling after screening, and require that participants be assured of the confidentiality of their test results (see Chapter 8). Enthusiasm turned to suspicion as many African-Americans concluded that the intent was to eradicate the sickle cell gene by preventing carriers from reproducing—thereby reducing the birth rate in the black community. These genetic testing programs were perceived by some as genocidal in intent.

Considerable time, effort, and money have been required to overcome these early mistakes. To promote research and develop high-quality programs of screening and counseling, the National Heart, Lung, and Blood Institute provided funding in the 1970s under the national act to establish 10 centers for sickle cell disease research and 25 clinics to carry out education, screening, and counseling in high-risk populations. Under these auspices, protocols for more effective education, screening, and counseling were developed and the criteria for appropriate management of sickle cell anemia were developed. Early studies by the Centers for Disease Control (CDC) found that the laboratories providing tests often made technical errors and were sometimes doing primary screening with a test that did not distinguish sickle cell trait from the disease. Federal support through the CDC proficiency testing and assistance program helped laboratories to improve the quality of testing. Similarly, federal support for community-based sickle cell programs included education of providers and consumers, improving the understanding of both groups. It was not until 1978 that sickle cell anemia could be diagnosed in amniotic fluid cells obtained by amniocentesis (Kan and Dozy, 1978). Prior to that time, diagnosis was possible on fetal blood, although obtaining it carried much greater risks to the fetus than amniocentesis (Hollenberg et al., 1971). And not until 1986, as the result of a collaborative nationwide randomized controlled trial, was it established that penicillin prophylaxis reduced infant and childhood mortality from sickle cell anemia (Gaston et al., 1986), thereby providing a therapeutic rationale for screening newborns for sickle cell anemia. Although 42 states now screen newborns for sickle cell disease (CORN, 1992), not all infants with the disease receive treatment.

Tay-Sachs Disease and Trait

That community-based programs could be effectively mounted was demonstrated by the development of Tay-Sachs carrier screening. Beginning in Baltimore, this program spread rapidly to Jewish communities across the country and around the world. Unlike sickle cell anemia, whose manifestations and severity vary considerably, the predominant form of Tay-Sachs disease in Jews of eastern European (Ashkenazi) origin was uniformly fatal in early childhood. The basic defect in this form of the disease—the absence of an enzyme—and the ability to identify carriers had been established shortly before screening was contemplated. Prenatal testing was also available—it was possible to detect fetuses with the disorder by assaying amniotic fluid cells for the missing enzyme. This meant that couples in which both partners were found to be carriers could avoid the birth of any child with this uniformly fatal disease without having to forgo childbearing.

Before Tay-Sachs disease screening started, intense discussions of the goals and methods, as well as means of publicizing the program, were held with rabbis, physicians in the community, and other community and religious leaders. Pilot studies were conducted to determine the validity and reliability of the automated serum enzyme assay to be used for screening, and a more definitive confirmatory test (leukocyte assay) was established. Organizers decided that screening would be most relevant to reproductive decision making and, therefore, would be targeted to young married couples; it was later expanded to include unmarried individuals 18 years and older. Screening was held in community sites—primarily community centers, religious schools, and synagogues—medical geneticists and genetic counselors were present, along with community volunteers, to provide on-

---

BOX 1-1 Tay-Sachs Disease: Chevra Dor Yeshorim Program

Preventing Tay-Sachs disease by avoiding reproduction between carriers was the option selected by Hasidic Jews, originally in New York City (Chevra Dor Yeshorim Program) (Merz, 1987). This community has a high risk of Tay-Sachs disease and also opposes abortion and contraception. The program is based on the community practice of arranged marriages. When a woman turns 18, or a man 20, a blood sample is tested anonymously for Tay-Sachs disease. The laboratory assigns a code number, which it retains (without names) with the results; the laboratory gives the code number but not the result to the person tested. When a marriage is planned, a matchmaker queries the registry by giving the code numbers of the two prospective partners. A couple considering marriage can also query the registry. Only if both partners are carriers will they be told that they should each seek another partner. This system was designed with a relatively high degree of anonymity to avoid possible stigmatization of carriers (Merz, 1987). Originating in New York, the program has spread to communities elsewhere in the United States, Canada, Europe, and Israel. This approach was designed for the particular religious beliefs and customs of ultra-Orthodox Jews.

---

site education and respond to questions. Results were mailed personally but, in addition, those with positive tests were usually informed by telephone. Couples in which both partners were found to be carriers were routinely referred for genetic counseling with a genetic counselor. Informed consent was obtained before all testing. The results were kept confidential and were made available only to the individuals tested by use of a self-addressed envelope filled out at testing.

Couples found by screening to be at risk for having a child with Tay-Sachs disease almost always decided to proceed with prenatal diagnostic testing and to terminate affected pregnancies when diagnosed (President's Commission, 1983). By 1992, more than 2,400 pregnancies at risk for Tay-Sachs disease were tested in programs throughout the world; nearly 500 fetuses were found to be affected by the fatal disorder, and virtually all of these pregnancies were terminated (Kaback, 1992). Of particular significance, more than 1,800 healthy offspring have been born to these at-risk couples; many of these children might never have been conceived or brought to term without genetic testing. Since 1971, screening in the Ashkenazi Jewish populations has led to more than a 90 percent reduction in Tay-Sachs disease in that population in the United States and Canada. By contrast, it is the committee's impression that the incidence of sickle cell anemia among African-Americans has not decreased since screening began.

We still have more to learn about education and counseling for a population. Even in the relatively well-educated population being screened for Tay-Sachs, there was occasional confusion about the meaning and implications of test results (Childs et al., 1976; Zeesman et al., 1984; Kaback, 1993). Nevertheless, this continues to be a highly effective genetic carrier detection effort in which more than a million people have been screened to date. The program has wide acceptance, with little evidence of personal, family, or community stigmatization of individuals found to be carriers or of couples at risk of Tay-Sachs disease in their offspring.

Thalassemia

Thalassemia screening began in 1976, based substantially on the Tay-Sachs disease model (early planning with the relevant communities, laboratory quality control, and prescreening and posttest education and counseling). With the availability of prenatal testing, thalassemia carrier screening has been organized in a number of Mediterranean countries and in communities in other countries with populations that are at high risk for thalassemia. In some of these countries, the frequency of thalassemia, and particularly the need for blood transfusions in patients with the disorder, was so high that a sizable fraction of the population suffered from the disorder and a significant fraction of health resources was consumed in management of the disorder. In Sardinia (Cao et al., 1981, 1989), Cyprus (Angastiniotis, 1990), and among Cypriots in London (Modell et al., 1980), after thalassemia screening, couples were offered prenatal diagnosis and if found to be carrying a fetus with thalassemia, the majority decided to abort; this has resulted in a 10-fold reduction in infants born with this disease. In Sardinia, for example, the incidence of thalassemia has declined from 1 in 250 births to one in 1,200 births since 1974, and because of the educational program and the follow-up screening of families, the majority of persons are now being screened before pregnancy (Cao et al., 1989). This model has also been adapted to high-risk populations in Canada and in the United States (Fisher et al., 1981; Rowley et al., 1984; Scriver et al., 1984).

Important lessons emerged from early screening programs. In PKU, screening was made mandatory at a time when neither the benefits of the therapy for PKU nor the sensitivity of the test had been clearly established. In sickle cell, screening was started hastily without a clear effort to distinguish screening for carriers from screening for disease, as well as without adequate education of the public. When problems such as these were analyzed and worked out in advance, as in Tay-Sachs disease and thalassemia screening, genetic screening programs were developed in a more appropriate way, and implementation raised fewer scientific, ethical, legal, and social issues.

UPDATING THE FINDINGS OF THE 1975 NAS COMMITTEE

The 1975 NAS committee concluded that it would be useful to elaborate some fundamental principles and rules of procedure for genetic testing. In reviewing these 1975 principles, the current Institute of Medicine (IOM) committee asked whether these principles and rules are still valid for the 1990s and beyond; whether changing conditions necessitate new principles; and whether specific actions are needed to ensure implementation of the principles. To a large extent, these questions guide the discussion in the chapters that follow. As mentioned earlier, the 1975 committee focused on population-based screening, although most of its principles apply equally to other forms of genetic testing.

Aims of Testing and Screening

The aims of testing and screening are multiple. The first is *management* (i.e., a search for people with treatable genetic disorders that could prove dangerous to their health if left untreated). A second is providing *reproductive options* to people with high probability of having children with severe, untreatable disease, for whom counseling could be helpful and prenatal diagnosis or abortion of interest, with Tay-Sachs disease as the prototypical example. A third is *enumeration of cases* (e.g., for some public health purpose such as determining the incidence and prevalence of congenital anomaly). Finally, *research* is an aim which might (1) involve the testing of hypotheses relating to human physiology or evolution, (2) serve to enumerate the incidence of other diseases, or (3) investigate the feasibility and value of new methods or tests.

(summarized from NAS, 1975)

The aims of screening remain the same, but the potential scope of screening has expanded remarkably as a result of the ability to test at the DNA level, and new aims have been identified. In screening for "management" of disease, newborns may now be screened for up to 11 disorders, depending on the policy of the state in which they are born. However, the treatment for some of these disorders may not always restore normal function (e.g., some cases of galactosemia and maple syrup urine disease), and, in some instances, may prolong life that many would view as of poor quality. In addition, screening of people of various ages for genetic predispositions to disease is on the verge of becoming a reality. If cholesterol screening is viewed as a search for genetic disease (since hypercholesterolemia often has a genetic basis), such screening is already here. As more is learned about the role of somatic cell mutations in the chain of events leading to malignant neoplasms, it is becoming possible to screen individuals for certain precancerous mutations (e.g., p53). All of these types of screening offer benefit through permitting the individual to reduce the risk of severe disease by taking medications, undergoing periodic monitoring, or altering behavior or life-style (see Chapter 2).

Opportunities have also expanded in screening for reproductive options. Maternal serum alpha-fetoprotein (MSAFP) is now widely used to screen pregnant women of all ages to determine if they are at higher risk of carrying a fetus with a neural tube or other serious birth defect, including increased risk of chromosomal abnormalities. Amniocentesis remains the principal technique for prenatal diagnosis, although chorionic villus sampling can be performed earlier in pregnancy (with a somewhat increased risk to the fetus). To increase a couple's reproductive options as early in pregnancy as possible, new technologies are being devised rapidly. Recently, highly experimental genetic tests have become possible prior to fertilization of the ovum and prior to implantation of the fertilized ovum, although not without the stress, cost, and other issues associated with in vitro fertilization. Work is also in progress in genetic testing of fetal cells isolated from the maternal blood-stream early in pregnancy (Bianchi et al., 1991; Elias et al., 1992).

Multiplex testing—using technologies that will concurrently test for dozens if not hundreds of disease-related mutations—was not considered in 1975 except to the extent that each test would have to satisfy the committee's criteria for screening. The sheer number of tests that could be performed at one time on a single sample raises serious issues of informed consent (see Chapter 8).

Genetic testing is also already being used for nonmedical purposes, such as forensic identification (OTA, 1990a; NAS, 1992). The U.S. Armed Forces Institute of Pathology is now collecting and storing blood samples from every member of the Armed Forces, and the Federal Bureau of Investigation has developed a national DNA profile data bank system for the identification of criminals. At least 17 states maintain DNA samples for criminal identification, and some states (see Virginia, 1990) require a sample for DNA identification as a condition of parole. Such nonmedical uses of genetic information may lead to breaches of privacy and confidentiality (see Chapter 8).

It has been conjectured that genetic testing may be able to predict an individual's intellectual capabilities and aptitudes. The committee doubts that—in the foreseeable future—genetic testing will permit an accurate assessment of a child's specific physical or mental capabilities; these traits are far too complex (in their genetic and environmental interactions) to enable a genetic test to predict them accurately. Consequently, any such use of testing is likely to result in mislabeling of individuals and will result in considerable harm.

Of much greater immediate concern is the use of genetic test results—intended for medical diagnosis or management—for purposes that may not be in the best interest of the person being tested. One such use is specifically to determine insurability or employability. Although this practice is not now widespread (OTA, 1990b, 1992), there is a growing danger that the results of genetic testing, obtained by an individual primarily for purposes of disease management or for reproductive options, may be used by an insurer or employer to deny health or life insurance or employment (see Chapters 7 and 8).

The 1975 committee indicated research purposes as another aim of screening. This report does not deal with such uses, except for investigations, including pilot programs, undertaken to assess the value of screening for management or the provision of reproductive options.

Criteria for Testing

Tests should be of benefit to the individual tested, and if offered to anyone they should be offered to everyone. Singling out of subpopulation groups for genetic testing raises the potential for stigmatizing such groups. The tests should be reliable and accurate, being reasonably specific and highly sensitive. Results should be communicated quickly and under circumstances that take into account the implications of the news and its impact on the feelings of those receiving it. Standards should be uniform throughout the Nation. Mechanisms to ensure consistency and continuous evaluation should be instituted. Centralization of screening laboratories is desirable to maintain standards. Screening should not be undertaken in the absence of pilot studies or facilities for follow-up.

(summarized from NAS, 1975)

The committee finds itself in strong agreement with these criteria, especially the principle that tests should be of benefit to the individual being tested. This principle has several applications. In newborn screening, it means that testing should be undertaken only to benefit the newborn. In screening for disease management, the interventions that follow the test should benefit those screened, and not be used against them. The committee was concerned that some uses of genetic test information may represent harmful and unwarranted intrusions on individual privacy. For example, in adoption cases, information from genetic screening programs should not be used in a detrimental way to determine suitability as adoptive parents or as a potential adopted child. Obviously, the use of genetic information, as well as other medical information, in adoption is a complex subject, and requires further study (see Chapter 9).

The committee also agrees that there should be equal access to testing, with the further condition that equal access should be provided for people *at approximately equal risk of having a genetic disorder.* If there are wide discrepancies in risks to subsegments of the population, there would be no need to screen those at lower risk; the committee believes that the mere availability of a genetic test should not mean that it should necessarily be offered to everyone. Such a policy might be difficult to implement, but—if a low-risk group can be delineated—the committee does not believe that it would be necessary to offer them testing. This will help to hold down the costs per case averted at a time when neither the states nor the federal government is as likely to finance an expansion of genetic testing or screening as they were for PKU and sickle cell anemia. Equal access may also depend on reforms in our health insurance system that will either pay for, or reimburse for, appropriate genetic tests and follow-up services regardless of an individual's ability to pay (see Chapters 7 and 8).

Quality of Testing

With the expansion of genetic testing, concern about its reliability and validity is greater today than it was in 1975. There are several reasons. First, the proliferation of laboratories and new tests may outpace the establishment of criteria for judging quality and even for deciding when the validity of the test warrants its use clinically. Second, defining what constitutes reasonable specificity and sensitivity is difficult and can be decided only when evidence is available on the performance characteristics of the tests under consideration, and criteria are likely to vary with different types of tests depending on the ratio of benefits to risks. Third, this proliferation of testing sites makes it more difficult to reach all sites with external quality assessment programs, and increases the chance of errors in testing. Fourth, greater concerns surround genetic testing performed to provide reproductive options, given the potential consequences of errors.

Like the earlier committee, we view high laboratory quality and demonstrated safety, quality control, and effectiveness of tests as critical principles with which there can be no compromises. Federal legislation is already in place both for assessing the characteristics of new tests before they are marketed and for assessing the quality of laboratories that are providing clinical services. However, these are not being fully applied to genetic testing. Although centralization of testing facilities could help to maintain standards of testing, that centralization may not be possible as long as companies compete with each other, and in some instances with academic centers, for the testing business. However, centralization is important and attainable for tests for rare disorders, which are less lucrative financially (see Chapter 3).

Conflicts of Interest

The proliferation of tests and extension of testing into commercial laboratories have led to new issues in conflicts of interests. A key new issue is the potential for conflict of interest on the part of those who are in a position to recommend tests. Such individuals, including geneticists and primary care physicians, may have a business or financial interest in laboratories or companies that provide testing and/or hold patents on genes from which royalties are generated through the testing process. The committee believes that all such holdings should be publicly disclosed and strongly discouraged. The American Medical Association recently voted overwhelmingly that it is unethical in most cases for a physician to send a patient for tests to a clinic owned by the physician (AMA, 1992). The committee believes that the same disclosure requirement should apply to genetics and laboratory personnel who have a financial interest in a labѵratory providing genetic tests.

Pilot Studies

This committee also agrees that pilot studies should precede routine testing, and it would emphasize the principle that pilot studies must have prespecified objectives, clear methods, defined end points, and outside evaluation. In the years since the 1975 report, this principle has not always been followed rigorously. In newborn screening, for example, "pilot studies" imperceptibly became part of routine testing (Holtzman, 1991). Even though pilot studies cannot replicate all aspects of the situation that would ensue if screening were to become routine, pilot programs can be very useful in helping to establish a standard of care. This is especially true as genetic screening becomes incorporated into routine medical practice, which the committee believes will happen increasingly. Medical follow-up will also become far less of a problem than it has been in past screening programs (organized on a state public health or community-wide basis), except for people without a regular source of medical care (see Chapter 7). However, ensuring adequate patient education and genetic counseling will pose new challenges (see Chapter 4).

Auspices and Settings

The sponsorship of state and local government is essential to provide guidance, facilities, and follow-up. The 1975 study suggested that states or other communities institute commissions with authority to recommend new tests and programs, to monitor those in place, and to ensure standards for education, counseling, follow-up, treatment, and test procedures, thereby mitigating public concern about the many ethical issues that arise.

(summarized from NAS, 1975)

It is in this area that the situation is changing greatly from the time of the earlier recommendations. As already indicated, neither state nor federal government is likely to organize screening, although state health agencies may require private physicians to offer such tests (e.g., the MSAFP screening program in California), and state insurance laws may ensure that charges for genetic tests are reimbursed. But today the concern is no longer that of ensuring that new genetic screening tests will be done, but rather that pretest education and counseling, the offering of tests, their performance, and the counseling and medical interventions that follow positive test results, will be done *appropriately*. As testing technology becomes more simplified, walk-in testing (e.g., at shopping malls), mail-order kits, and home test kits become real possibilities; because of the importance of education and counseling and current deficiencies in public understanding, the committee believes that testing at nonmedical sites is inappropriate at this time. There are not now, nor in the future are there likely to be, sufficient numbers of medical geneticists and individuals trained primarily as genetic counselors to explain genetic tests and test results to all who might want them. Thus, it seems likely that much of genetic testing will be incorporated into the mainstream of medical care and provided particularly by primary care practitioners (family physicians, internists, obstetrician-gynecologists, and pediatricians). More problematic is the lack of time and inclination to provide counseling among primary care practitioners. The committee notes that, in many instances, primary care physicians, by virtue of having continuing contact with their patients, are better suited in several respects to provide counseling than specialists who are likely to first encounter patients only after positive test results have been obtained. Physicians' knowledge of genetics currently has serious deficiencies, and more attention to genetics and genetic testing is needed in medical education (see Chapter 6). Genetic counselors can help in the training of physicians, and in the training of nurses and social workers, who in turn can assist primary care physicians in genetic education and counseling (see Chapters 4 and 6).

Standards of Care

If testing is to be provided primarily by primary care physicians, how will these providers know when to adopt genetic tests? One protection will be afforded by ensuring that new tests and the laboratories performing them have been rigorously examined before they are approved by the appropriate federal agencies (see pilot studies above, Chapters 3 and 9). The committee believes, moreover, that in considering genetic tests, agencies must also consider problems of test interpretation, so that physicians receiving the results have a thorough and understandable explanation of their major implications and limitations. In addition, those providing reimbursement for testing should also require evidence of their safety and validity before reimbursement is provided (see Chapter 7). Of paramount importance is the role of professional organizations, such as the American Society of Human Genetics, American College of Medical Genetics, the American Academy of Pediatrics (AAP), and the American College of Obstetricians and Gynecologists, that can establish expert review panels to collect and review the evidence for deciding whether or not specific genetic tests should be designated "standard of care" and under what conditions. These panels should be guided by the principles enumerated in this chapter and by the criteria for specific types of testing outlined in Chapter 2. Objective, professional input is particularly important as physicians are increasingly bombarded by advertisements and other promotional material from laboratories providing tests or from companies selling various products.

The committee recognizes that successful litigation against physicians for failing to provide prenatal tests (Holtzman, 1989; Andrews, 1992) probably accelerated the adoption of some genetic tests and may induce physicians to adopt tests whose limitations are unclear to them. The committee would hope that prospective standard setting—and making physicians aware of such standards—will reduce the chance of poor practices and, consequently, of liability suits.

The committee believes that the standard is for *offering* the test, not actually providing it, and that no genetic test should be done without the consent of the persons being tested or, in the case of newborns, the consent of their parents, as discussed below and in depth in Chapter 8.

The committee strongly supports continued attention to scientific, ethical, legal, and social issues in genetics at all levels. The committee sees a particular need for advisory bodies—with grass roots consumer representatives—to guide state health departments or legislatures on such issues as deciding when tests should be added to state-run screening programs and to ensure that the offering, testing, and associated education and counseling are always conducted in accord with the principles suggested in this report. The committee also sees the need for continuing national oversight for the evaluation of existing and new genetic tests, and of pilot projects for the use of such tests, to help states decide what tests to adopt, to advise federal agencies with responsibilities related to genetic testing, and to provide broad policy advice on genetic testing (see Chapter 9 for the committee's recommendations).

Age for Testing

The optimal age for testing depends on the aims of the test. If the test is performed for disease management, the time to test is sometime before the age at which treatment must be started in order to be effective. If the test is performed for reproductive counseling, the time to test is when reproduction is being considered.

(summarized from NAS, 1975)

The committee agrees with this principle: there is little point, and possibly some harm, to testing at an age earlier than necessary to prevent irreversible damage. For instance, at the moment, there is considerable controversy about screening children for hypercholesterolemia. It is not clear that screening per se, or even lowering of cholesterol in children, is without harmful effects (Holtzman, 1992). Nor is it clear that lowering cholesterol in childhood confers any additional benefit of reducing the risk of future coronary artery disease over lowering cholesterol in early adulthood. However, getting accustomed to a prudent diet relatively early may be an advantage.

The committee rejects the assertion that the timing of screening should be determined primarily by when people come for health care and much prefers reform in the health care system to improve access so that many more people will come for care at optimal times. Because many women who contemplate pregnancy will not come for care until they are pregnant, some have argued that there is little point in providing carrier screening until pregnancy. The committee rejects this notion. First of all, some women will come for care too late in pregnancy to obtain any benefit from carrier testing in that pregnancy (see Chapter 2). Second, by delaying screening until pregnancy, women are deprived of options other than prenatal diagnosis and abortion. Nevertheless, when testing must first be done in pregnancy, it should be done in accord with the principles and criteria stated in this report.

Education of the Public

> Screening programs cannot fulfill their aims unless the public is aware of the purpose of the test, the disease it is intended to detect, its availability, its benefits to individuals, and its limitations.
>
> (summarized from NAS, 1975)

The principle of having an informed public takes on added importance as the scope of genetic testing increases. A recent survey (March of Dimes, 1992) shows that whereas members of the public have strong opinions about both genetic testing and gene therapy, they report little knowledge or understanding of either. Even when sufficient information is provided when tests are being offered, people with little familiarity with genetics will find it difficult to understand all of the ramifications. Informed decision making will be helped by improved teaching of genetics, probability, human variation, and ethical issues, beginning in the elementary grades, and increased attention to the issues in genetic testing in the media, so people will be better prepared to make informed decisions (see Chapter 5).

Ethical Issues

> People should know that their presence at the place of testing and the results of testing will be held in confidence. With this knowledge, people should be free to decide whether or not they want to be tested or screened. The only possible exception is newborn screening leading to effective treatment "if it were found that nonmandatory screening leaves many babies unscreened because of parental noncooperation or physicians' ignorance or oversight" (NAS, 1975, p. 191). People asking for tests should understand clearly that the test will be done *only* for the intended purposes and that there is no element of discrimination or of eugenic purpose.
>
> (summarized from NAS, 1975)

The expansion of testing heightens the importance of these ethical principles and the need to address others. In fact, much of this report is an exposition of what is needed for the principle of autonomy, in particular, to be taken seriously. The chapters on genetic counseling (see Chapter 4) and public education (see Chapter 5) emphasize the need for effective education before testing, which in turn depends on the client's ability to understand as much as possible about the basic concepts of genetics and probability (see Chapter 4). The instrument for ensuring the principle of autonomy is informed consent: whether or not a person should be tested is for him or her to decide after giving explicit consent based on adequate information. This is especially important in the case of reproductive choices and in prenatal diagnosis, where the growing range of technological options associated with genetic testing is placing increasing pressures on women to make difficult and unprecedented decisions (see Chapters 2, 4, and 9). Individuals also need to be assured that the results of a test will not be disclosed to others without their explicit permission, although there may be *rare* occasions when such disclosures can be justified (see Chapter 8).

Allocation of Resources

It is becoming common in health care to make decisions regarding programmatic support and reimbursement based on cost-benefit determinations. The committee explored cost-benefit and cost-effectiveness issues to a limited degree. There are troubling implications of cost-benefit analysis of genetic testing at this stage in the development of such testing, especially when effective treatment exists for relatively few diagnosable disorders. The implication of such analysis— that if an economic benefit were to be established, testing should be encouraged— violates the principle of patient autonomy, with particularly grave consequences in testing for reproductive options.

Most—but certainly not all—people who undergo prenatal testing have chosen to avoid having children with very severe disorders (especially those that cause extreme retardation or early death) without any degree of directiveness. However, some degree of coercion would probably be needed to gain widespread testing for carriers of defects that are less severe, but entail high costs (perhaps because survival is longer). It will, moreover, be difficult for people to agree on what is severe. If directiveness is accepted for any form of testing for which a safe, effective, and widely accepted treatment is not available, this compromises a critically held tenet: patient autonomy. The decision to support or reimburse genetic tests should be based on how well they meet the criteria and principles stated here and in Chapters 2 and 8, not on economic considerations. The committee believes that cost-effectiveness analyses may be appropriate when safe, effective, and widely accepted treatment is available, but additional research is needed on how to apply these techniques appropriately to genetic testing issues (see Chapter 9).

*Recognition of Human Diversity and Respect and Tolerance
for People with Disabilities*

The committee heard powerful and moving testimony from individuals with disabilities who believe that genetic testing and the consequent increase in abortion promote the premise that individuals with disabilities (whether tests exist for early detection or not) have less intrinsic worth. They pointed out that many people with disabilities lead full and productive lives and that society's negative view of disabilities is sometimes of greater harm to them than the disabilities themselves (Waxman, 1992). Some people with disabilities would resist any expansion of genetic testing. The committee recognizes the weight of these concerns and urges broad public education to dispel myths about people with disabilities—genetic or otherwise—and to reduce barriers to their participation in society (see Chapter 5). The committee rejects the notion of restricting any expansion of genetic testing based on the concerns of persons with disabilities that the technologies are inherently harmful. Such a restriction would undermine individual autonomy as much as the view that people should be urged or forced to use genetic tests and abortion to prevent disabilities. Nevertheless, the concerns of persons with disabilities are critical ones for our society. The committee is concerned that society may be moving closer to adopting the view that people should be urged or forced to use genetic tests and abortion to prevent disabilities; steps must be taken to counteract this tendency by decreasing pressures to test and increasing education and understanding of disabilities. If testing becomes widespread, efforts to urge people to undergo genetic testing might engender a greater intolerance for persons with disabilities—even though most disabilities are not the result of genetic causes. Avoiding the social pitfalls of intolerance based on genetic testing will require continuing vigilance.

REFERENCES

American College of Obstetrics and Gynecology (ACOG). 1988. Ultrasound in Pregnancy (Technical Bulletin No. 116), Washington, D.C.

American Medical Association (AMA). 1992. Resolution of the AMA House of Delegates on Physician Ownership and Self-Referral. December 12, 1992.

Andrews, L. 1992. Torts and the double helix: Malpractice liability for failure to warn of genetic risks. 29 Houston Law Review 149.

Angastiniotis, M. 1990. Cyprus: Thalassemia programme. Lancet 336:119-120.

Baron, M., et al. 1992. Diminished support for linkage between manic depressive illness and X-chromosome markers in three Israeli pedigrees. Nature Genetics 3:49-55.

Bianchi, D., et al. 1991. Fetal cells in maternal blood: Prospects for non-invasive prenatal diagnosis. Paper presented at the International Congress of Human Genetics, Washington, D.C.

Botstein, D., et al. 1980. Construction of a genetic linkage map in man using restriction fragment length polymorphisms. American Journal of Human Genetics 32:314-331.

Cao, A., et al. 1981. Prevention of homozygous beta-thalassemia by carrier screening and prenatal diagnosis in Sardinia. American Journal of Human Genetics 33:592-605.

Cao, A., et al. 1989. The prevention of thalassemia in Sardinia. Clinical Genetics 36:277-285.

Chelly, J., et al. 1989. Illegitimate transcription: Transcription of any gene in any cell type. Proceedings of the National Academy of Sciences USA 86:2617-2621.

Childs, B., et al. 1976. Tay-Sachs screening: Motives for participating and knowledge of genetics and probability. American Journal of Human Genetics 28:537-549.

Clow, C., and Scriver, C. 1977. The adolescent copes with genetic screening: A study of Tay-Sachs screening among high school students. In Kaback, M. (ed.) Tay-Sachs Disease: Screening and Prevention. New York: Liss.

Collins, F. 1992. Cystic fibrosis: Molecular biology and therapeutic implications. Science 256(5058):774-779.

Collins, F., et al. 1989. Genetic and physical maps come into focus. American Journal of Human Genetics 44(1):1-5.

Committee on Genetics. 1982. New issues in newborn screening for phenylketonuria and congenital hypothyroidism. Pediatrics 69:104-106.

Council of Regional Networks for Genetic Services (CORN). 1992. Newborn Screening Report: 1990 (Final Report, February 1992). New York: CORN.

Cutting, G., et al. 1992. Analysis of four diverse population groups indicates that a subset of cystic fibrosis mutations occur in common among Caucasians. American Journal of Human Genetics 50(6):1185-1194.

Donis-Keller, H., et al. 1987. A genetic linkage map of the human genome. Cell 51:319-337.

Donis-Keller, H., et al. 1992. A genetic linkage map of the human genome. Science 258:67-86.

Egeland, J., and Kidd, K. 1989. Re-evaluation of the linkage relationship between chromosome 11p loci and the gene for bipolar affective disorder in the Old Order Amish. Nature 342(6247):238-243.

Elias, S., et al. 1992. First trimester prenatal diagnosis of trisomy 21 in fetal cells from maternal blood. Lancet 340:1033.

Farfel, M., and Holtzman, N. 1984. Education, consent, and counseling in sickle cell screening programs: Report of a survey. American Journal of Public Health 74:373-375.

Fearon E., and Vogelstein B. 1990. A genetic model of colorectal tumorigenesis. Cell 61:759-767.

Filly, R., et al. 1987. Fetal spine morphology and maturation during the second trimester. Journal of Ultrasound in Medicine 6(11):631-636.

Fisher, L., et al. 1981. Genetic counseling for beta-thalassemia trait following health screening in a health maintenance organization: Comparison of programmed and conventional counseling. American Journal of Human Genetics 33:987-994.

Fuchs, F. 1966. Genetic information from amniotic fluid constituents. Clinical Obstetrics and Gynecology 9:565.

Gaston, M., et al. 1986. Prophylaxis with oral penicillin in children with sickle cell anemia. New England Journal of Medicine 314:1593-1599.

Goate, A., et al. 1991. Segregation of a missense mutation in the amyloid precursor protein gene with familial Alzheimer's disease. Nature 348:704-706.

Goldstein, J., and Brown, M. 1989. Familial hypercholesterolemia. Pp. 1215-1245 in Scriver, C., et al. (eds.) The Metabolic Basis of Inherited Disease (6th edition). New York: McGraw Hill.

Goldstein, M. et al. 1977. Health behavior and genetic screening for Tay-Sachs disease: A prospective study. Journal of Social Sciences and Medicine 11:515-520.

Goldstein, R., et al. 1989. Sonography of anencephaly: Pitfalls in early diagnosis. Journal of Clinical Ultrasound 17(6):397-402.

Greenberg, D. 1993. Linkage analysis of "necessary" disease loci versus "susceptibility" loci. American Journal of Human Genetics 52:135-143.

Gusella, J., et al. 1983. A polymorphic DNA marker genetically linked to Huntington's disease. Nature 306:234-238.

Haddow, J., et al. 1992. Prenatal screening for Down's syndrome with use of maternal serum markers. New England Journal of Medicine 327:588-593.

Hahneman, N., and Mohr, J. 1968. Genetic diagnosis in the embryo by means of biopsy from extraembryonic membrane. Bulletin of the European Society of Human Genetics 2:23-29.

Hampton, M., et al. 1974. Sickle cell "non-disease." American Journal of Diseases of Children 128:58-61.

Hollenberg, M., et al. 1971. Synthesis of adult hemoglobin by reticulocytes from the human fetus at midtrimester: Possible applications to prenatal detection of sickle cell anemia and other disorders. Science 171:689-702.

Holtzman, C., et al. 1986. PKU newborn screening in descriptive epidemiology of missed cases of phenylketonuria and congenital hypothyroidism. Pediatrics 78(4):553-558.

Holtzman, N. 1970. Dietary treatment of inborn errors of metabolism. Annual Review of Medicine 21:335-356.

Holtzman, N. 1977. Anatomy of a trial. Pediatrics. 60:932-934.

Holtzman, N. 1989. Medical professional liability in screening for genetic disorders and birth defects. In Rostow, V., and Bulger, R. (eds.) Medical Professional Liability and the Delivery of Obstetrical Care. Vol. II: An Interdisciplinary Review. Washington, D.C., National Academy Press.

Holtzman, N. 1991. What drives neonatal screening programs? New England Journal of Medicine 325:802-804.

Holtzman, N. 1992. The great god cholesterol. Pediatrics 89(4):686-687.

Holtzman, N., et al. 1986. Effect of age at loss of dietary control on infant performance and behavior of children with phenylketonuria. New England Journal of Medicine 314:593-598.

Huntington Disease Collaborative Research Group. 1993. A novel gene containing a trinucleotide repeat that is expanded and unstable on Huntington's disease chromosomes. Cell 72:971-983.

Jacobson, C., and Barter, R. 1967. Intrauterine diagnosis and management of genetic defects. American Journal of Obstetrics and Gynecology 99:769.

Kaback, M. 1992. In Scriver, C., et al. (ed.) The Metabolic Basis of Inherited Disorders. New York: Liss.

Kaback, M., and Leonard, C. 1971. Control studies in the antenatal diagnosis of human genetic-metabolic disorders. In Harris, M. (ed.) Early Diagnosis of Human Genetic Defects: Scientific and Ethical Considerations. Fogarty International Center Proceedings 6:169-178.

Kaback, M., and Zeiger, R. 1972. Practical and ethical issues in an adult genetic screening program: The John F. Kennedy Institute Tay-Sachs Program. In Hilton, B. (ed.) Ethical Issues in Human Genetics. New York: Plenum Press.

Kaback, M., et al. 1986. Tay-Sachs disease: A model for the control of recessive genetic disorders. Pp. 248-262 in Motulsky, A., and Lenz W. (eds.) Birth Defects. Amsterdam: Excerpta Medica.

Kan, Y., and Dozy, A. 1978. Antenatal diagnosis of sickle cell by DNA analysis of amniotic fluid cells. Lancet 2:910-912.

Klinger, K. 1992 (published in 1994). New clinical and laboratory procedures: Fluorescence in situ hybridization. In Fullarton, J. (ed.) Proceedings of the Committee on Assessing Genetic Risks. Washington, D.C.: National Academy Press.

Lancet. 1992. Screening for fetal malformations (editorial). 340:1006-1007.

Levi, S., et al. 1991. Sensitivity and specificity of routine antenatal screening for congenital anomalies by ultrasound. Ultrasound in Obstetrics Gynecology 1:102-110.

March of Dimes Birth Defects Foundation News Release. 1992. White Plains, N.Y. September 29.

Massarik, F., et al. 1977. Community-based genetic education, communication channels and knowledge of Tay-Sachs disease. Pp. 353-366 in Kaback, M. (ed.) Tay-Sachs Disease: Screening and Prevention: Progress in Clinical and Biological Research. Vol. 18. New York: Alan Liss.

Medical Research Council. 1968. Present status of different mass screening procedures for phenylketonuria. British Medical Journal 4:7-13.

Meryash, D., et al. 1981. Prospective study of early neonatal screening for phenylketonuria. New England Journal of Medicine 304:294.

Merz, B. 1987. Matchmaking scheme solves Tay-Sachs problem. Journal of the American Medical Association 258:2636-2639.

Modell, B., et al. 1980. Effect of introducing antenatal diagnosis on reproductive behavior of families at risk for thalassemia major. British Medical Journal 280:1347-1350.

Nadler, H. 1968. Antenatal detection of hereditary disorders. Pediatrics 42:912.

National Academy of Sciences (NAS). 1972. Sickle Cell Disease in the Armed Forces. Washington, D.C.: NAS.

National Academy of Sciences (NAS). 1975. Genetic Screening: Programs, Principles and Research. Washington, D.C.: NAS.

National Academy of Sciences/National Research Council (NAS). 1992. DNA Technology in Forensic Science. Washington, D.C.: National Academy Press.

National Institutes of Health Centre d'Etude du Polymorphisme Humain (NIH/CEPH) Collaborative Mapping Group. 1992. A comprehensive genetic linkage map of the human genome. Science 258:67-86; 148-162.

National Institutes of Health (NIH) Consensus Conference. 1984. Diagnostic Ultrasound Imaging in Pregnancy. Public Health Service. U.S. Department of Health and Human Services. NIH Publication No. 84-667. Washington, D.C.: U.S. Government Printing Office.

Office of Technology Assessment (OTA). 1990a. Genetic Witness: Forensic Uses of DNA Tests. OTA-BA-438. U.S. Congress. Washington, D.C.: U.S. Government Printing Office.

Office of Technology Assessment (OTA). 1990b. Genetic Screening in the Workplace. OTA-BA-456. U.S. Congress. Washington, D.C.: U.S. Government Printing Office.

Office of Technology Assessment (OTA). 1992. Cystic Fibrosis and DNA Tests: Implications of Carrier Screening. OTA-BA-532. U.S. Congress. Washington, D.C.: U.S. Government Printing Office.

President's Commission for the Study of Ethical Problems in Medicine and Biomedical and Behavioral Research. 1983. Screening and Counseling for Genetic Conditions. Washington, D.C.: U.S. Government Printing Office.

Reilly, P. 1977. Genetics, Law and Social Policy. Cambridge, Mass: Harvard University Press.

Rommens, J., et al. 1989. Identification of the cystic fibrosis gene: Chromosome walking and jumping. Science 245:1059.

Rothman, B. 1992 (published in 1994). Early prenatal diagnosis: Unsolved problems. In Fullarton, J. (ed.) Proceedings of the Committee on Assessing Genetic Risks. Washington, D.C.: National Academy Press.

Rowley, P., et al. 1984. Screening and genetic counseling for beta-thalassemia trait in a population unselected for interest: Comparison of three counseling methods. American Journal of Human Genetics 36:677-689.

Sarkar, G., and Commer, S. 1989. Access to a messenger RNA sequence or its protein product is not limited by tissue or species specificity. Science 244:331-334.

Schellenberg, G., et al. 1992. Genetic linkage evidence for a familial Alzheimer's disease locus on chromosome 14. Science 258:668-671.

Scriver, C., et al. 1984. Beta-thalassemia disease prevention: Genetic medicine applied. American Journal of Human Genetics 36:1024-1038.

Scriver, C. 1989. Phenylketonuria. In Scriver, C., et al. (ed.) The Metabolic Basis of Inherited Disease (6th ed.). New York: McGraw Hill.

Sidransky, D., et al., 1992. Identification of *ras* oncogene mutations in the stool of patients with curable colorectal tumors. Science 256:102-105.

Simpson, J., and Carson, S. 1992. Preimplantation genetic diagnosis (editorial). New England Journal of Medicine 327(13):951-953.

Stamatoyannopoulos, G. 1974. Problems of screening and counseling in the hemoglobinopathies. Pp. 268-276 in Motulsky, A., and Lenz, W. (eds.) Birth Defects. Amsterdam: Excerpta Medica.

Steele, M., and Breg, W. 1966. Chromosome analysis of human amniotic fluid cells. Lancet 1:383.

Verlinsky, Y., and Kuliev, I. (eds.) 1992. Pre-Implantation Diagnosis of Genetic Diseases. New York: Alan Liss.

Verlinsky, Y., and Pergament, E. 1984. Preimplantation diagnosis by embryonic biopsy. American Journal of Human Genetics 36:199S.

Virginia Code Annotated. 1990. Section 19.2-310.6.

Waxman, B. 1992 (published in 1994). Human Genome Program: A disability perspective. In Fullarton, J. (ed.) Proceedings of the Committee on Assessing Genetic Risks. Washington, D.C.: National Academy Press.

Weissenbach, J., et al. 1992. A second-generation linkage map of the human genome. Nature 359:794-801.

Wilson, J., and Jungner, Y. 1968. Principles and practice of mass screening for disease. Bol. Oficina Sanitaria de Panama 65(4):281-293.

Zeesman, S., et al. 1984. A private view of heterozygosity: Eight-year follow-up study on carriers of the Tay-Sachs gene detected by high school screening in Montreal. American Journal of Human Genetics 18:769-778.

2

Genetic Testing and Assessment

Genetic disease or genetic predisposition to disease is present in gametes before conception; therefore, theoretically it can be detected from that point on. If the capability exists for identifying a specific mutation, one can do so in gametes, in the zygote immediately after conception, in the early embryo, prenatally throughout pregnancy, in the newborn period, in childhood or adolescence, as part of reproductive planning in adulthood, or thereafter. A variety of technologies are used for genetic testing, including chromosomal, biochemical, or DNA-based techniques. The biological test sample may come from blood, amniotic fluid, or other tissue. In addition, DNA must sometimes be obtained from more than one family member for the test to be informative for a disorder when testing is done by a linked marker gene. The purpose of the following sections is to illustrate how genetic tests are used in practice and to identify issues raised by their use in various types of testing and in various populations.

This chapter briefly describes the fundamentals of human genetics and genetic testing and their application to human health—from reproduction and conception through the life span. Specifically, genetic tests are discussed in different settings and for different types of disorders: in newborn screening (e.g., phenylketonuria (PKU), sickle cell anemia), heterozygote or carrier testing (e.g., Tay-Sachs disease), identification of signs or symptoms (e.g., myotonic dystrophy), prenatal diagnosis (e.g., neural tube defects), predictive testing for monogenic late-onset disorders (e.g., Huntington disease), and susceptibility testing for late-onset disorders of complex genetic and environmental interaction (e.g., coronary heart disease). Principles to be considered in the use of genetic tests in various populations are discussed. More detailed discussions—of genetic counseling and education; laboratory quality control; and social, legal, and ethical issues—can be found in later chapters of the report. Genetic disorders are discussed because they illustrate issues in genetic testing; the list of genetic disorders is not intended to be encyclopedic.

BASIC HUMAN GENETICS AND GENETIC ANALYSIS

Genetics explores the manner by which specific traits are passed from generation to generation and how they are expressed. Genetics can be studied at many levels. For example, study of an individual's phenotype, or observable properties, can provide information about modes of inheritance, allowing estimates for risks of recurrence. Studies of an individual's chromosomes, or cytogenetics, provide information about the person's gender and about certain diseases that are directly related to abnormal numbers or configurations of the 23 pairs of chromosomes found in humans (e.g., Down syndrome, fragile X syndrome). Genetic testing may involve studies of a physiological, immunological, or biochemical function, or may involve direct study of the genes in the individual's genome. Assessment of the molecular basis for inheritance is done by examining the specific structure and function of genetic material, or DNA. Locating a disease-causing gene on a chromosome and isolating it are an important goal of research. Elucidating the gene's structure and function may provide opportunities for diagnosis and may lead to treatment of the disorder. Molecular biology is being integrated into genetics and medicine at a rapid pace.

Understanding the associations between a gene's information and the physical manifestation of its instructions is accomplished by studies of gene expression (i.e., how the organism carries out the instructions of the DNA to create products that are essential for structure and function of all cells in the body). Understanding gene expression and its regulation is the key to understanding genetic disease and hereditary variation. Hereditary variation is the result of changes—or mutations—in DNA.

Changes that occur in germ cells (egg or sperm) are inherited by offspring. Changes that occur in somatic cells (body cells other than egg or sperm) are not passed to future generations but can result in disease for the individual possessing them (e.g., cancer). Changes—sometimes called *mutations*—can occur as a result of mistakes in coding in the coding nucleotides, rearrangements within the gene, insertion of new genetic material into the gene, or duplication or deletion of parts or all of a gene. Disorders resulting from changes in one gene alone are called *monogenic* (e.g., cystic fibrosis, sickle cell anemia, Duchenne muscular dystrophy). Disorders resulting from changes in several genes, usually in combination with an environmental influence, are called *multifactorial*. Multifactorial disorders (e.g., common types of coronary heart disease and most forms of diabetes) tend to affect far more individuals than do monogenic disorders.

In human monogenic disorders, the altered gene can be located on any one of the 22 autosomal chromosomes or on a sex chromosome. Modes of inheritance of the altered gene can be autosomal dominant, autosomal recessive, or X-linked. In an *autosomal dominant* disorder, a single abnormal gene causes the trait to be expressed, even though the corresponding gene (all autosomal genes are paired) is normal. Thus, an individual with an autosomal dominant disorder will have one mutant gene and one normal gene (unless both parents are affected), and the person will usually be symptomatic at some level, although symptoms might vary in severity and age of onset. In autosomal dominant disorders, an affected individual generally has an affected parent. Each child of an affected individual with an autosomal dominant disorder has a 50 percent chance of inheriting the mutant gene, with the same risks for both males and females. In some cases, however, the mutation arises spontaneously (also called *sporadic mutations*) and is not inherited from either parent. The proportion that is due to a new mutation varies greatly for various disorders and is highest for the most severe diseases; this is because those most severely affected usually do not reproduce.

In contrast, *autosomal recessive disorders* result in illness only if a person receives two copies of the mutant gene, one from each parent who is a carrier. Such a person is considered *homozygous* for the gene and is affected with the disorder. Individuals who carry only one copy of the mutated gene are called *heterozygotes*, or *carriers*, and are clinically asymptomatic. Examples of autosomal recessive disorders are cystic fibrosis (CF), Tay-Sachs disease, phenylketonuria, sickle cell anemia, and thalassemia. Autosomal recessive disorders tend to occur with varying frequencies among different racial and ethnic populations. If both parents are carriers of the same recessive trait, each pregnancy carries a 1 in 4 risk of producing an affected child (homozygous affected) and a 1 in 2 chance of producing an asymptomatic carrier, such as themselves. A 1 in 4 chance also occurs with each pregnancy that the child with be neither a carrier nor affected by the disease.

Each individual has two sex chromosomes in the normal condition; males have an X and a Y chromosome, females have two X chromosomes. Theoretically, altered genes can occur on either the X or the Y chromosome, but the Y chromosome carries few genes. In X chromosomal recessive disorders (*X-linked*), males are disproportionately affected by these disorders because they possess only one X chromosome, which carries the mutation. Carrier females have one normal chromosome and one carrying the altered gene. Recessive diseases caused by alterations in genes on the X chromosome include Duchenne muscular dystrophy, fragile X syndrome, and hemophilia. In X-linked dominant diseases, men and women are affected equally since the abnormal gene dominates its normal partner; there can never be male to male transmission, however, because an affected father only passes a Y chromosome to his sons.

A phenomenon called *heterogeneity* sometimes adds to the complexity of determining inheritance within and across families. For example, different genes located on different chromosomes can independently give rise to the clinically identical phenotype, as is the case for retinitis pigmentosa, an inherited form of blindness. Another form of heterogeneity, *allelic heterogeneity,* is caused by different mutations in a single gene that give rise to manifestations of a disease. In the case of CF, more than 300 mutations have been found in the same gene. To complicate matters further, a mutation that expresses itself clinically in one person may produce no detectable effect in another (*reduced penetrance*) or, if it does appear, it may have a wide range of symptomatology or severity (*variable expressivity*). Both of these phenomena may be due to other genes that ameliorate the effect of the mutated gene.

Some genetic conditions do not manifest clinically until adulthood and may only become apparent in middle age or later. Predictive testing aims at predicting diseases before they are clinically expressed. Although some monogenic disorders of late onset are not particularly rare (e.g., polycystic kidney disease, hemochromatosis), they do not make up a large fraction of the disease load of the population. In contrast, common diseases of more complex etiology that include genetic factors comprise the bulk of diseases producing ill health.

We are learning that many common diseases may be due to the presence of a variable number of susceptibility genes. Thus, in coronary heart disease, a yet-unknown number of genes related to fat and cholesterol metabolism, clotting susceptibility, and other effects, interacts with environmental factors such as smoking and diet, to lead to the clinical end result. The relative contribution of genes and environment varies between individuals and families. This general pattern of interaction between heredity and environment appears to apply to many common diseases such as hypertension, diabetes, and allergies. Such conditions are not commonly considered genetic diseases, but genetic factors are thought to play a significant role in their development. Since elucidation of various genetic factors can often detect those at greatest risk, genetic testing for susceptibility might be useful in identifying groups of persons who could benefit from appropriate preventive measures. Understanding the genetic components of these disorders may lead to the development of new therapies as well.

In addition to the classical patterns of monogenic and multifactorial inheritance, several novel mechanisms of inheritance have been described in recent years. The severity and nature of the disease may depend on which parent provided the faulty gene. This phenomenon, called *genomic imprinting*, has recently been detected in rare disorders and is currently under intensive study. In *uniparental disomy*, both members of a chromosomal pair are transmitted from one parent (instead of the one chromosome that would ordinarily be transmitted from each parent); this rare event allows a recessive disorder to be expressed in a child when only *one* parent is a carrier for the mutant gene.

In another recent development, research has focused on the diseases resulting from the DNA transmission of *mitochondrial disorders*. Mitochondria are energy-generating organelles (components inside the cytoplasm of every cell) and carry their own chromosomal DNA. They are thought to be descendants of ancient bacteria that migrated into animal cells and became essential functional parts of those primitive cells. Sperm lose their mitochondria when they penetrate the egg; thus, mitochondrial genes (and any mutations in them) are passed only from the mother. Mutations in mitochondrial genes can be detected by molecular techniques and have been positively associated with certain types of blindness (Leber optic atrophy), muscle diseases, a type of epilepsy, and dementias associated with aging.

Another type of inheritance is known as *allelic expansion*. Here, instead of DNA remaining constant over the generations, as is usually the case, a gene segment expands in size when transmitted from parent to child. The expanded gene may cause a characteristic disease such as Huntington disease, myotonic dystrophy, spinal bulbar muscular atrophy, or fragile X mental retardation syndrome. Disease severity may be related to the size of the expanded gene. Allelic expansion accounts for a phenomenon called *anticipation*, in which there is earlier onset and/or increasing severity of disease as the expanding gene is transmitted from generation to generation. Molecular tests for allelic expansion are already available.

Mosaicism is the existence of cells with different genetic constitution in the same organism and is of greatest clinical importance in cancer. Cancer cells usually carry genetic mutations not shared by the normal cells. The organism affected with such a mutation is a somatic mosaic, where the cancerous tissue often has a different genetic constitution from the rest of the body. Germinal mosaicism affecting gonadal cells (sperm- and egg-forming tissue) also occurs. The finding of several affected siblings with an unexpectedly nonaffected parent in diseases that are transmitted by autosomal dominant inheritance may be due to germinal mosaicism. In such cases a section of the parent's gonad carries the disease-producing mutation.

Technologies for Detecting Genetic Disorders

Technologies to detect genetic disorders have existed for some time but have expanded dramatically in their scope, accuracy, and speed over the past 20 years. The earliest forms of genetic diagnosis, still frequently practiced, were based on observation of an individual's clinical findings or constellation of anomalies, and on an assessment of the family history. Later, biochemical assays were developed to test for inborn errors of metabolism, such as phenylketonuria or sickle cell disease. These earlier techniques remain useful today. Chromosomal analysis has been in use for more than 30 years to diagnose errors in number or shape of chromosomes that can result in genetic disorders and disease. Chromosomal analysis is most often practiced in the evaluation of newborns with malformations and for prenatal diagnosis for advanced maternal age. (As a female ages, the eggs she carries are more likely to produce errors in meiosis, leading to an increased risk of bearing a child with a chromosomal anomaly.) Advances in DNA technology have greatly advanced our ability to directly examine the genetic basis for disease. Today, DNA-based tests encompass a variety of diagnostic techniques that allow examination of markers very near the genes (e.g., some forms of polycystic kidney disease) or direct examination of the genes themselves for the characteristic mutations (e.g., CF, sickle cell anemia). DNA can be extracted from any tissue containing nucleated cells, including the white blood cells in a blood sample. Once extracted, the DNA is stable and can be stored indefinitely so that samples from individuals with genetic disorders can be collected and saved for future investigation or diagnostic tests.

Two major approaches are currently used in DNA diagnosis and study of genetic disease—direct tests and indirect tests (known as *linkage analysis*). In *direct analysis* of the gene or gene variant, family members need not be tested. Direct tests are now being conducted for cystic fibrosis, the thalassemias, and Duchenne muscular dystrophy, to name just a few. In disorders like CF, for which more than 300 mutations have been identified, screening for all mutations is not feasible. In most cases, only the more common mutations are searched for in testing. The second approach—*linkage analysis*—is used in cases where the gene has been localized to a region of a chromosome, but the gene has not been cloned; tracking the inheritance of linked DNA markers provides a means of predictive testing. In this situation, DNA from family members, including at least one affected family member, is essential to the determination of the genetic status of an individual.

Diagnosis using *linkage analysis* is limited for the following reasons: (1) DNA from at least one affected family member is required (taken either from a living individual or from stored DNA from blood or other tissues), together with DNA from other unaffected family members; (2) undetected (*nonallelic*) genetic heterogeneity may confound the analysis unless the disease in the family is known to be due to a mutation at a specific locus; (3) maternity and paternity must be known; and (4) a phenomenon known as *crossing over* can occur between the marker and the gene, which can lead to erroneous diagnostic conclusions. Crossing over can be detected if multiple markers in the region of the disease locus are available. In the past, gene tracking by this method has been successfully used for Huntington disease, Duchenne muscular dystrophy, CF, and neurofibromatosis. For disorders in which the gene has been cloned but all mutations cannot be detected or are not completely known, a combination of direct testing and linkage analysis can be employed.

Technology such as the polymerase chain reaction (PCR) has greatly magnified these capabilities because it allows for rapid DNA analysis using minute amounts of DNA. PCR and other advances in automation have great potential value for increasing the speed and accuracy of diagnosis in carrier screening programs, as well as lowering costs. These advances also present new challenges for quality control (see Chapter 3). Finally, even with the increased accuracy of direct tests, variable expressivity, incomplete penetrance, and heterogeneity can interfere with the ability to make correct predictions regarding the extent and severity of disease.

Genetic tests include the many different laboratory assays used to diagnose or predict a genetic condition or disease susceptibility. *Genetic testing* encompasses the use of specific assays to determine the genetic status of individuals already suspected to be at increased risk for a particular inherited condition because of family history or clinical symptoms. *Genetic screening* is defined as the use of various genetic tests to evaluate populations or groups of individuals independent of a family history of a disorder or symptoms. (However, although the committee has distinguished genetic testing from genetic screening, these terms are often used elsewhere interchangeably when discussing techniques for diagnosing or predicting a genetic condition or disease susceptibility.) Ideally, genetic counseling is provided in conjunction with both kinds of genetic tests. *Genetic counseling* refers to the communication process by which information about the nature, recurrence risk, burden, and reproductive options of a genetic condition, as well as empathic counseling and support concerning the implications of such genetic information, is provided to individuals and their family members.

Genetic testing services—in the context of the delivery of medical care to individuals and families who are either self-referred or referred by other physicians—have included services offered by specialized genetics centers (provided at medical and research centers by medical geneticists and genetic counselors). Primary genetic services are also provided by pediatricians (for childhood disorders), obstetricians (for prenatal diagnosis), and family physicians, internists, and specialists (for late-onset disorders) in the course of their regular practice. Genetic screening, on the other hand, has also been offered on a population basis in communities at higher risk. Lessons learned from past experiences in newborn screening, carrier detection, prenatal diagnosis, and testing for late-onset genetic disorders are instructive in designing strategies for the future (these are discussed here and in Chapter 1).

NEWBORN SCREENING

Newborn screening is a preventive health measure that, once proven to be beneficial, can be made available to all neonates. Screening tests are designed to speedily and inexpensively evaluate a large number of test samples. Newborn screening tests are now performed on blood samples from just over 4 million babies born annually in the United States; these blood samples are collected on filter paper *spots* obtained from "heel-sticks" of newborn infants. These blood spots serve as the basis for newborn screening in the United States, making newborn screening the most common type of genetic testing today (Holtzman, 1991; CORN, 1992). These screening tools are not definitive diagnostic tests, however, and positive results must be confirmed through specific testing for the disease in question.

The nature of the biochemical tests now in use requires that a trade-off be made between false positive and false negative results. False positives may have serious consequences (Tlucek et al., 1990), and the occurrence of false negatives will also be devastating to the infant and the family. Because newborn screening initially produces a high rate of false positives, parental anxiety and uncertainty can be created. Thus, accurate and timely confirmatory tests are essential to a beneficial screening program.

The first population-based newborn screening program was for the purpose of presymptomatic treatment of infants with PKU. PKU is an inborn error of metabolism characterized by a deficiency in the enzyme phenylalanine hydroxy-lase that results in high phenylalanine levels, which if not diagnosed and corrected early in life can lead to severe, progressive mental retardation. PKU occurs in about 1 in 10,000 Caucasian births. Dietary restriction of phenylalanine, if started early in infancy and continued throughout early life, is highly effective in preventing mental retardation (Holtzman, 1991).

Newborns are usually screened today for several inborn errors of metabolism and for some other disorders as well. Screening of newborns for PKU and congenital hypothyroidism—two treatable disorders—is mandatory in many states. Some states screen for as many as 11 conditions, including 42 states that screen routinely for sickle cell anemia (Table 2-1). Colorado and Wyoming added CF to their mandatory newborn screening program in 1989. Newborn screening for genetic disease is one area of genetics services that, because of its public health history and justification, has remained almost exclusively within the province of state control, although private laboratories perform newborn screening tests in eight states (CORN, 1992; also Table 3-1 in Chapter 3).

Chapter 1 reviews problems that arose in the development of newborn screening, particularly for phenylketonuria and sickle cell anemia. Although these problems were well documented and addressed in the 1975 National Academy of Sciences report (NAS, 1975), the committee found evidence that the basic principles that should guide newborn screening have not been followed consistently since 1975. Since the 1975 NAS report, new tests have been added to newborn screening programs without careful assessment of benefits and risks, often without the review of institutional review boards, and generally without concern for obtaining informed parental consent or even the opportunity for "informed refusal." Colorado, for example, added screening for CF to its program in 1982, despite statements by professional societies that the benefits of newborn screening for CF had not been demonstrated (Taussig et al., 1983). After Colorado adopted its newborn screening program, the National Institutes of Health and the Cystic Fibrosis Foundation funded a prospective randomized controlled study in Wisconsin to assess the benefits and risks of CF newborn screening (Fost and Farrell, 1989); after eight years of study, no clear evidence of benefit had been found in the treatment group. Nevertheless, Colorado made its CF newborn screening program mandatory in 1989, based on the belief that CF screening at birth would improve health outcomes (Hammond et al., 1991).

Typically, state health departments have broad discretion to introduce such tests (Cunningham, 1992), often with little oversight. Examples include testing for histidinemia and iminoglycinuria, genetic conditions that were later determined to have little clinical significance and, for which the screening itself provides little opportunity for benefit but has the potential harm of possible stigmatization. The committee is concerned that the Human Genome Project raises the prospect of the availability of multiplex testing for a number of diseases and disorders for which there is no clear beneficial treatment.

The justification for requiring clear benefit to the newborn (as developed further in Chapter 8) derives from the general principle that a person should not be used as a means for the benefit of others. This principle led the committee to the conclusion that newborn screening should not be done for the purpose of identifying newborns who are heterozygous for autosomal recessive disorders, or for *the purpose of* helping parents determine their own carrier status.

Newborn screening programs may also lack adequate attention to education and counseling of parents who are informed that their child is affected with a genetic disorder, including cases of false positive and false negative results. Newborn screening for sickle cell anemia provides an example of the need for adequate education and counseling.

Sickle cell screening, as presently conducted, identifies newborns who are carriers as well as those affected with the disease; carriers for the sickling trait will be identified about 40 times as often as an infant with sickle cell anemia in sickle cell screening programs for newborns. In contrast, in PKU, the nature of the test used for neonatal screening does not identify carrier status. There is no medical benefit to the newborn of knowing its carrier status.

If a newborn is determined to be a carrier, one parent must be a carrier; if the infant is determined to be affected with sickle cell anemia, both biological parents must be obligate carriers. There are ways other than newborn screening in which couples can determine their carrier status and reproductive risks without using the newborn as a means to that end, through voluntary testing in the preconception or prenatal setting.

The committee deliberated at length about the dilemma posed when a newborn is unintentionally discovered to be a carrier as in newborn tests for sickle cell anemia. On the one hand, informing parents about carrier status in the newborn (1) does not meet the principle that newborn screening be of benefit to the newborn; and (2) may result in harmful stigmatization by labeling children as carriers without any clear compensating benefits for the child. On the other hand, there is a dilemma in not communicating newborn carrier status to parents, since parents would not then have the potential advantage of learning that one of them is a carrier, so that they could consider carrier screening for themselves and genetic

TABLE 2-1 Disorders for Which Newborns Were Screened in 1990

State	Phenyl-keton-uria	Hypo-thyroid-ism	Galactos-emia	Maple Syrup Urine Disease	Homo-cystin-uria	Biotin-idase Defic-iency	Cystic Fibrosis	Adrenal Hyper-plasia	Tyrosin-emia	Toxo-plas-mosis	Hemo-globin-opathy
Alabama	X	X									X
Alaska	X	X	X	X	X			X	X		X
Arizona	X	X	X	X	X	X					X
Arkansas	X	X									X
California	X	X	X								X
Colorado	X	X	X	X	X	X	X				X
Connecticut	X	X	X								X
Delaware	X	X	X	X	X	X					X
District of Columbia	X	X	X	X	X						X
Florida	X	X	X								X
Georgia	X	X	X	X	X			X	X		X
Hawaii	X	X									
Idaho	X	X	X	X	X	X			X		X
Illinois	X	X	X			X		X			X
Indiana	X	X	X	X	X						X
Iowa	X	X	X	X				X			X
Kansas	X	X	X								X
Kentucky	X	X	X								X
Louisiana	X	X									
Maine	X	X	X	X	X					X	
Maryland	X	X	X	X	X	X					X
Massachusetts	X	X	X	X	X			X		X	X
Michigan	X	X	X	X		X					X
Minnesota	X	X									X
Mississippi	X	X									X

State											
Missouri	X	X	X								X
Montana	X	X	X								
Nebraska	X	X	X			X					
Nevada	X	X			X	X			X		X
New Hampshire	X	X	X	X	X					X	X
New Jersey	X	X	X	X							X
New Mexico	X	X	X								X
New York	X	X	X	X	X	X					X
North Carolina	X	X						X			
North Dakota	X	X									
Ohio	X	X	X		X						X
Oklahoma	X	X									X
Oregon	X	X	X	X	X	X			X		
Pennsylvania	X	X									X
Rhode Island	X	X	X	X	X						X
South Carolina	X	X									X
South Dakota	X	X									
Tennessee	X	X									X
Texas	X	X	X					X			X
Utah	X	X	X								X^a
Vermont	X	X	X	X	X						X
Virginia	X	X	X	X	X	X					X
Washington	X	X						X			
West Virginia	X	X	X								
Wisconsin	X	X	X	X	X		X^b				X
Wyoming	X	X	X	X	X	X	X				X
Puerto Rico	X	X									X
Virgin Islands	X	X									X
Total	52	52	38	22	21	14	3	8	5	2	42

^{a}Hemoglobinopathy pilot study, June 1, 1990-March 31, 1991 (now discontinued).
^{b}Cystic fibrosis screening for research purposes only.

counseling to aid them in making more informed reproductive choices regarding subsequent pregnancies. However, if both parents elect to be tested for carrier status, misattributed paternity can also be unwittingly exposed. Since states generally do not obtain informed consent for testing, the discovery of misattributed paternity is usually unexpected and unanticipated. Despite these real and complex side effects of newborn screening, which require intensive genetic counseling, few states conducting sickle cell screening in the newborn period have adequate resources for genetic counseling for the many parents whose infants will be found to be sickle cell carriers.

Furthermore, mandatory screening has not been shown to be essential to achieve desired public health benefits (Faden et al., 1982) and screening may not be sufficient to achieve intended health benefits. Nevertheless newborn screening programs have tended to become institutionalized. Previously established newborn screening programs need to be continually evaluated to ascertain whether the goals have been realized (Holtzman, 1989). For example, a test for maple syrup urine disease, a rare, fatal, autosomal recessive condition (1 in 200,000 births), has been included in the newborn screening panel by most states for many years. The potential efficacy of such screening may not be realized since affected newborns are often seriously ill before test results are available (Kaplan et al., 1991). This may also occur in screening newborns for galactosemia (also an autosomal recessive disorder occurring in 1 in 60,000 births) because mental function is least impaired if a galactose-free diet is begun prenatally. Although early diagnosis and therapeutic intervention by 3 weeks of age can essentially eliminate mental retardation in galactosemia (Donnell et al., 1980), if newborn diagnosis is delayed or results of testing are delayed, the central nervous system will already have sustained damage.

Finally, future uses of stored newborn blood spots deserve careful attention. Filter paper with newborn blood spots can now be used for DNA analysis as well (Matsubara et al., 1991; McCabe, 1992). This new development has raised many new issues, including the reuse of newborn blood spots for research purposes, issues of consent for such reuse, problems raised by efforts to recontact families if other genetic conditions are found, and questions surrounding who owns and controls access to the blood spots themselves (Knoppers and LaBerge, 1990; Clayton, 1992; LaBerge and Knoppers, 1992; McCabe, 1992) (see Chapter 8 for further discussion).

CARRIER TESTING AND SCREENING

We are all potential carriers of several deleterious recessive genes that would prove lethal to our offspring if they received a double dose (McKusick, 1992). For most of these genes, the likelihood of one's mate carrying the identical mutation is very small. However, for a small number of autosomal recessive disorders, the mutant version of the gene is more common in certain ethnic and racial groups.

The most common autosomal recessive disorders include CF (1 in 25 carriers in the Caucasian population), sickle cell anemia (1 in 12 carriers in the African-American population), thalassemia (variable high carrier rates in Asian, Mediterranean, and Middle Eastern populations), and Tay-Sachs disease (1 in 30 carriers in Jews of Ashkenazic descent).

Genetic drift, or variation in the frequency of genetic traits due to chance, is one of the reasons for a higher than average frequency of specific recessive diseases in a specific ethnic group. Another reason may be some unknown protective benefit of the carrier state (e.g., sickle cell trait conferring resistance to malaria), or the origin of the trait in a common ancestor (*founder effect*), or a combination of both mechanisms, a well-known example of which is the high frequency of Tay-Sachs disease in Ashkenazi Jewish populations. As a result of the higher population frequency of these disorders, much effort has been expended in search of the genes for these diseases. In some cases, the altered gene has been identified; in other cases, biochemical assays serve as indirect indicators of the carrier or disease state.

Carrier testing can also be conducted for X-linked recessive disorders, such as hemophilia, Duchenne muscular dystrophy, or fragile X syndrome (see Box 2-1 for discussion of fragile X syndrome). In these cases, the mother of an affected son—who has no other affected relatives—might desire carrier testing to confirm whether the disease is a heritable trait or a "fresh" or new mutation (more common in X-linked recessive disorders than in autosomal recessive disorders); the sister, aunt, or female cousin of an affected individual might also seek carrier testing.

Heterozygote detection is intended to identify carriers of one copy of the mutant gene. Persons who carry a single copy of the gene for a recessive disorder do not have that disease, nor are they symptomatic. *Carrier testing* involves individuals known to be at high risk of being carriers because of family history; it is almost always conducted in a specialized medical setting. *Carrier screening* involves individuals with no previous family history in order to determine their risk; such screening programs are usually not conducted in a specialized medical setting. Testing and screening to detect carrier status for autosomal recessive disorders are used primarily to aid in informed reproductive planning and decision making.

When at-risk couples are both identified as carriers for autosomal recessive disorders, they have several options available to them:

- they can take their chances, understanding there is a 75 percent likelihood with each pregnancy that the child would *not* be affected with the disease, or a 25 percent likelihood that each child will be affected;
- they can avoid reproduction, consider adoption, and be fully informed about contraception or sterilization;
- they can conceive through gamete donation, which ideally includes screening of a potential sperm or ovum donor to rule out carrier status for the same trait;

BOX 2-1   Diagnostic Testing for Fragile X Syndrome

One of the most common monogenic causes of mental retardation is fragile X syndrome, so named because of an unusual constriction of the X chromosome. The syndrome affects all ethnic groups and has a disease prevalence of more than 1 in 2,000 males and a carrier prevalence of 1 in 1,000 females (Shapiro, 1991). About one-third of female carriers show mental impairment that is usually milder than the retardation seen in affected males, although learning disabilities have been noted with normal intelligence, and severe retardation has also been observed in carrier females. The disorder has posed numerous challenges to geneticists because of unusual recurrence risks in families, imprinting effects, variable expressivity, nonpenetrance, and imperfect diagnostic tests. The molecular origin of the disorder is due to mutations in the length of a trinucleotide repeat element (CGG) located within an exon of coding sequence near the beginning of the fragile X gene (FMR-1) (Fu et al., 1991; Kremer et al., 1991; Oberle et al., 1991; Verkerk et al., 1991). In the normal population the range of allele sizes varies from 6 to 54 repeats with an average of 29 repeats (Fu et al., 1991). However, in fragile X families, repeats ranging from 52 to 200 have been found not only in carrier females but also in the novel category of carrier males; these lengths represent a predisposition for the disorder. The transition to the full mutation (alleles with more than 200 repeats) occurs with high frequency when the parent transmitting the premutation chromosome is female, and the transition frequency depends on the size of the premutation (Fu et al., 1991; Yu et al., 1991; Heitz et al., 1992). Recent evidence indicates that a small number of founder chromosomes carrying the upper-normal number of repeats may explain the current mutations present in the fragile X population (Richards et al., 1992; Oudet et al., 1993).

Direct DNA analysis offers a more rapid and accurate test for the identification of normal, premutation, and fragile X (i.e., full mutation) chromosomes (Fu et al., 1991; Rousseau et al., 1991; Sutherland et al., 1991) than the previously available cytogenetic or linkage-based methods. Direct DNA analysis has also been shown to be more informative in predicting mental impairment, and testing is currently performed for confirmatory diagnosis in suspected affected males, carrier testing for at-risk females, and prenatal diagnosis for at-risk pregnancies. The DNA test may be most helpful to persons with concerns about the accuracy of cytogenetic detection methods or who have had inconclusive results in the past.

The practitioner counseling a family with fragile X must take these complexities into consideration when discussing which family members might wish to be tested for carrier status and deciding which diagnostic test to order. Furthermore, pilot projects are already under way in some schools (in Pennsylvania). Proposals have also been made to screen persons in institutions.

- they can undergo prenatal diagnostic testing using amniocentesis or chorionic villus sampling (CVS) and selectively abort an affected fetus;
- they can undergo prenatal diagnostic testing using amniocentesis or chorionic villus sampling and make preparations for the birth of an affected child; or
- although still experimental, it may soon be possible to undergo in vitro studies in gametes (ova and polar bodies) or in early blastomeres to permit selective uterine implantation of embryos that are not homozygous for currently diagnosable genetic disorders.

Sickle cell anemia, CF, and Tay-Sachs disease are examples of recessive disorders for which carrier testing and screening are available. Carrier detection for each of these disorders raises unique issues (described in Chapter 1). Sickle cell and Tay-Sachs screening programs of the past have illuminated the following issues: (1) the need to recognize social and cultural differences in screening high-risk populations; (2) the need for reliable, easy, and relatively inexpensive carrier tests; (3) the importance of people understanding the benefits and risks from participating in screening; and (4) the importance of pre- and posttest education and counseling. The setting of carrier screening programs may also be a critical factor in their success because it may affect community trust and confidence in such screening programs.

Population carrier screening for cystic fibrosis would be unprecedented in the United States in terms of the number of individuals who could potentially be tested. CF is the most common, potentially lethal autosomal recessive genetic disorder in the United States. Current population data indicate that 1 in 2,500 newborns of European ancestry is affected by CF (about 30,000 persons), and that 1 in 25 (about 15 million Americans) is an unaffected carrier of a single copy of the gene for CF (Collins, 1992; OTA, 1992). CF causes chronic lung disease and pancreatic insufficiency, characterized by excessive production of thick mucus, primarily in the lungs, and increased risk of infection, although there is a wide range in severity of symptoms. Men with CF are usually sterile; women with CF have low fertility rates and pregnancy may exacerbate their disease. In the past, many children with CF died in early childhood. There is currently no cure available, but with improved treatments, median survival for persons born with CF in 1964 has increased to age 29 (OTA, 1992). Some individuals with CF are living into their forties and fifties. Intensive research efforts are under way to develop a variety of drug and gene therapy approaches, including gene replacement, to the treatment of CF, but the success of these efforts is still being studied at this time (ASHG, 1992).

The most common mutation causing CF is known as delta F508, a deletion of an amino acid at the 508 codon in the gene (Collins, 1992). It accounts for about 70 percent of CF mutations among those of European ancestry. Six to twelve other mutations account for an additional 15 to 20 percent of all mutations. More than 230 mutations have already been identified (ASHG, 1992), and experts suggest that there may be many more, some of which may be extremely rare, but some that might account for 1 to 3 percent of CF carriers (Collins, 1992).

The large number of CF mutations greatly complicates carrier detection and counseling. Even with the best tests, which can detect 85 to 95 percent of CF mutations in those of northern European Caucasian descent, the possibility of false negative tests remains (erroneously identifying persons as not being carriers when they are). The differential frequency of the various mutations in other ethnic populations—even in the Caucasian population—makes practical screening difficult. The variable expression of severity in CF is related to the particular mutation (a few mutations are associated with much milder CF than the classic type) and adds significantly to the difficulty in interpreting the results of genetic testing and in counseling individuals and families, because it is not possible to predict how severe the CF disorder will be in any given person.

In response to these complexities, the American Society of Human Genetics (ASHG) has developed a policy statement supporting testing of couples with a family history of CF, but opposing routine screening of pregnant women and other individuals in the general population for CF genes (Caskey et al., 1990). A similar policy emerged from a 1990 National Institutes of Health (NIH) consensus conference (NIH Workshop, 1990). Pilot studies were recommended to gather more data on laboratory, educational, and counseling aspects of screening; these studies were initiated and funded by the NIH National Center for Human Genome Research, the National Institute of Child Health and Human Development, and others in 1992. Opposition to *routine* screening of pregnant women was reviewed and reaffirmed by the ASHG in 1992, with some additional language, including recognition that "testing of highly motivated individuals in the general population may occur and should only be provided by knowledgeable health care professionals after appropriate education and counseling" (ASHG, 1992).

The central reasons for the restraint urged by the ASHG and the NIH statements regarding CF carrier screening can be found in the principle that such tests must be accurate, sensitive, and specific (Lappe et al., 1972; NAS, 1975; President's Commission, 1983). In 1989, the CF test could identify only 70 percent of carriers; thus, only 49 percent of the couples at risk would be detected. About 1 in 12 couples would have one member test positive and the other negative, with no way of knowing if the negative partner was truly negative. A consensus has been developing that routine screening should be offered only (1) when the test is 90 to 95 percent sensitive, and (2) when experience with appropriate education, counseling, setting(s), etc., for such screening has been evaluated (ASHG, 1992). At the same time, there is general agreement that testing to detect carrier status is appropriate in families with a history of the disorder because of the high risk of being a carrier. However, while new drugs and devices are subject to strict federal regulation requiring demonstration of safety and effectiveness, new genetic testing interventions and mass screening programs are generally not held to such standards.

PRENATAL DIAGNOSIS

Prenatal diagnosis is now available for hundreds of conditions, ranging from profound mental retardation and early death (e.g., trisomies 13 and 18, Tay-Sachs), to disorders that affect daily living and shorten life span but do not cause serious mental incapacity (e.g., CF and hemophilia), and includes disorders that cause serious mental and physical deterioration but do not begin until middle age (e.g., Huntington disease). For many couples, the option of prenatal diagnosis offers the potential benefit of enabling them to have children they might not otherwise have been willing to bear because of the fear of severe birth defects or serious genetic disorders. In the vast majority of pregnancies in which it is used, the availability of information from prenatal diagnosis relieves parental anxiety (Platt and Carlson, 1992).

The most common indication for women seeking prenatal diagnosis is advanced maternal age historically at age 35 years and older. The incidence of chromosomal abnormalities increases gradually with maternal age. Prenatal diagnosis in advanced maternal age is a form of genetic testing generally provided in the United States by obstetricians as part of prenatal care during pregnancy. In a policy statement, the American College of Obstetrics and Gynecology has determined that *offering* prenatal diagnosis is part of the medical "standard of care" for women age 35 and older (ACOG, 1985). Pregnant women are increasingly being offered maternal serum alpha-fetoprotein (MSAFP) screening, which is a blood test that can indicate the possible presence of a neural tube defect (NTD) (an opening in the fetal brain or spinal cord), Down syndrome, and an array of other fetal malformations. In addition, some fetal malformations of the heart, kidney, urinary tract, and stomach can be identified prenatally by using ultrasonography.

Prenatal diagnosis has focused largely on chromosomal abnormalities in pregnancies in women of advanced maternal age, couples with a family history of genetic disease, MSAFP screening for fetal neural tube defects and Down syndrome, diagnosis of hemoglobin disorders and hemophilia, and some biochemical abnormalities (WHO, 1983; NERGG, 1989; Medical Research Council, 1991; Modell, 1992). Some experts estimate that as many as 2.1 million pregnant women are now screened annually in the United States using MSAFP to determine increased risk of fetal genetic disorders (Haddow et al., 1992; J. Haddow, personal communication, 1993). Prenatal diagnosis is available for those couples identified through carrier screening as high risk. Rapid advances in genetic testing technology, especially with the advent of DNA testing (see Chapter 3), make it increasingly likely that a panel of prenatal genetic tests will soon be available, providing information on a large number of genetic disorders in the fetus—all at a relatively low cost (see Chapters 3, 4, and 8).

Chromosomal, biochemical, and increasingly, DNA-based laboratory methods are used for detecting genetic disease in the fetus (see Box 2-2). There are some important additional health risks associated with obtaining samples for anal-

BOX 2-2   Current Prenatal Diagnostic Technologies

• Traditional genetic *amniocentesis* is performed at 14 to 16 weeks gestation. The technique was first developed in the 1950s for monitoring pregnancies at risk for Rh incompatibility. It has since become widely accepted as a safe and accurate procedure where medically indicated (NICHD, 1979; Tabor et al., 1986; Rhoads et al., 1989; Medical Research Council, 1991). Cells shed by the developing fetus are extracted from a sample of amniotic fluid that has been withdrawn from the mother's uterus by a needle. The cells are then cultured, and chromosomal, biochemical, or DNA analyses are conducted, depending on the condition for which the procedure is being performed. The procedure carries an estimated risk of fetal loss of 0.5 percent in the United States to 1.0 percent and higher elsewhere (NICHD National Registry, 1976; NICHD, 1979; WHO, 1983; Tabor et al., 1986; Canadian Collaborative Trial, 1989; Rhoads et al., 1989), but great variability can exist among operators.

There are no good estimates of the number of amniocenteses performed in the United States. There are no comprehensive reporting systems for these or other prenatal diagnostic procedures, particularly because many of these procedures are performed in individual physician's offices. The Council of Regional Networks for Genetic Services (CORN) has estimated, on a very limited sample of reporting centers, that over 1 million amniocenteses were performed in the United States in 1990 (Meaney, 1992). Since this would imply that nearly 25 percent of all pregnancies in the United States undergo amniocentesis, the committee believes that this estimate is too high. Basic data are needed on this and other genetics services (see discussion of basic data set on genetics services in Chapter 9); of all genetic testing, relatively comprehensive data exist only on newborn screening (CORN, 1992).

Limitations of amniocentesis are the relatively advanced gestational age at which it is performed and the waiting period associated with the culture of the amniotic cells before test results are available. These delays can result in increased patient anxiety and might limit the options available to some patients as a consequence of religious beliefs, ethical concerns, or legal restrictions concerning midtrimester abortion. Thus, patients, their genetic counselors, and physicians have sought safe methods of earlier, more rapid diagnosis.

• *Chorionic villus sampling* (CVS) has, in part, met that need (Mennuti, 1989). CVS, first developed over 20 years ago (Steele and Breg, 1966), is now performed between 9 and 12 weeks of gestation but can be performed as early as 8 weeks of gestation (Jackson et al., 1992). Rapid reporting of results in 24 hours is also an advantage compared to the 10 to 14 days required to grow cells from traditional second trimester amniocenteses (Lancet, 1991), but cells are still cultured for karyotyping. CVS can be performed transcervically (a catheter is passed through the cervix into the uterus of the pregnant woman with the aid of ultrasound) or transabdominally (a needle is passed through the mother's abdominal wall and through the wall of the uterus) (Lancet, 1991).

Because CVS addresses some of the important limitations of amniocentesis, initial response to it was positive. A number of major international comparative trials of CVS and amniocentesis have been undertaken to determine the safety and diagnostic accuracy of these two forms of prenatal diagnosis. A 1989 study found CVS to have a slightly higher rate of fetal loss (1 percent over background rate) (Rhoads et al., 1989). CVS is considered slightly less successful in obtaining fetal cells than amniocentesis, but comparable in accuracy (Canadian Collaborative Trial, 1989; Mennuti, 1989). Not all conditions, however, can be reliably diagnosed as early as 8 weeks of fetal development (such as some neural tube defects) (Mennuti, 1989), and follow-up anmiocentesis is still necessary in approximately 1 percent of cases (D'Alton and DeCherney, 1993).

A significant increase in fetal damage following CVS has been reported by some centers, along with scattered reports of subsequent abnormal limb development in fetuses tested using CVS techniques compared to amniocentesis (Firth et al., 1991; Hsieh et al., 1991; Medical Research Council, 1991). However, a recent report of a World Health Organization expert panel (1992) suggests that fetal limb disorders were associated with CVS done at less than 9 weeks, and may be related to the expertise of the practitioner, especially the number of procedures previously performed (Modell, 1992).

In deciding on prenatal diagnosis by CVS versus amniocentesis, the clinical disadvantages of a slightly increased risk of fetal loss or injury and potential for diagnostic error must be weighed against the benefits derived from earlier results, which can result in reduced anxiety and potentially more acceptable options for selective termination of the pregnancy. In addition, if chosen, abortion is earlier and safer.

• *Percutaneous umbilical blood sampling* (PUBS) is another method for obtaining fetal cells for prenatal diagnosis. Fetal blood can be obtained at approximately 18 weeks gestation with a needle inserted, under ultrasound guidance, into the umbilical cord. Initially developed for the diagnosis of toxoplasmosis, the procedure allows access to the fetal circulation for evaluation of hematologic abnormalities and diagnosis of some inborn errors of metabolism. PUBS may be used in efforts to clarify ambiguous chromosomal analysis resulting from amniocentesis or CVS. Prenatal diagnosis using the PUBS technique has been reported to be associated with a 5 percent rate of fetal loss and should therefore be reserved for situations in which rapid diagnosis is essential or in which diagnostic information cannot be obtained by safer methods (D'Alton and DeCherney, 1993).

• *Ultrasound* (or ultrasonography) was developed more than 25 years ago and has long been used alone and as an adjunct to other forms of prenatal diagnosis. Ultrasound is noninvasive and can assess gestational age and position of the fetus, evaluate fetal growth and development, guide the instruments in amniocentesis and CVS prenatal testing, identify certain structural birth defects (such as missing limbs, some cleft lip, and spina bifida), and can help identify certain high-risk pregnancies for which cesarean (surgical) delivery would be appropriate, for example, with some neural tube defects such as hydrocephalus (Nicolaides et al., 1992). Although no long-term studies have ever established clinical harms to the fetus from *routine* ultrasonography, concerns have been raised about its use in pregnancy. A 1984 NIH consensus development conference concluded that because long-term studies were lacking, ultrasound should be used only when medically indicated (NIH, 1984). More recently, randomized clinical trials have not demonstrated any significant reduction in perinatal mortality or other benefits from

continued

BOX 2-2—Continued

intrauterine therapy or from routine use of ultrasonography (Purkiss et al., 1988; Nicolaides et al., 1992). The low sensitivity, specificity, and predictive value of ultrasound examinations for congenital abnormalities, as well as the time and expertise needed for the procedure (Gowland, 1988; Manchester et al., 1988), have also dampened scientific enthusiasm for routine ultrasound screening for congenital abnormalities in the United States (U.S. Preventive Services Task Force, 1989; Holtzman, 1990). Although prenatal ultrasonography is not considered "standard of care" for routine obstetrical practice in the United States by the American College of Obstetrics and Gynecology, it has generally become a routine part of obstetrical practice. However, standards for ultrasound equipment and for the training and certification of personnel have not yet been developed. Some ultrasonography experts (Filly et al., 1987; Gowland, 1988; Manchester et al., 1988; Townsend et al., 1988; Goldstein et al., 1989; Lancet, 1992) report a substantial error rate (as high as 10 percent wrong diagnoses with both false positives and false negatives) among obstetricians and some centers in reading ultrasound images, and large variations in image quality associated with equipment and its maintenance.

Ultrasound is a tool commonly used by primary care providers in routine obstetrical practice where an individual practitioner will see few abnormalities. Consultation with genetics professionals and highly specialized ultrasonographers is essential when fetal abnormalities are suspected because of the inherent difficulty of interpretation and the need for experience in recognizing abnormalities. When ultrasound is performed by highly skilled operators, the sensitivity of this screening device in detecting congenital malformations can be as high as 90 percent (Manchester et al., 1988).

ysis for prenatal diagnosis. Many of the concerns that exist regarding the specificity or sensitivity of particular tests apply to prenatal diagnosis, as well as newborn screening and heterozygote detection (see above). The key difference is that the mother must undergo an invasive procedure that puts the fetus at risk in order to obtain this information. The risks to the fetus of a prenatal screening or diagnostic procedure need to be weighed in decisions about prenatal diagnosis, along with the risk of the birth of an affected child. There must be a much lower tolerance for false positive test results in prenatal diagnosis because of the undue anxiety that can be raised by the uncertainty (Juengst, 1988), as well as the potential for erroneously aborting an unaffected fetus.

A variety of techniques are currently in use for obtaining fetal cells for genetic analyses, including midtrimester amniocentesis, chorionic villus sampling, and the less common percutaneous umbilical blood sampling (PUBS). Ultrasonography is used for guidance of the needle in all three techniques. It is also used for fetal visualization and gestational dating, and can detect gross fetal anomalies (see Box 2-2).

In use now for nearly 20 years, MSAFP screening illustrates some of the dilemmas and potential complexities of determining increased risk of genetic disorders in the fetus (Brock and Sutcliffe, 1972). It is often the first screening test used to begin the process of identifying high-risk pregnancies, and can be followed by multiple prenatal diagnostic technologies, which may include further blood testing, ultrasound, and amniocentesis. An MSAFP test is a simple maternal blood test administered between 15 and 20 weeks of gestation as a first-step *screening test* to detect those pregnancies at possible *increased risk for a variety of conditions*; the MSAFP test does not *diagnose* fetal disorders.

The MSAFP screening test serves as a basis for appropriately referring, for more definitive tests, women who exhibit elevated or decreased levels of the fetal protein in their blood. High levels of AFP in the mother's blood might be associated with failure of the neural tube to close around the spinal column of the developing fetus. If the neural tube does not close completely, a variety of structural abnormalities may result, ranging from spina bifida (an open area on some part of the cover of the spinal column with varying degrees of disability) to anencephaly (the absence of the brain above the brain stem). The use of the MSAFP test for screening for *increased risk* of neural tube defects was approved by the U.S. Food and Drug Administration (FDA) in 1983. Although use of MSAFP for screening for increased risk of fetal Down syndrome (Cuckle and Wald, 1984; Merkatz et al, 1984; Hook, 1988) has also become widespread, this application of MSAFP testing has never been approved by the FDA (see Chapter 3). In 1985, the American College of Obstetrics and Gynecology distributed a professional liability "alert" advising obstetricians about the professional liability implications of AFP testing and advising them that "it is imperative" for them to discuss the availability of such screening with their patients and to document the discussion in the patient's chart (ACOG, 1985).

In addition, single and multiple fetal malformations, including heart, kidney, and gastric wall defects, or urinary and abdominal wall abnormalities, may be present when MSAFP is elevated (Crandall, 1992). An apparent abnormal MSAFP level may also result from misdating the pregnancy, multiple births, errors in determining or reporting race/ethnicity, diabetes mellitus, and body weight in the mother—all of which require adjustment of MSAFP levels for correct interpretation. Errors in reporting such critical information by the referring physician can result in additional laboratory errors in interpreting MSAFP results (Holtzman, 1992).

Several concerns have been raised regarding the routine use of MSAFP in prenatal care. ASHG has issued a policy statement recognizing that MSAFP testing was becoming part of routine obstetrical practice but stating that the test was not simply an office test (ASHG, 1987, p. 75). Among the concerns identified were (1) the complexity of setting cutoff levels for interpreting results due to the high rate of false positives and false negatives, doubts about the predictive value of the test results, and wide variability in the severity of the disorders for which the screening is being conducted; (2) social controversy surrounding the fact that no treatment exists for most of the conditions for which the screening is being done and that prevention of the disorders involves termination of pregnancy; (3) the critical importance of a qualified MSAFP testing laboratory (and essential criteria for quality control in such laboratories); and (4) the need for adequate education of physicians or other health professionals, as well as for facilities and personnel for follow-up of abnormally high or low MSAFP results, as well as for those whose initial results are false positive, and patient education (ASHG, 1987, 1989). In addition—with the use of folate supplements prior to or early in pregnancy—the risk of NTDs may be reduced (Laurence, 1990; Scott et al., 1991); research is continuing (McPartlin et al., 1993).

Several new research techniques have been developed that may hold promise for prenatal diagnosis in the future, including genetic tests on fetal cells isolated from maternal blood and genetic tests associated with preimplantation diagnosis. These techniques are still experimental, however, and have not been thoroughly studied and evaluated for safety, reliability, and effectiveness. Despite their early stage of development, some of these techniques are already beginning to be used in clinical diagnosis (see Box 2-3).

An experimental test that is already widely used, called the "triple-marker screening test," has been reported to increase the effectiveness of MSAFP screening alone in predicting increased risk of a variety of fetal trisomies in pregnancy (Crandall, 1992; Haddow et al., 1992). The new screening test involves the analysis of the combined measurements of AFP, plus serum human chorionic gonadotropin and unesterified estriol (a component of estrogen), in maternal blood. These tests can be used between approximately 15 and 20 weeks of gestation. This triple-marker screening is reported to be more reliable than MSAFP alone in identification of pregnancies at increased risk of Down syndrome (60 percent detection versus 20 percent detection, respectively), and of some cases of trisomy 18 (a severe form of physical disability and mental retardation). Triple-marker screening is also reported to improve identification of twins, correct determination of gestational age, and improve identification of women at increased risk of late-pregnancy complications (those with unexplained high levels of MSAFP) compared with MSAFP alone. As with MSAFP alone, confirmatory amniocentesis and ultrasound are required.

Critical Issues in Prenatal Diagnosis

Many people believe that prenatal diagnosis can assure them of having a baby healthy in every respect (Wertz, 1992). However, most disorders cannot now be diagnosed prenatally, and there are few possibilities for primary prevention of most congenital abnormalities. DNA technology offers the prospect of gene therapy and genetic engineering at some time in the future, but the more immediate application of this technology is the expansion of the number of disor-

BOX 2-3 New Techniques in Prenatal Diagnosis

Early amniocentesis is being used as early as 9-14 weeks of pregnancy, the time in which CVS is now used. The procedure is the same as described earlier in the chapter; just the timing of its use is different. Its safety and accuracy have not yet been adequately evaluated.

Fluorescence in situ hybridization (FISH) is a modified cytogenetic technique intended for more rapid detection of chromosomal disorders in the fetus (Klinger, 1992). Originally a research tool like many other DNA technologies, FISH is rapidly being adopted as a diagnostic tool in prenatal diagnosis as well as in cancer and infectious disease diagnosis (Caskey, 1991). FISH allows rapid cytogenetic assays based on in situ hybridization of chromosome-specific DNA probes that can be visualized by fluorescence methods (Cremer, 1988; Lichter et al., 1988; Klinger et al., 1990, 1991).

Karyotyping (analysis of chromosomes) is accurate and can often detect subtle chromosome rearrangements. However, chromosome analysis is time consuming (often taking from one to as much as two weeks); it is also labor intensive and requires highly skilled operators. The time delay is a source of anxiety for many patients, particularly for those not tested until the second trimester of pregnancy and when ultrasound has detected possible fetal abnormalities. Thus, many people have perceived a need for simple methods for the rapid detection of chromosome abnormalities (Lichter et al., 1988).

FISH can be used to count the number of copies of a specific chromosome present (aneuploidy detection), to identify unknown (marker) chromosomes present in metaphase spreads, and to identify predefined chromosome translocations (Klinger, 1992). Proficiency testing does not now exist for FISH, nor have any of the available probes been approved by the FDA (see Chapter 3). FISH analysis is now available from at least one laboratory upon physician request, and only in conjunction with a complete karyotype analysis (Klinger, 1992). This technique has also been the source of recent controversy about "a rapid (but wrong) prenatal diagnosis" (Benn et al., 1992) in which a prenatal diagnostic error resulted from a test whose accuracy is said to exceed 99 percent (see Chapter 3).

Diagnosis using fetal cells isolated from maternal blood holds the promise of noninvasive prenatal diagnosis by genetic analysis of fetal cells isolated from a sample of the mother's blood (Bianchi et al., 1991). Techniques have been developed to isolate or concentrate genetic material from the very few fetal cells circulating in maternal blood. These techniques include fluorescence-activated cell sorting using monoclonal antibodies, polymerase chain reaction, and in situ hybridization of fetal cells. Once concentrated, selected genetic components need to be multiplied so they can be analyzed correctly. Fetal cells have been detected in maternal blood as early as 9 weeks of gestation. First trimester prenatal diagnosis of Down syndrome has now been reported in fetal cells from maternal blood (Elias et al., 1992). PCR has been used to amplify a sample for prenatal testing from a single fetal cell. One limitation of this technique is that some fetal cells may be left from previous pregnancies (Bianchi et al., 1991). The slightest contamina-

continued

BOX 2-3—*Continued*

tion can result in incorrect diagnosis (both false positives and false negatives). This technique is still being evaluated.

Preimplantation Diagnosis. Techniques described here require removal of ova (eggs) from a woman's ovaries, involving some risk to the woman. When fertilized eggs have divided into four to eight as yet undifferentiated cells, one of these cells can be removed for genetic testing. Because there is very little DNA to work with, amplification by polymerase chain reaction makes prenatal diagnosis possible prior to implantation (Handyside et al., 1990, 1992). There is some research on testing of ova and sperm before fertilization, but these techniques are relatively early in their development and are still experimental; they have technical hazards and may have biological hazards as well. In one method, a nonfunctioning product of cell meiotic division (polar body) may be tested (Verlinsky and Kuliev, 1992), or cells destined to become placenta may be tested (Simpson and Carson, 1992).

The appeal of this earliest form of prenatal diagnosis is that it could avoid many of the difficult decisions and potential psychosocial consequences of decisions to selectively terminate a fetus affected with a genetic disorder. Couples at risk of having children affected by diagnosable genetic disorders might be spared repeated decisions in each pregnancy about possible termination of affected fetuses identified at a later stage in fetal development (Simpson and Carson, 1992). Very little is known about the technical and biological safety of these techniques.

In vitro fertilization (IVF) is the process for implantation following preimplantation diagnosis, generally six days after ovulation. It is being offered by some commercial diagnostic laboratories for as many as eight conditions, including muscular dystrophy, hemophilia, and fragile X and Down syndromes. In IVF, after hormonal stimulation, eggs (ova) are removed from the ovaries of the woman by needle aspiration under local anesthesia and placed in a culture medium. Sperm from the man is then used to fertilize these eggs. Successfully fertilized eggs begin cell division in the culture medium.

There are limitations to in vitro fertilization to which are added the limitations of preimplantation diagnosis. In the United States, only 14 percent of women deliver a live-born infant after one cycle of in vitro fertilization, and the rate of live births is no better than 1 for every 10 embryos transferred at the centers with the best records (SART, 1992). The emotional burdens of in vitro fertilization and the physical techniques for removal of eggs from the woman (i.e., by needle aspiration from the ovaries under local anesthesia) limit the appeal of this experimental method of prenatal diagnosis.

In addition to the extremely high cost of IVF (more than $15,000 per cycle), there are also substantial resource limits related to the use of these technologies, including a team highly experienced in assisted reproductive technology, experience in recovering embryonic cells in an environment free of DNA contaminants, and the ability to perform the necessary analysis with a very small amount (one cell) of DNA (Simpson and Carson, 1992). Frequently, multiple embryos will be implanted with these techniques, and the need for "fetal reduction" (an invasive procedure to reduce the number of fetuses carried to term) also diminishes the applicability of this technique.

ders for which prenatal diagnosis will be possible (Holtzman, 1989, 1990; D'Alton and DeCherney, 1993). Prenatal diagnosis has potential benefits, but it also "brings new challenges" with it (Milunsky, 1985; Mennuti, 1989). These challenges were highlighted by a recent NIH Workshop on Reproductive Genetic Testing (1991) (also see Box 2-4 for recommendations of this NIH conference).

> Reproductive genetic testing, counseling and other genetic services can be a valuable component in the reproductive health care of women and their families. These services have the potential to increase knowledge about possible pregnancy outcomes that may occur if a woman decides to reproduce; provide reassurance during pregnancy; enhance maternal-infant bonding and other relationships; allow a woman an opportunity to choose whether or not to continue a pregnancy in which the expected child has a birth defect or a genetic disorder; and if continuing, facilitate prenatal or early infant therapy for their expected child when possible and prepare for bearing and rearing of a child with special needs. Conversely, these services have the potential to increase anxiety; place excessive responsibility, blame, and guilt on a woman for her pregnancy outcome; interfere with maternal-infant bonding; and disrupt relationships between a woman, family members and her community.
>
> The challenge is to provide each woman with an opportunity to have access to desired genetic services in a way that will improve her control over the circumstances of her reproductive life, her pregnancies, childbearing and parenting, within a framework that is sensitive to her needs and values and minimizes the potential for coercion. The value placed on these services by women and their families depends heavily on a mixture of psychological and ethno-cultural influences, religious and moral values, and legal and economic considerations that are unique to each woman. As a consequence, women in different circumstances may weigh the merits of reproductive genetic services quite differently.

Psychological effects, including increased anxiety associated with amniocentesis and other forms of prenatal diagnosis, have been studied extensively (Blumberg and Golbus, 1975; Black and Furlong, 1984; Beeson and Golbus, 1985; Rothman, 1986, 1992, 1993; Rapp, 1988a,b, 1991; Black, 1989, 1990; Mennuti, 1989; Press and Browner, 1992, 1993). Some studies have found that women who underwent amniocentesis did not exhibit high levels of anxiety or depression in the period following amniocentesis (Rapp, 1987). Other studies, incorporating intensive interviewing techniques, found more significant impacts of the use of prenatal diagnosis, leading one commentator to coin the phrase "the tentative pregnancy" (Rothman, 1986, 1992, 1993; Tymstra, 1991) to describe the conditional relationship that some women feel is imposed between them and their developing fetus. It is difficult to measure the extent to which prenatal diagnosis increases anxiety because baseline anxiety levels differ and individual expectations vary among couples (Tymstra et al., 1991; Wexler, 1992).

**BOX 2-4   Recommendations of the NIH Workshop on
Reproductive Genetic Testing: Impact on Women**

In November 1991, the NIH conference "Reproductive Genetic Technologies:
Impact on Women" made recommendations for a research and policy agenda related to reproductive genetics services. A summary of those recommendations
follows (NIH Workshop on Reproductive Genetic Testing, 1991, pp. 1-8):

1. Reproductive genetic services should not be used to pursue "eugenic" goals,
but should be aimed at increasing individual control over reproductive decisions.
Therefore, new strategies need to be developed to evaluate the success of such
services . . . . Reproductive genetic services must ultimately serve personal, not
public interests in improving the overall reproductive options of women . . . . The
ideals of self-determination in family matters and respect for individual differences
that lie behind the client-centered view of reproductive genetic services are jeopar-
dized whenever the primary goal of these services becomes the prevention of the
birth of individuals with a disorder or a disability. Such a goal has the potential to
constrain the choices available to women and to further stigmatize those individuals affected by a particular disorder or disability. To the extent that voluntary genetic services are evaluated even indirectly in "eugenic" terms, societal pressures
have the potential to threaten the important interests and desires of individual
women and their families.

2. Reproductive genetic services should be meticulously voluntary.

3. Reproductive genetic services should be value-sensitive.

4. Standards of care for reproductive genetic services should emphasize genetics information, education and counseling rather than testing procedures alone.

5. Social, legal and economic constraints on reproductive genetic services
should be removed.

6. Increasing attention focused on the development and utilization of reproductive genetic testing services may further stigmatize individuals affected by a particular disorder or disability: The values that some place on health and disabilities,
what people may be told about disabilities and even the use of certain language to
describe the benefits of reproductive genetic testing has the potential to place a
value on the worth of individuals with disabilities in society. Increased sensitivity to
these issues and improved communication between the biomedical and the disabilities communities is urgently needed in order for the true impact of these developing technologies to become known. Individuals with disabilities, whose lives
may be significantly influenced by these technologies must be involved in the development and implementation of further research to be carried out in the future.

The primary options now available following the identification of an affected
fetus are to terminate the pregnancy or to prepare for the birth of an affected child.
Given the limited but real hazards of prenatal diagnostic procedures, many experts initially recommended using prenatal diagnosis only if all the options it could
offer were actually going to be utilized (Littlefield, 1970). However, a broad
consensus developed in the intervening years that requiring parental commitment

to follow through with abortion if the fetus is identified as affected with a genetic disorder is ethically inappropriate as a criterion for selecting candidates for amniocentesis or other prenatal genetic tests (NICHD, 1979). Recent data of Wertz and Fletcher (1989a,b; Wertz et al., 1990) showed that 96 percent of the responding geneticists would perform prenatal diagnosis for a couple who requested it but who opposed abortion. There may be benefits in knowledge from prenatal diagnosis if the pregnancy is continued; for example, detection of a neural tube defect may help to evaluate the need for prelabor delivery by cesarean section.

One further issue deserves particular attention—prenatal diagnosis for early determination of the sex of the fetus. Historically, prenatal diagnosis for identification of fetal sex was used where pregnancies were at risk of X-linked genetic disorders such as muscular dystrophy. In some cultures, such as India and China, however, sex identification has also been sought for planning the birth order of children of a particular sex, or for the preferential selection of children of one sex, usually males (Wertz and Fletcher, 1989b; Wertz et al., 1990; Wertz, 1992). In a recent survey in the United States, only a very small percentage (5 percent) of the public reported that they favored prenatal diagnosis for sex selection (Singer, 1991). Such practices have been called "homemade eugenics" (Kevles, 1985, 1991).

In the surveys reported by Wertz and Fletcher, slightly less than one-third (32 percent) of responding geneticists in the United States reported that they were willing to perform prenatal diagnosis for sex selection or other non-disease-oriented traits, and another 28 percent were willing to refer patients to someone who would perform prenatal diagnosis for sex selection. In most cases their decision was governed by respect for parental autonomy; others wished to avoid paternalism and to preserve nondirectiveness. Thus, sex selection was the genetic dilemma that respondents said gave them the greatest ethical conflict, attempting to balance *autonomy* (the right of patients to decide) with *nonmalificence* (the moral obligation not to harm) (Wertz et al., 1990).

There have been several international policy statements opposing prenatal diagnosis for sex selection or for other non-disease-related traits. A policy statement from the European Council of International Organizations of Medical Sciences (CIOMS) opposes prenatal diagnosis for sex selection (Niermeijer, 1988, p. 93):

> The working group considers it a misuse of new genetic technologies to use chorionic villus sampling to make a diagnosis of sex in the eighth or tenth week of pregnancy. Since sex is no disease, the use of fetal diagnosis for knowledge of fetal sex is to be discouraged, at least in European and American cultures.

The report of the Privacy Commission of Canada (1992, p. 40) also raises concern on this subject:

> To what extent should genetics be employed to generate information for decisions that are repugnant to some, like abortion, as a means of sex

selection? . . . The issue of genetic testing for sex selection requires further analysis . . . the [Canadian] Royal Commission on New Reproductive Technologies is examining issues surrounding sex selection.

The British Medical Association (BMA, 1992) advises its physicians not to participate in sex selection in the absence of medical need. The ethics committee of the Royal College of Obstetricians has a policy statement under discussion (Choo, 1993). The Canadian Royal Commission on New Reproductive Technologies is preparing a statement on genetic testing for sex selection scheduled to be issued later in 1993.

TESTING FOR LATE-ONSET DISORDERS

Many diseases do not manifest clinically until adulthood and may become apparent only in middle age or later. *Predictive* or *presymptomatic* testing and screening can provide clues to which people may later develop one or more of these disorders. Often such tests will give information regarding a genetic susceptibility or predisposition, rather than providing definitive prediction. In some cases, a family history of a monogenic disorder in a close relative informs others in the family that they are at high risk for developing the disease. Appropriate testing might then resolve whether the mutant gene is present. Examples include Huntington disease and polycystic kidney disease. Sometimes a certain percentage of people with a particular disease have the genetic form. Genes have been found for familial Alzheimer disease and familial amyotrophic lateral sclerosis, two devastating, fatal, late-onset disorders. Even though the majority of those with these disorders have the nonfamilial form (e.g., Alzheimer disease), understanding the flaw in the gene that causes the familial form may lead to new treatments for all who are affected.

More frequently a disorder is multifactorial—or complex—in its causation, including both multiple genetic factors and environmental effects. Many common diseases of adulthood fall in this category, including coronary artery disease, some cancers, diabetes, high blood pressure, rheumatoid arthritis, and some psychiatric diseases (King et al., 1992). Different sets of genes can operate in different families (genetic heterogeneity), and environmental factors may interact with only one set of genes and not with another. There may also be interaction between the various genes involved, so that the effects of multiple gene action cannot be predicted by separate analyses of each of the single genes. In such cases, definitive prediction will rarely, if ever, be possible, and it will be impossible to group individuals into two distinct categories—those at no (or very low) risk and those at high risk (Risch, 1992).

On the other hand, the availability of presymptomatic and predispositional testing can provide an opportunity for physicians and patients to work toward prevention of disease. Since environmental factors are often essential for the manifestation of complex diseases, the detection of those at high risk will identify some individuals who are more likely to benefit more from certain interventions (e.g., dietary measures in coronary heart disease). The newly acquired ability to identify some persons at high risk for certain cancers now permits more frequent monitoring for the earliest manifestations of cancer (e.g., bowel cancer). Further research and the unfolding of the Human Genome Project are very likely to reveal the underlying genes mediating predisposition to numerous common diseases, and genetic susceptibility testing will be increasingly possible. The current state of knowledge of some disorders illustrates some of the complexities of genetic testing for disorders of late onset.

Monogenic Disorders of Late Onset

Huntington Disease

The problems posed by monogenic diseases of late onset vary considerably. Huntington disease has received the most study, since indirect DNA testing has been available for nearly a decade (Gusella et al., 1983; Conneally et al., 1984; Martin and Gusella, 1986) (see Box 2-5). Indirect DNA diagnosis requires testing of an affected family member and other relatives in order to diagnose the disease in a person at risk. The identification of the genetic defect for Huntington disease as a trinucleotide expansion (Huntington's Disease Collaborative Research Group, 1993) now permits direct DNA testing and eliminates the many difficulties and the measure of uncertainty that accompanies indirect DNA testing using linkage analysis. However, since this late-onset, lethal disorder is not treatable, direct genetic testing—even without involving other family members—continues to raise many complex ethical, legal, and social issues that must be addressed through education and counseling.

Alzheimer Disease

Monogenic adult early-onset Alzheimer disease raises similar considerations to those raised by Huntington disease in that there is no effective treatment or cure (Marx, 1992). Approximately 5 percent of all cases of Alzheimer disease are transmitted as an autosomal dominant trait, and several different genes have been implicated in various families (St. George-Hyslop et al., 1990; Goate et al., 1991; Schellenberg et al., 1992), requiring a different test probe for indirect DNA testing for each of these genes. When these genes and the corresponding mutations responsible for Alzheimer disease are identified, a direct DNA test may become feasible. When a better test is developed, however, difficult decisions will still have to be made about whether, if ever, to offer testing. These dilemmas will affect many more people should predictive testing become available for the more common Alzheimer disease that starts late in life (70 to 80 years of age).

BOX 2-5 Presymptomatic Testing for Huntington Disease

Huntington disease (HD) is an autosomal dominant neurodegenerative disorder of late adult onset with a prevalence of 1 in 10,000. In the United States, 30,000 persons are symptomatic and another 150,000 individuals are at risk. HD causes involuntary movements of all parts of the body, including chorea and dystonia, cognitive impairment including failures of organizational capacities and memory, and psychiatric disturbances, particularly severe suicidal depression, apathy, or obsessive-compulsive disorders. Symptoms usually manifest between the ages of 30 and 50 but can appear as early as age 2 or as late as 80 years of age (Farrer and Conneally, 1985). Once symptoms take hold, there is a 10-20 year unremitting and inexorable progression toward death. Children progress more rapidly and are more severely affected in motor function and behavior. There is no effective treatment or cure.

HD was the first autosomal disorder to be localized to a chromosome using novel recombinant DNA techniques. In 1983, it was discovered to be in the telemeric region of the short arm of chromosome 4 (Gusella et al., 1983).

The existence of DNA markers tightly linked to the gene made presymptomatic and prenatal testing possible in 1986. The test was offered in only a limited number of settings, primarily universities specializing in HD or neurogenetics, in the United States, Canada, and Europe. Because the test was based on the observation of DNA-linked markers and not the gene itself, it could be used only by those with genetically informative families.

Prior to the existence of the test, many surveys of family interest indicated a strong desire for predictive testing but when the possibility of actually seeing the future became a reality, only a tiny fraction of those at risk chose to utilize the test. Even many people who contacted testing centers decided not to pursue the test after learning more about it and considering the possible consequences of learning whether one is free of, or destined to die from, this disease.

There have been fewer than 300 individuals tested in the United States, and it is too early and the numbers are still too small to know the long-term effects of presymptomatic testing. Not surprisingly, a wide range of reactions has been observed. Some of the people have found the information useful to help shape their lives, even if they were found to be gene carriers; others have been severely traumatized to learn that they have escaped the disease since they have built an identity around the certainty that Huntington disease was in their future. Some have had babies secure in the knowledge that the illness would never strike them; others were so devastated by their experience of the testing process and by the news that their own risk had increased to almost 100 percent that they proceeded to have children and not test the pregnancy. Some families found that all the siblings were diagnosed; others none, and still other families had to cope with a mix of positive and negative outcomes. Some have been hospitalized for depression on learning that Huntington disease was to be their fate; others felt more tranquil after resolving the uncertainty. Some people coped with the news of a diagnosis by deciding that the test was wrong or that they represented a recombination event or that God or science would find an answer in time for them.

The linkage test to date has been given in sophisticated centers familiar with Huntington disease. The test was initially made available under the aegis of pilot research projects to assess the best way to deliver it. A uniform protocol has been adopted in all centers giving the test. It requires three to six sessions of pretest counseling and education, and as many or more hours of posttest counseling and follow-up. Extensive neurological, neuropsychological, and psychiatric evaluations are performed to determine if the person is already symptomatic and to learn more about a person to help him or her cope better with either possible outcome. People are requested to select a therapist—prior to getting diagnostic information—who can be available as necessary. They are also asked to bring a companion with them to the counseling sessions and particularly to the outcome session.

On March 26, 1993, after 10 arduous years of searching for the Huntington disease gene, it was finally isolated by the Huntington's Disease Collaborative Group. Although the protein it makes is still unknown, the mutation was found to be a small expanded repeat of CAG, coding for glutamine. Children with HD have the highest numbers of repeat, but below a certain number, the correlation between numbers of repeat and age of onset is too loose to be diagnostically useful.

The discovery of the gene permits a direct presymptomatic diagnostic test for HD. Anyone in the population can be screened. The PCR-based test is significantly less expensive than the previous test. It is also more subject to laboratory error. The diagnostic information one learns from this new test, however, is the same as the old: HD is still a fatal, progressive, neurodegenerative disease. Technological ease at the bench should not diminish the intensive education and counseling both prior to and following testing. The technological imperative should not sweep people into being tested without very careful consideration of its consequences. HD is also a disorder for which people are frequently denied insurance, have difficulties obtaining employment, are turned down for adoptions, and which can be otherwise socially stigmatizing.

The World Federation of Neurology Research Group on Huntington's Disease and the International Huntington's Disease Association, representing family organizations throughout the world, joined together to develop guidelines for presymptomatic testing for HD. These guidelines have been recently revised to take into account the discovery of the gene and availability of direct testing for HD.*

---

*Revised guidelines for testing for Huntington disease are available from the Hereditary Disease Foundation, 1427 Seventh Street, Suite 2, Santa Monica, CA 90401; 301-458-4183

Hemochromatosis

Unlike Huntington and Alzheimer disease, hemochromatosis is a treatable condition (see Box 2-6). In *autosomal recessive hemochromatosis* (iron storage disease), a significant portion, but not all of those who carry the double dose of the mutant gene (about 1 in 500 of the Caucasian population), will develop symptoms and be at risk of death from liver cirrhosis, heart muscle failure, diabetes, and liver cancer (Bothwell et al., 1989). The excess iron can be removed by frequent bloodletting, and the disease is then completely curable, with a normal life span, provided that treatment starts before clinical manifestation (Niederau et al., 1985). Al-

---

BOX 2-6   Hemochromatosis

Hemochromatosis is a common autosomal recessive disorder characterized by excessive iron deposits in the liver, heart, pancreas, and other organs, caused by increased iron absorption over many years. Functional organ impairment characteristically begins in middle age and, once developed, is usually fatal (see Bothwell et al., 1989 for extensive references). Symptoms may be nonspecific, such as lethargy and weakness, or atypical arthritis. Cardiomyopathy, cirrhosis and liver cancer, skin pigmentation, and diabetes are late manifestations of hemochromatosis.

Men are 10 times more frequently affected clinically than women, presumably because periodic blood loss during menstruation removes excess iron. The condition can easily and successfully be treated by periodic bloodletting to rid the body of excess iron. While the abnormal gene has been mapped to the short arm of chromosome 6 in close vicinity to the HLA-A locus, the basic defect causing increased iron absorption has not yet been discovered. About 1 in 300 to 1 in 800 Caucasians carries the double dose of the mutant gene and, therefore, may potentially become clinically affected. The actual frequency of clinically significant overload is not well defined. Between 8 and 12 percent of the population are single-dose carriers of the gene or heterozygotes. The heterozygous status for hemochromatosis is clinically benign and does not cause significantly increased iron storage.

Laboratory tests for the condition currently rely on assessment of the phenotypical consequences of abnormal iron metabolism (serum iron, the extent of serum iron binding by transferrin, and serum ferritin levels) since no DNA test exists. A combination of these tests is required for diagnosis of iron overload due to hereditary hemochromatosis. There are many false positive and false negative tests, depending on the cutoff for laboratory values that are selected as abnormal. A definitive diagnosis currently requires liver biopsy to demonstrate the characteristic deposits of iron in hepatic parenchymal cells.

The detection of hemochromatosis among family members (but not in the population) can be aided by a linkage study using the closely linked HLA locus. Such linkage analysis requires a blood sample from an affected homozygous relative. Siblings will have a 25 percent chance of being homozygotes and will share both HLA haplotypes of the affected sibling. Various DNA markers linked to the hemochromatosis locus are also beginning to be used for family linkage studies. However, whether DNA testing has advantages over HLA testing is not clear.

Diagnosis of the heterozygous state currently requires family studies with linked genetic markers such as HLA types. Various tests of iron status are often slightly abnormal in heterozygotes, sometimes making it difficult to distinguish between carrier heterozygotes and affected homozygotes. The current complexity of testing highlights the importance of the search for the basic defect in hemochromatosis. Once found, more direct genetic testing should be possible.

Early diagnosis of hemochromatosis, followed by treatment, is essential to prevent liver cirrhosis and early death; the life expectancy of hemochromatosis patients without cirrhosis is identical to the normal control population (Niederau et al., 1985). A potentially fatal disease, therefore, can be transformed into one with a normal life expectancy. Once liver cirrhosis has developed, iron depletion does not reduce the frequency of liver cancer often seen in hemochromatosis. These facts emphasize the importance of early detection among family members once a patient has been diagnosed, and the possible use of population screening in the future if a practical test system has been determined to be effective in pilot studies.

though not all persons who are homozygous for the mutant gene for hemochromatosis will develop clinical disease, frequent bloodletting might be the preferred course of action because the risk of treatment is less than the risk of developing the disease. The availability of therapy favors efforts aimed toward testing first-degree relatives of affected individuals. Many physicians and medical geneticists would recommend informing siblings that they are at high risk (25 percent) of developing a potentially fatal but treatable disease (see Chapter 8 for discussion of issues in informing relatives).

Familial Hypercholesterolemia

Familial hypercholesterolemia (Goldstein and Brown, 1989; Motulsky, 1989) associated with coronary artery disease illustrates issues in predictive testing for a disease for which preventive treatment is available. Familial hypercholesterolemia (frequency of about 1 in 500) results from a monogenic defect that causes elevated LDL (low-density lipoprotein) cholesterol levels that lead to heart attacks in 50 percent of male heterozygotes by the age of 50 years and in 50 percent of female heterozygotes by the age of 65 years. There are almost 200 different mutations at the locus causing familial hypercholesterolemia (Hobbs et al., 1990). Diagnosis by biochemical techniques can be difficult since cholesterol and LDL cholesterol levels may not be definitive. Physical findings can be absent. Differentiation from the more common types of hypercholesterolemias that are associated with complex gene action interacting with environmental factors is often difficult (see below). Because of the large number of mutations, a clinically useful DNA test for this entity is not yet available. Effective treatments that reduce cholesterol levels exist and decrease the probability of heart attacks. In the event that an accurate predictive test is developed, high-risk individuals (by virtue of high cholesterol levels or family history) could be tested and, if affected, treated, even though not all persons who carry the gene will develop coronary heart disease (Motulsky and Brunzell, 1992).

Polycystic Kidney Disease

Predictive testing for *autosomal dominant polycystic kidney disease* (PKD) raises additional issues (Grantham and Gabow, 1988; Gabow, 1992). This condition has a frequency of 1 in 500 to 1 in 1,000. The most common gene is mapped to chromosome 16p but has not yet been cloned; the site of the other gene is not known. At least 50 percent of those carrying the more common of the two genes that can cause this condition will develop renal failure by the age of 70 (Parfrey et al., 1990). Many individuals will develop renal failure in middle age, and 8 to 10 percent of end-stage renal disease is caused by this disorder. There is no definitive treatment that has been shown to defer the onset of renal failure, although treatment of hypertension and urinary infections may help to do so (Ravine et al., 1991). In the absence of dialysis or kidney transplant, renal failure leads to death.

The positive advantages of knowing whether one carries the gene and the potential advantages of symptomatic treatment must be weighed against problems with discrimination in occupation, insurance, and other areas of life (Sujansky et al., 1990). Full discussion of such issues should be carried out before testing is initiated for the presence of polycystic kidneys. Phenotypic testing by ultrasound and indirect testing through family linkage studies are currently available (Ravine et al., 1992). When both ultrasound and DNA diagnosis are offered to well-informed at-risk patients, most chose ultrasound testing alone. The DNA test can indicate if one is a carrier and will develop the disease in the future while the ultrasound reveals one is affected at that time. People seem more interested in determining current status than future probabilities (Gabow, 1992).

Inherited Susceptibility to Cancers

It has been speculated for some time that genetic factors influence susceptibility to cancer; in fact, rare but highly heritable familial forms of specific cancers have been identified as constituting approximately 5 percent of all cancers (see Box 2-7) (Schimke, 1992). Specific genes that are inherited have already been localized in breast cancer (Hall et al., 1990) and identified in colon cancer (Nishisha, 1991). Indirect DNA testing in at-risk families by tracing the coinheritance of the linked marker and the cancer gene is already possible in some instances, such as inherited breast carcinoma, and direct testing for the responsible gene can be carried out in a few instances (e.g., testing for retinoblastoma or for the p53 gene in Li-Fraumeni syndrome—see Box 2-8). While most cancers are not caused by such Mendelian or monogenic cancer genes, the total number of affected persons with inherited cancer in the population is large. Screening for inherited susceptibility to cancers raises many issues, including appropriate therapy, access, intense anxiety, and discrimination.

Another set of diseases for which predictive testing is now being investigated is cancers of complex origin. In addition to the cancer genes that have a large effect in predisposed individuals, other genes affecting DNA repair and the metabolism of carcinogenic substances may have a significant effect in determining who will be at greatest risk of developing cancer (Caporaso et al., 1990; McLemore et al., 1990; Nazar-Stewart et al., 1993). Population screening is not yet feasible for common cancer predispositions.

Much attention is currently being given to a very rare syndrome, Li-Fraumeni syndrome, in which mutations of a common tumor suppressor gene (p53) are transmitted by autosomal dominant inheritance and may cause tumors in multiple organs, including breast cancers and sarcomas, sometimes beginning in childhood (Malkin et al., 1990; Hollstein et al., 1991). Recent guidelines on predictive test-

BOX 2-7   Determining Susceptibility to
Breast Cancer of Early Onset

For some years it has been inferred that a heritable gene that predisposes women to breast cancer is responsible for about 5 percent of cases—specifically the rare inherited form that strikes women in their thirties and forties. Approximately one woman in 200 inherits the defective gene, and those who do face an 80 to 90 percent risk of developing the disease. The same altered gene seems also to predispose to ovarian cancer. Identification of this gene could lead to new methods for detection far earlier than is currently possible, with the advantage of earlier and more aggressive treatment. Linkage studies in affected families are already providing some women with predictive tests. Current technology is available in some large families to identify family members at risk for breast cancer by testing DNA markers co-segregating with the cancer gene. For early detection of the gene to be beneficial, individuals carrying the inherited cancer gene may need, in the future, to undergo further periodic screening using biomarker approaches in the target organ. At the present time, women at risk can be closely monitored with physical examinations and mammograms for signs of malignancy. Presented with the options, however, many will choose bilateral preventive prophylactic mastectomy and often also removal of their ovaries after completion of childbearing as a preventive measure.

The development of this predictive test has raised numerous questions regarding wide-scale screening and testing (Marshall, 1993). It is currently impossible to identify women at high risk of inherited breast cancer by general population screening. Identification of the normal and mutant sequence(s) of the critical susceptibility gene(s) would be necessary for this purpose. For now, testing is limited to large families at risk. With anticipated discovery of the gene(s) in the near future, however, it is conceivable that efforts would be made to screen the general population. The psychosocial consequences of receiving such loaded information have not yet been fully evaluated, nor has the effect of such information on insurability. Pilot studies will be needed to determine to whom the test should be offered, including where and when. Current research protocols provide intensive counseling by genetic counselors and physician geneticists. This process is very costly and may not be feasible economically or in terms of available trained personnel if large-scale genetic screening interventions in breast cancer or other forms of cancer are developed.

ing for p53 (see Box 2-8) were developed in NIH consensus conferences (Li et al., 1992, p. 1160):

> An overall benefit of predictive p53 testing cannot be assumed and should be evaluated along with harmful effects in research protocols. Potential psychological, economic, and social benefits to those who test negative should be weighed against the increased distress to those who test positive.

BOX 2-8 Predictive p53 Testing Among Cancer-Prone Individuals

Recent NIH consensus conferences have made the following recommendations for predictive p53 testing for germline mutations in clinically healthy individuals from cancer-prone families (Li et al., 1992). With recent reports of germline mutations in families with Li-Fraumeni syndrome (multiple cancers in families, often occurring early in life), there is the possibility of genetic testing of healthy persons from high-risk families. This possibility of such testing also raises issues about the appropriate use and protection of genetic information, including issues of autonomy, privacy, confidentiality, and equity, and may raise complex family issues as well, including the testing of minors.

- The p53 carriers should be counseled to seek early medical attention for signs and symptoms of cancer, and their changes in patterns of utilization of health services should be evaluated.
- Evaluation should be made of psychosocial effects, both beneficial and harmful, that result from predictive testing. Effect of support services to ameliorate harmful consequences should be monitored.
- The p53 carriers should be counseled and urged to pursue a healthier lifestyle and diet, with avoidance of cigarette smoking, excess alcohol use, and exposures to other carcinogens; compliance should be evaluated.
- Pilot chemoprevention research studies should be considered in p53 mutation carriers, such as a tamoxifen trial to prevent breast cancer.
- Physicians of test subjects need to be educated about the extraordinary risk of cancer in p53 carriers, the need for confidentiality, and the importance of attention to complaints that might be attributed to cancer.
- Because reduction in cancer morbidity and mortality will require many years to evaluate, test subjects should have *long-term* follow-up.
- Evaluation of benefits and harm will be hampered by the limited numbers of eligible study subjects. Large effects, whether beneficial or harmful, might be detectable with as few as 10-15 subjects. However, smaller effects are likely to require study of 100 or more subjects. Therefore, test centers should be encouraged to use protocols with some similar elements so that these results can be pooled to increase statistical power.
- Registries should be established to collect data on Li-Fraumeni families and collate findings from p53 testing programs worldwide.
- A national advisory group should be established to address additional issues, such as professional and public education, that are generic to predictive testing for mutations in cancer-susceptibility genes.

Testing for Multifactorial Genetic Disorders

Coronary Heart Disease

Coronary heart disease is a common cause of morbidity and death. Various genes are often predisposing factors and are better understood than the genetic etiology of many other complex disorders. In most cases, no single gene can be identified; a variety of genes (mostly affecting lipid-related proteins) as well as environmental factors such as high-fat and cholesterol diets have been defined (Motulsky and Brunzell, 1992). Other more poorly understood factors are also involved, such as those affecting blood coagulation and vessel wall response. Genetic susceptibility testing for coronary heart disease requires the assessment of a variety of predisposing genes. Only occasionally will a single gene such as that causing familial hypercholesterolemia (Goldstein and Brown, 1989) be the major factor. Most affected persons will carry a combination of the underlying predisposing genes, but the specific set of genes accounting for susceptibility is likely to vary from family to family.

A surrogate for genetic testing reflecting the action of *both* genetics and environment is already being used. The finding of elevated cholesterol levels (Motulsky and Brunzell, 1992) constitutes a probabilistic measure of risk for coronary heart disease. However, cholesterol levels alone remain an imperfect predictor of coronary heart disease since many patients with "normal" cholesterol levels develop coronary heart disease. Furthermore, many individuals with high cholesterol levels will not be clinically affected. Other predictors of coronary heart disease are already known, such as low levels of high-density lipoprotein (HDL) and high lipoprotein (a) (Lp(a)) levels. Ongoing work is likely to elucidate the role of various genes and their interaction in the pathogenesis of coronary heart disease. Based on this knowledge, it is likely that a small battery of tests reflecting the major susceptibility genes and their biochemical correlates (which also reflect environmental interaction) will be developed to predict the probability of coronary heart disease better than current tests. High-risk individuals in the population could, therefore, be identified who could take preventive actions by dietary and possibly pharmaceutical interventions.

Hypertension

Familial aggregation, twin, and adoption studies have shown that genetic factors play a role in high blood pressure (Burke and Motulsky, 1992a). Multiple genes interacting with environmental factors are likely to be involved, since monogenic inheritance is not observed. Hypertension does not exist in individuals in primitive populations but may develop when such individuals are translocated to a Western environment with more salt intake and stress. Salt sensitivity (i.e., raised blood pressure associated with salt intake) may be under genetic control. Several candidate genes for predisposition to hypertension are under study (Burke and Motulsky, 1992b); these include genes controlling sodium ion transport and other metabolic processes affecting the renin-angiotensin system.

Hypertension is a risk factor for strokes, kidney failure, heart failure, and certain eye diseases. Genetic tests that predict the development of hypertension would be useful once preventive measures to avoid high blood pressure are clearly defined. Since the genetic causes of hypertension are likely to differ among individuals, definition of the genetic-biochemical defect(s) in a given person may lead to more rational therapy directed to the underlying cause. Thus, salt restriction might be advisable for salt-sensitive persons but not for all individuals, and a specific class of drug to lower blood pressure could be selected when drug therapy becomes indicated. Medications that lower blood pressure are currently used empirically, without defining the specific cause of high blood pressure. There is now some evidence that hypertension among African-Americans is less likely to respond to certain classes of drugs (beta-blockers) than hypertension among Caucasians, suggesting genetic heterogeneity in the mechanism of hypertension in these populations. Much more work will be needed before genetic tests can be useful as practical tools for predicting high blood pressure and directing therapy.

Cancers of Complex Origin

Unlike those cancers with inherited susceptibility, discussed earlier, most cancers have complex etiology; they are caused by alteration of the genetic material (DNA) in somatic cells of various organs (such as breast and colon) that occur after birth. Most cancers, therefore, may be classified as *somatic* genetic disease. Unlike classic heritable diseases where every body cell carries the altered DNA, the characteristic molecular and cellular alterations in cancer affect only the descendants of the original cancer cell in a given organ, which grow in an unregulated fashion and may spread to other organs.

Detection of the somatic mutations of cancer is becoming increasingly possible by genetic techniques, and many of these techniques are already coming into clinical use. In hematologic cancers, different specific alterations characteristic of a given disorder were initially observed in the chromosomes of the involved tissue (IOM, 1992). The genes affected by these cytogenetic anomalies are being identified and can sometimes be utilized for molecular diagnosis. Occasionally, detection of a specific chromosomal or molecular abnormality is helpful in predicting the clinical severity of the cancer and in a few cases may aid in selecting the most appropriate treatment (IOM, 1992). In colon cancer and probably in many other cancers, a sequential series of different mutations of the involved somatic tissue is required for the ultimate development of the malignant tumor (Fearon and Vogelstein, 1990). Once characteristic genetic alterations have been recognized, increased monitoring may make possible early diagnosis of a tumor in the affected organ and provide the appropriate treatment.

Better still, a tumor may be recognized in its premalignant stages, allowing prevention of its growth by life-style changes, chemoprevention, or a variety of other interventions. Mutations of common tumor suppressor genes such as the p53 gene are often involved (Frebourg and Friend, 1992). Screening of the general population for common somatic cancers for which everyone is at risk may become feasible using such tumor biomarkers by examining DNA from cells in stool, blood, sputum, and urine, and in breast, cervical, and prostatic fluids. This kind of screening for tumors promises to be a major application of genetic screening tests in the future. It cannot yet be done, and the exact applications in practice require more research. Once available, extensive pilot studies will be required to assess the value of such investigations, their potential impact on reducing cancer mortality, and their cost-effectiveness. Generally, this type of screening is similar to current screening by mammography for breast cancer or search for occult blood in stool for colon cancer. Specifically, the search detects an abnormality *already present*. It should be contrasted to screening for cancers where an inherited mutation transmitted from one or both parents makes individuals more susceptible and therefore warrants additional screening (discussed earlier), although they may not yet have developed a neoplasm.

Diabetes

Two principal varieties of diabetes exist: early-onset or insulin-dependent diabetes, and late-onset or non-insulin-dependent diabetes (Rotter et al., 1992). Both types have unrelated genetic determinants. Insulin-dependent diabetes usually starts early in life and is associated with severe insulin deficiency. Genes of the HLA complex on chromosome 6 have been implicated as etiologic factors in this form of diabetes associated with autoimmune destruction of the pancreas; other genes are likely to be involved but have not been clearly elucidated. However, even in family testing, 75 percent of siblings identified to be at risk by HLA testing never develop clinical diabetes. Although preventive therapy of high-risk persons by immunosuppressive drugs is being considered, the drugs currently available are too toxic for general use. Predictive tests may become practical in the future when better methods of testing and less toxic therapies are available to prevent diabetes. Population testing cannot be recommended at this time, and even family testing has limited use because of low prediction rates and the absence of preventive treatment.

Non-insulin-dependent diabetes tends to manifest in middle age and is usually milder clinically. This form of diabetes has much stronger genetic determinants, based on identical twin studies in which concordance is almost 100 percent. Unfortunately, the specific genes causing the disease are unknown. Since transmission patterns do not fit monogenic inheritance, different interacting genes are likely to be at work; it is likely that different genes are operative in different families, and genes affecting the biochemical action of glucose and insulin are being investigated (Leahy and Boyd, 1993; Mueckler, 1993). No definitive measures are currently known that will prevent clinical non-insulin-dependent diabetes. Definition of the involved genes may lead to such preventive measures. Since this form of diabetes is very common (affecting 3 percent of the population) and the disease is associated with a wide range of related health effects, the development of accurate predictive testing and effective prevention and therapy would be a major health advance. Although a number of genes are under active study, predictive testing is not feasible at this time.

Rheumatoid Arthritis

Rheumatoid arthritis is a common, often disabling disease that in severe cases can shorten life expectancy markedly (King et al., 1992; Winchester, 1992). Certain genes in the HLA system help to determine susceptibility, and other HLA alleles help to determine the severity of the illness. However, other poorly defined genetic and environmental factors are also involved in the etiology of rheumatoid arthritis.

Infectious Diseases

Genetic host factors affecting susceptibility and resistance to many different microbial infections, including viruses, have been recognized for many years in experimental animals (Childs et al., 1992). Genetic variation also occurs in the offending microorganism. The effect of genetic variation in both host and microorganism on mortality has become well recognized, although mechanisms governing susceptibility and resistance are often specific for a given infection and may not be related to immunity. Twin and adoption studies show some evidence of genetic influences in infectious disease mortality. Genetic factors affecting cellular HLA immunity have been implicated in many different infections. Associations of HLA alleles have been claimed for immunologic responses to a variety of vaccines (e.g., tetanus, influenza, hepatitis A and B) and for infectious diseases (tuberculosis, leprosy, measles, AIDS, and malaria).

The clearest evidence for specific gene involvement in the host—unrelated to immune factors—comes from malaria. Lack of expression of the Duffy gene in red blood cells is a common genetic trait in Africans and their descendants in the United States. Lack of expression of this gene provides complete resistance to vivax malaria and is an example of how an altered gene prevents entry of a microorganism into cells. Genes for hemoglobin S, alpha- and beta-thalassemia, and glucose-6-phosphate-dehydrogenase (G6PD) deficiency are all involved in conferring relative resistance to falciparum malaria in respective gene carriers.

It has already been shown that HLA alleles are involved in influencing the course of HIV (human immunodeficiency virus) infection. The interplay of genetically influenced immunologic responses together with more specific genetic variation affecting inborn resistance could affect the natural history of HIV infections. The search for genetic variation among appropriate populations (e.g., persons with short versus long latency periods, individuals resistant to HIV infection despite exposure, and identical and fraternal twins) may ultimately uncover the specific mechanisms, and such findings might be useful in devising novel approaches to prevention and therapy in the future.

Psychiatric Diseases

Nowhere is the need for caution more apparent than in predictive testing for psychiatric diseases. The most common psychiatric diseases are schizophrenia and manic depressive disorders. Based on extensive family, twin, and adoption studies, there is agreement that genetic factors play an important role in the causation of these diseases (Goldin et al., 1992; Hanson and Gottesman, 1992). However, the nature and number of the underlying genes are entirely unknown. Mendelian inheritance is rarely observed, and the mechanisms of transmission are generally obscure. There was much excitement when genetic linkage studies using anonymous DNA markers appeared to map specific genes in schizophrenia (Sherrington et al., 1988) and manic depressive disorders (Egeland et al., 1989), but repeated tests to replicate this work have, to date, yielded negative results (Kelsoe et al., 1989; Baron et al., 1993). Some other neuropsychiatric disorders in which genetic factors have been implicated include panic disorders (Crowe, 1992), Tourette syndrome, and certain types of alcoholism (Propping, 1992). However, no specific genes have been mapped or otherwise identified in any of these disorders.

It is likely that multiple genes, often interacting with yet poorly understood environmental factors, will be operative in many psychiatric disorders. As with other complex conditions, predictive testing in psychiatric diseases is unlikely to be as accurate as prediction in monogenic diseases. Prediction will always be more probabilistic, and there will be uncertainty regarding whether the disorder will ever manifest and, if so, at what age. The implications of predictive testing for mental disorders raise even more problems than those for other complex medical diseases, because of the heightened potential for stigmatization and discrimination.

CONCLUSIONS AND RECOMMENDATIONS

Newborn Screening

The benefits of screening have been demonstrated in diseases such as PKU and congenital hypothyroidism, because of the overall benefit of early diagnosis of diseases for which effective treatment is available. Screening may offer no benefit if no treatment exists or services are not available. **The committee recommends that newborn screening only take place (1) for conditions for which there are indications of clear benefit to the newborn, (2) when a system is in place for confirmatory diagnosis, and (3) when treatment and follow-up are available for affected newborns.** The committee recommends that states with newborn screening programs for treatable disorders also have programs to ensure that necessary treatment and follow-up services are provided to affected children identified through newborn screening.

The committee recommends that newborns not be screened for disorders that have no beneficial treatment available, and that newborns not be screened using multiplex testing for many disorders unless those disorders are treatable (see also Chapter 8). To determine clear benefit, well-designed, peer-reviewed studies will be required to demonstrate the safety and effectiveness of the proposed screening program. Proposals for new population-based newborn screening programs should be subject to the same standards as other experimental interventions on nonconsenting subjects. Although DNA typing will provide new tools for newborn screening, in general, the committee recommends that these tools be employed only when genetic heterogeneity is small; when the ability to detect disease-causing mutations is high; when a high percentage of such mutations for a given disease is known; when costs are reasonable; and when the benefits to newborns of early detection are clear.

The committee recommends that couples in high-risk populations who are considering reproduction seek carrier screening for themselves. When newborn screening might lead to the identification of carrier status in an infant, parents should be informed in advance about this possibility and about the benefits and limitations of genetic information and genetic counseling, including that the information has no bearing on the health of their child. If the parents wish information on the infant's carrier status for consideration in their reproductive decision making in the future, this information should be communicated to them; the decisions of the parents about whether or not they wish to receive such information should be respected. Ideally, this information should only be conveyed within the context of genetic counseling.

For a variety of reasons, including problems associated with carrier detection in newborn screening, the committee recommends that informed consent be an integral part of newborn screening. Disclosure should include (1) benefits and risks of the tests and treatments; (2) the possibility of uncovering misattributed paternity; and (3) the policy of not *volunteering* results that offer no benefit for the infant. States should, at the least, anticipate the problems discussed above and have in place protocols, including genetic counseling, for dealing with such potential crises as the inadvertent discovering of misattributed paternity. Genetic testing should not be used in ways that disrupt families. The committee recognizes the complexities of identifying information about misattributed paternity, but on balance, the committee recommends that such information be revealed to the mother but *not* be volunteered to the mother's partner. There may be *rare* special circumstances that warrant such disclosure, but these situations present difficult counseling challenges (see Chapters 4 and 8).

The committee believes that mandatory *offering* of established tests (e.g., PKU, congenital hypothyroidism) that lead to the diagnosis of treatable conditions is appropriate. If there is no other way to ensure that affected newborns will be identified and have access to effective treatment (e.g., in PKU, congenital hypothyroidism), then mandatory newborn screening is accept-

able. In the rare instance where parents would be considered negligent for refusing an indicated test, established legal procedures should be used to obtain necessary parental authorization.

Newborn screening programs should include provision for counseling of all parents who are informed that the child is affected with a genetic disorder, including those for whom the diagnosis in the child proves to be false in later testing.

Since some existing programs may not have been subject to careful evaluation, the committee recommends that ongoing programs be reviewed periodically, preferably by a body independent of the program or laboratory performing the testing, such as a broadly representative state commission or advisory council (see Chapter 9). The evaluation should include technical issues such as the sensitivity and specificity of the tests, quality control procedures, and evidence that early detection actually improves outcome. Furthermore, once tests are instituted, newborn screening laboratories should have strict standards for quality control and proficiency testing (see Chapter 3 for further discussion). Detailed statutory requirements for specific tests may be unduly inflexible; the committee recommends that the states would be better served by an advisory mechanism that is authorized to add, eliminate, or modify existing programs, and to provide guidance for standards.

The committee recommends that stored newborn blood spots should be made available for additional research only if identifiers have been removed; as with other research involving human subjects, such research proposals should be reviewed by an appropriate institutional review board. If identifiable information is to be disclosed beyond the immediate purpose of an approved service program, informed consent of the infant's parent or guardian should be obtained prior to use of the specimen (see Chapter 8 for further discussion).

Carrier Testing and Screening

Determination of carrier status involves decisions concerning significant reproductive issues (i.e., abortion, medically assisted conception, adoption, sterilization, etc.). **There was consensus among committee members that pregnancy is not the preferred time for carrier screening because reproductive options are limited.** Because of the significant anxiety that may be raised by learning of carrier status for the first time during pregnancy, testing to determine carrier status before pregnancy is optimal. **Carrier testing and screening must be voluntary and must be preceded by education and counseling.** High standards of explicit informed consent must be met, with attention to ensuring that a couple is told, in easily understood terms, the medical and social choices available to them should one or both of them be determined to be carriers. Some members of the committee realized that much of carrier screening would be pushed back into pregnancy because of inertia, lack of education, and the difficult logistics of widespread testing of young adults prior to childbearing. In general, however, the committee had reservations about carrier screening programs in the high school setting in the context of the health and educational systems of the United States, or carrier testing of persons younger than age 18; the committee was dubious that sufficient education, counseling, and follow-up would be provided in such settings. Research is needed to develop innovative methods for carrier detection in young adults at a time before pregnancy, and to evaluate these methods through pilot studies.

The committee believes that, until benefits and risks have been demonstrated, genetic screening programs are a form of human experimentation. Therefore, such programs should be preceded by pilot studies demonstrating their safety and effectiveness. Standard safeguards such as institutional review, requirements for demonstrated safety and effectiveness, voluntariness, and informed consent should be applied in initiating a new carrier detection program. In addition, the nature of the disorder for which testing is to be carried out must be of sufficient severity, impact, frequency, and distribution to warrant population-based screening. Since it seems likely that screening will be done increasingly as part of routine medical care, the same principles should apply regardless of the setting of testing or screening.

The committee is unaware of any additional autosomal recessive disorders that have a sufficiently high frequency in the general population to be recommended for heterozygote screening for reproductive purposes at this time. Carrier screening has been suggested in females to detect carriers of fragile X, the most common form of serious mental retardation. The availability of a DNA test for this condition is likely to lead to more extensive testing before or during pregnancy for reproductive decisions since no treatment is available, but pilot studies are needed before such programs are implemented for fragile X (see Box 2-1). Hemochromatosis is a high-frequency, common autosomal recessive disease, but its onset is usually later in life and reproductive decisions are rarely, if ever, raised; heterozygote detection, therefore, is not indicated, and testing for the homozygote state, which occurs in about 1 in 500 Caucasians, is best deferred until adulthood (see Box 2-6).

Finally, the committee recommends that multiplexed tests should be grouped into categories of tests and disorders that raise similar issues and implications, both for informed consent and for genetic education and counseling. If found to be a carrier in such multiplex testing, individuals should be informed of their carrier status to allow testing and counseling to be offered to the partner (who usually will be found not to be a carrier). However, if both partners are carriers, they should be referred for genetic counseling to help them understand available reproductive options, including the possibility of abortion of an affected fetus. **Once multiplex testing of this kind becomes possible, pilot studies of its appropriate use need to be carried out.**

Prenatal Diagnosis

Prenatal diagnosis can provide the context in which to choose whether or not to continue a pregnancy in which the expected child has a birth defect or a genetic disorder. It can allay anxiety and, in some cases, may allow high-risk couples to undertake a pregnancy they previously would have avoided. If, following identification of a fetus at high risk for a genetic disorder through prenatal diagnosis, a decision is made to continue the pregnancy, such information can, in some cases, facilitate prenatal or early infant therapy, as well as prepare for the delivery of an infant who may need special care at birth or delivery by cesarean section. These services also have the potential to (1) increase anxiety; (2) place excessive responsibility, blame, and guilt on a woman for her pregnancy outcome; (3) interfere with maternal-infant bonding; and (4) disrupt relationships among a woman, her family members, and her community.

Autonomous decision making should be the goal in prenatal diagnosis and the committee recommends that health professionals, society, and the state be neutral on the outcome of individual reproductive choices. Reproductive genetic services should be aimed at increasing individual control over reproductive options and should not be used to pursue eugenic goals. The committee recommends that *offering* prenatal diagnosis in circumstances associated with increased risk of carrying a fetus with a diagnosable genetic disorder, including for advanced maternal age, be considered an appropriate standard of care. The committee recommends that a family history of a diagnosable genetic disorder warrants comprehensive genetic counseling, including offering of prenatal diagnosis, regardless of maternal age, as does determination of carrier status in one or both parents of a disorder for which prenatal diagnosis is available. Prenatal diagnostic services for detection of genetic disease for which there is a family history, as well as genetic counseling, should be reimbursed by insurers as medically indicated or "necessary" (see Chapter 7). Within these categories of increased risk for genetic disorders, the ability to pay should not restrict appropriate access to prenatal diagnosis, with the recognition that this recommendation has implications for the delivery of genetics services and the cost of such medical care.

However, the recommendation that prenatal diagnosis be offered should not be taken to mean that prenatal diagnosis should be undertaken without the woman's prior consent based on adequate information, even if it becomes possible in the future to perform prenatal diagnosis with simple, less invasive techniques such as the use of fetal cells isolated from maternal blood (see Box 2-3). In addition, the committee believes that prenatal diagnosis and selective abortion for carrier status for an autosomal or X-linked recessive disorder are not generally appropriate.

The benefits of maternal serum alphafetoprotein (MSAFP) screening are its low physical risk (using only a blood sample from the pregnant woman) and its ability to identify, at an early gestational age, fetuses at increased risk of neural tube defects or Down syndrome for further follow-up prenatal diagnosis, including a second MSAFP test, ultrasound, and amniocentesis. However, a serious drawback in the use of this screening test in a broad population is the anxiety it creates for women and their families. Generally, the women being tested had no reason to be concerned about genetic disorders in their fetus based on family history or other indications of high risk; when test results are negative, parental anxiety created by the screening can often be relieved. On the other hand, the committee heard testimony about the significance of the anxiety raised by MSAFP screening, as well as evidence that the *initial screening* nature of the test may not be well understood by pregnant women to whom it is offered (Faden et al., 1985; Hoyt, 1992; Press and Browner, 1992a,b). Given the nature of MSAFP screening, with its high rate of initial positives and the variety of conditions that aberrant levels might indicate, the committee recommends intensive follow-up, both to confirm predictive value and to ensure counseling for women with abnormal screening results.

Thus, the committee recommends that anyone considering prenatal diagnosis be informed about the risks and benefits of the testing procedure, and the possible outcomes, as well as alternative options to testing and other reproductive options that might be available. Principles of disclosure for informed consent, whether for routine or experimental prenatal screening or diagnosis, should include (1) fair and balanced explanation of the procedures and their safety; (2) a description of the risks and benefits; (3) consideration of all possible outcomes, including the possibility that one option might be termination of the pregnancy; (4) knowledge of the potential need for and availability of psychosocial counseling; (5) documentation of consent; and (6) full information concerning the spectrum of severity of the genetic disorders for which prenatal diagnosis is being offered (e.g., CF, Down syndrome, fragile X). Furthermore, invasive prenatal diagnosis is justified only if the pursuant diagnostic procedures are accurate, sensitive, and specific for the disorder(s) for which prenatal diagnosis is being offered. All candidates being offered prenatal screening and diagnosis should be informed about all of the risks and benefits described above to ensure that participation is voluntary.

The committee recommends that standards of care for prenatal screening and diagnosis should include education and counseling before and after the test. Thus, prenatal diagnosis should always be provided in conjunction with genetic counseling, either directly or by referral. **Furthermore, the committee recommends that third-party insurers and payers should reimburse for appropriate prenatal diagnostic services** (see Chapter 7) **for those at increased risk of serious genetic disorders, or screening to determine increased risk, including genetic counseling as an essential service, and that third-party payers should be neutral on the reproductive outcome of the prenatal diagnosis and subsequent reproductive decision making; third-party payers should not be informed of the results of prenatal screening and diagnosis.**

If and when such techniques as fluorescence in situ hybridization (FISH), triple-marker screening, or fetal cells isolated from maternal blood are validated for genetic testing, the committee recommends that (1) their use in prenatal diagnosis should be reviewed with the same careful considerations as those that were applied to current prenatal diagnostic techniques; and (2) professional groups work together to develop standards for the use of these technologies. Nevertheless, even when simpler, safer methods of testing are available, prenatal diagnosis will continue to raise significant social and ethical issues for individuals and for society, and these issues and consequences need to be weighed carefully in prenatal education and counseling.

The committee recommends that prenatal diagnosis not be used for minor conditions or characteristics. In particular, the committee felt strongly that the use of fetal diagnosis for determination of fetal sex or use of abortion for the purpose of preferential selection of the sex of the fetus is a misuse of genetic services that is inappropriate and should be discouraged by health professionals. However, the committee recognizes the desire to use prenatal diagnostic technology for identifying the sex of the fetus at high risk for an X-linked disorder where direct testing is not available. The committee is concerned that entrepreneurial pressures may expand the offering of prenatal diagnosis for preferential selection of one sex over the other, and that this practice may become a greater problem in the future. The committee believes this issue warrants careful scrutiny over the next three to five years as the availability of genetic testing becomes more widespread, and especially as simpler, safer technologies for prenatal diagnosis are developed.

Testing for Late-Onset Disorders

The committee recommends caution in the use and interpretation of a predispositional or predictive test, especially for multifactorial diseases. The dangers of stigmatization and discrimination are areas of concern, as is the potential for harm due to inappropriate preventive or therapeutic measures.

Quality assurance in both testing and test interpretation is crucial in predictive testing with special attention to conditions for which effective interventions exist. The committee recommends that—in the current state of knowledge—reproductive interventions, including prenatal diagnosis and termination of the fetus, not be conducted for increased genetic susceptibility to multifactorial disorders. Testing in later life for these conditions may be appropriate. The benefits of the various presymptomatic interventions should be weighed against the potential anxiety, stigmatization, and other possible harms to individuals who are informed that they are at increased risk of developing future disease.

The principles for predictive testing of inherited cancer susceptibility are identical to those suggested for other late-onset genetic disorders: before any

widespread application of such tests is undertaken, the committee recommends that their predictive value be thoroughly validated in prospective studies of sufficient size and statistical power. If no effective preventive or therapeutic measures exist, the dilemma of whether to test for a cancer predisposition is somewhat similar to the problems raised by predictive testing for monogenic and other conditions that are only possibly treatable. Some individuals would want to have the test while others would not, and extensive counseling is required to aid in decision making. If partially effective prevention (such as frequent monitoring) or treatment is available, extensive counseling will be required to consider the benefits and harms that may be associated with testing and possible treatment interventions. If effective prevention or treatment is available, genetic testing should be offered. The decision about the point at which treatment or prevention is so efficacious that testing becomes routine will vary for different cancers and will require extensive deliberation. The appropriate time for initiation of testing will often vary. **The committee believes that presymptomatic screening in children for adult cancers would rarely be appropriate unless effective preventive or therapeutic measures exist and require early implementation for effectiveness.** In addition, the optimal time to start screening in adults may vary for different cancers. In the future, prenatal screening may become possible, and the possibility for prenatal diagnosis of many late-onset conditions raises troubling issues when the condition is potentially curable.

    The committee recommends that, if predictive tests for mental disorders become a reality, results must be handled with stringent attention to confidentiality to protect an already vulnerable population. If no effective treatment is available, testing may not be appropriate since more harm than good could result from improper use of test results. On the other hand, future research might result in psychological or drug treatments that could prevent the onset of these diseases. Carefully designed pilot studies should be conducted to determine the effectiveness of such interventions and to measure the desirability and psychosocial impact of such testing. Interpretation and communication of predictive test results in psychiatry will be particularly difficult. To prepare for the issues associated with genetic testing for psychiatric diseases in the future, all psychiatrists will need more training in genetics and genetic counseling; such training should include the ethical, legal, and social issues in genetic testing.

    The committee recommends that population screening for late-onset monogenic diseases be considered only for treatable or preventable conditions of relatively high frequency. Under such guidelines, population screening should only be offered after appropriate, reliable, sensitive, and specific tests become available. The committee also recommends extensive *pretest* counseling, to ensure voluntariness and informed consent, as well as counseling *after testing*, and medical management where appropriate for those identified with potentially deleterious genes. Providers who conduct such testing should be well schooled in the principles of genetics and genetic counseling, including the ethical, legal, and social issues in genetic testing (see Chapters 4, 6, and 8).

The availability of presymptomatic testing for Mendelian disorders and the possibility of predispositional testing for complex disorders, such as cancers and heart disease, raise unique issues not evident in genetic testing of newborns or for reproductive planning, particularly pertaining to confidentiality—both inside and outside the family—and create new challenges for the physician-patient relationship. The availability of presymptomatic and predispositional testing provides an opportunity for physicians and patients to work toward prevention of disease. Thus, the goal of nondirective counseling (as discussed in Chapter 4), so crucial in genetic services pertaining to reproductive planning, may not always be appropriate when primary prevention or effective treatments are available. In such instances, it is considered appropriate for practitioners to give guidance to patients regarding the relevant interventions after fully explaining what is known about the potential benefits and harms of testing and of following such advice. **In considering the use of presymptomatic tests, the committee recommends that the patient be the ultimate decision maker.**

One concern about genetic tests for common, high-profile, complex disorders is that the potential number of such tests is likely to make them widely available; for-profit testing facilities may not be equipped to deal with the complexities of testing, interpretation, communication of results, and genetic counseling. **The committee recommends strict guidelines for efficacy and standards for use to prevent premature introduction of this technology in disorders of late onset; this would be an appropriate role for the recommended national advisory body and its Working Group on Genetic Testing** (see Chapter 9).

REFERENCES

American College of Obstetricians and Gynecologists (ACOG). 1985. Professional Liability Implication of AFP Testing (Liability Alert). Washington, D.C., May.

American Society of Human Genetics (ASHG). 1987. Statement on maternal serum alpha-fetoprotein screening programs and quality control for laboratories performing maternal serum and amniotic fluid alpha-fetoprotein assays. American Journal of Human Genetics 40:75-82.

American Society of Human Genetics (ASHG). 1989. Update [on MSAFP Screening]. American Journal of Human Genetics 45:332-334.

American Society of Human Genetics (ASHG). 1992. Statement of the American Society of Human Genetics on cystic fibrosis carrier screening. American Journal of Human Genetics S1:1443-1444.

Baron, M., et al. 1993. Diminished support for linkage between manic depressive illness and X-chromosome markers in three Israeli pedigrees. Nature Genetics 3:49-55.

Beeson, D., and Golbus, M. 1985. Decision making: Whether or not to have prenatal diagnosis and abortion for X-linked conditions. American Journal of Medical Genetics 20:107-114.

Benn, P., et al. 1992. A rapid (but wrong) prenatal diagnosis; A reply from Integrated Genetics. New England Journal of Medicine 326(24):1638-1640.

Bianchi, D., et al. 1991. Fetal cells in maternal blood: Prospects for non-invasive prenatal diagnosis. Presented at the International Congress of Human Genetics, Washington, D.C., October.

Black, R. 1989. A one and six month follow-up of prenatal diagnosis patients who lost pregnancies. Prenatal Diagnosis 9:795-804.

Black, R. 1990. Prenatal diagnosis and fetal loss: Psychosocial consequences and professional responsibilities. American Journal of Medical Genetics 35:586-587.

Black, R., and Furlong, R. 1984. Prenatal diagnosis: The experience in families who have children. American Journal of Medical Genetics 20:369-384.

Blumberg B., and Golbus, M. 1975. Psychological sequelae of elective abortion. Western Journal of Medicine 123:188-193.

Bothwell, T., et al. 1989. Hemochromatosis. Pp. 1433-1462 in Scriver, C., et al. (eds.) The Metabolic Basis of Inherited Disease (6th ed.). New York: McGraw Hill.

British Medical Association (BMA). 1992. Our Genetic Future: The Science and Ethics of Genetic Technologies. London: British Medical Society.

Brock, D., and Sutcliffe, R. 1972. Alpha-fetoprotein in the antenatal diagnosis of anencephaly and spina bifida. Lancet 2:197.

Burke, W., and Motulsky, A. 1992a. Hypertension. In King, R., et al. (eds.) The Genetic Basis of Common Diseases. New York: Oxford University Press.

Burke, W., and Motulsky, A. 1992b. Molecular basis of hypertension. Monographs in Human Genetics 14:228-236.

Canadian Collaborative CVS-Amniocentesis Clinical Trial Group. 1989. Multi-centre randomised clinical trial of chorionic villus sampling and amniocentesis: First report. Lancet 1:1-6.

Caporaso, N., et al. 1990. Lung cancer and the debrisoquine metabolic phenotype. Journal of the National Cancer Institute 82:1264-1272.

Caskey, T. 1991. New molecular techniques for DNA analysis. Contemporary OB/GYN 36:(5):27-49.

Caskey, T., et al. 1990. Statement of the American Society of Human Genetics on cystic fibrosis screening. American Journal of Human Genetics 46:393.

Childs, B., et al. 1992. Pp. 71-91 in King, R., et al. (eds.) Genetic Basis of Common Diseases. New York: Oxford University Press.

Choo, V. 1993. Sex selection. Lancet 341:298-299.

Clayton, E. 1992 (published in 1994). Issues in state newborn screening programs. In Fullarton, J. (ed.) Proceedings of the Committee on Assessing Genetic Risks. Washington, D.C.: National Academy Press.

Collins, F. 1992. Cystic fibrosis: Molecular biology and therapeutic implications. Science 256(5058):774-779.

Conneally, P., et al. 1984. Huntington disease: Genetics and epidemiology. American Journal of Human Genetics 36:506-526.

Council of Regional Networks for Genetic Services (CORN). 1992. Newborn Screening Report: 1990 (Final report). February.

Crandall, B. 1992 (published in 1994). Triple-marker screening. In Fullarton, J. (ed.) Proceedings of the Committee on Assessing Genetic Risks. Washington, D.C.: National Academy Press.

Cremer, C. 1988. Detection of chromosome aberrations in metaphase and interphase tumor cells by in situ hybridization using chromosome-specific library probes. Human Genetics 80:235-246.

Crowe, R. 1992. Panic disorder. Pp. 866-875 in King, R., et al. (eds.) The Genetic Basis of Common Diseases. New York: Oxford University Press.

Cuckle, H., and Wald, N. 1984. Maternal serum alpha-fetoprotein measurement: A screening for Down syndrome. Lancet 1:926-929.

Cunningham, G. 1992 (published in 1994). Statewide governmentally administered prenatal blood screening: A case study in cost-effective prevention. In Fullarton, J. (ed.) Proceedings of the Committee on Assessing Genetic Risks. Washington, D.C.: National Academy Press.

D'Alton, M., and DeCherney, A. 1993. Current concepts: Prenatal diagnosis. New England Journal of Medicine 328(2):114-120.

Donnell, G., et al. 1980. Clinical aspects of galactosemia. In Burman, D., et al. (eds.) Inherited Disorders of Carbohydrate Metabolism. Baltimore, Md.: University Park Press.

Egeland, J., et al. 1989. Bipolar affective disorder linked to DNA markers on chromosome 11. Nature 325:783-787.

Elias, S., et al. 1992. First trimester diagnosis of Down syndrome using fetal cells from maternal blood. Lancet 340:1033.

Faden, R., et al. 1982. A survey to evaluate parental consent as public policy for neonatal screening. American Journal of Public Health 72:1342-1350.

Faden, R., et al. 1985. What participants understand about a maternal serum alpha-fetoprotein screening program. American Journal of Public Health 75(12):1381-1384.

Farrer, L., and Conneally, P. 1985. A genetic model for age of onset in Huntington disease. American Journal of Human Genetics 37:350-357.

Fearon, E., and Vogelstein, B. 1990. A genetic model for colorectal tumorigenesis. Cell 61:759-767.

Filly, R., et al. 1987. Fetal spine morphology and maturation during the second trimester: Sonographic evaluation. Journal of Ultrasound in Medicine 6(11):631-636.

Firth, H., et al. 1991. Severe limb abnormalities after chorion villus sampling at 56-66 days gestation. Lancet 337:762-763.

Fost, N., and Farrell, P. 1989. A prospective and randomized trial of early diagnosis and treatment for cystic fibrosis: A unique ethical dilemma. Clinical Research 37:495-500.

Fraser, F., and Pressor, C. 1977. Attitudes of counselors in relation to prenatal sex determination for the choice of sex. Pp. 109-120 in Lubs, H., and De la Cruz, F. (eds.) Genetic Counseling. New York: Raven.

Frebourg, T., and Friend, S. 1992. Cancer risks from germline p53 mutations. Journal of Clinical Investigation 90:1637-1641.

Fu, V., et al. 1991. Variation in the CGG repeat at the fragile site results in genetic instability: Resolution of the Sherman Paradox. Cell 67:1047-1058.

Gabow, P. 1992 (published in 1994). Autosomal dominant polycystic kidney disease. In Fullarton, J. (ed.) Proceedings of the Committee on Assessing Genetic Risks. Washington, D.C.: National Academy Press.

Gelertner, J., et al. 1993. Exclusion of close linkage of Tourette's syndrome to D1 dopamine receptor. American Journal of Psychiatry 150(3):449-453.

Goate, A., et al. 1991. Segregation of a missense mutation in the amyloid precursor protein gene with familial Alzheimer's disease. Nature 349:704-706.

Goldin, L., et al. 1992. The major affective disorders: Bipolar, unipolar, and schizoaffective. Pp. 801-815 in King, R., et al. (eds.) The Genetic Basis of Common Diseases. New York: Oxford University Press.

Goldstein, J., and Brown, M. 1989. Familial hypercholesterolemia. Pp. 1215-1245 in Scriver, C., et al. (eds.) The Metabolic Basis of Inherited Disease (6th Edition). New York: McGraw-Hill.

Goldstein, R., et al. 1989. Sonography of anencephaly: Pitfalls in early diagnosis. Journal of Clinical Ultrasound 17(6):397-402.

Gowland, M. 1988. Fetal abnormalities diagnosed from early pregnancy. Clinical Radiology 39:106-108.

Grantham, J., and Gabow, P. 1988. Polycystic kidney disease. Pp. 583-614 in Schrier, R., and Gottschalk, C. (eds.) Diseases of the Kidney. Boston: Little Brown.

Gusella, J., et al. 1983. A polymorphic DNA marker genetically linked to Huntington's disease. Nature 306:234-238.

Haddow, J., et al. 1992. Prenatal screening for Down's syndrome with use of maternal serum markers. New England Journal of Medicine 327:588-593.

Hall, J., et al. 1990. Linkage of early-onset familial breast cancer to chromosome 17q21. Science 250:1684-1689.

Hammond, K., et al. 1991. Efficacy of statewide neonatal screening for cystic fibrosis by assay of trypsinogen concentrations. New England Journal of Medicine 325:769-774.

Handyside, A., et al. 1990. Pregnancies from biopsied human preimplantation embryos sexed by Y-specific DNA amplification. Nature 344:768-770.

Handyside, A., et al. 1992. Birth of a normal girl after in vitro fertilization and preimplantation diagnostic testing for cystic fibrosis. New England Journal of Medicine 327:905-909.

Hanson, D., and Gottesman, I. 1992. Schizophrenia. Pp. 816-836 in King, R., et al. (eds.) The Genetic Basis of Common Diseases. New York: Oxford University Press.

Heitz, D., et al. 1992. Inheritance of the fragile X syndrome: Size of the fragile X premutation is a major determinant of the transition to full mutation. Journal of Medical Genetics 29:794-801.

Hobbs, H. et al. 1990. The LDL receptor locus in familial hypercholesterolemia: Mutational analysis of a membrane protein. Annual Review of Genetics 24:133-170.

Hollstein, M., et al. 1991. p53 mutations in human cancers. Science 253:49-53.

Holtzman, N. 1980. Public participation in genetic policy-making: The Maryland Commission on Genetic Disorders. Pp. 247-258 in Milunsky, A., and Annas, G. (eds.) Genetics and the Law II. New York: Plenum Press.

Holtzman, N. 1989. Proceed with caution: Predicting genetic risks in the recombinant DNA era. Baltimore: Johns Hopkins University Press.

Holtzman, N. 1990. Prenatal screening: When and for whom? Journal of General Internal Medicine 5:S42-S46.

Holtzman, N. 1991. What drives neonatal screening programs? New England Journal of Medicine 325:802-804.

Holtzman, N. 1992. Testimony before the Subcommittee on Intergovernmental and Human Resources, House Committee on Government Operations. U.S. Congress, Washington, D.C., July 23.

Hook, E. 1988. Variability in predicted rates of Down syndrome associated with elevated maternal serum alpha-fetoprotein levels in older women. American Journal of Human Genetics 43:160-164.

Hoyt, H. 1992. Testimony before the Subcommittee on Intergovernmental and Human Resources, House Committee on Government Operations. U.S. Congress, Washington, D.C., July 23.

Hsieh, F., et al. 1991. Limb-reduction defects and chorion villus sampling. Lancet 337:1091-1092.

Huntington Disease Collaborative Research Group. 1993. A novel gene containing a trinucleotide repeat that is expanded and unstable on Huntington's disease chromosomes. Cell 72:971-983.

Institute of Medicine (IOM). 1992. Advances in Understanding Genetic Changes in Cancer: Impact on Diagnosis and Treatment Decisions in the 1990s. National Academy of Sciences. Washington, D.C.: National Academy Press.

Jackson, L., et al. 1992. A randomized comparison of transcervical and transabdominal chorionic-villus sampling. New England Journal of Medicine 327(13):594-598.

Juengst, E. 1988. Prenatal diagnosis and the ethics of uncertainty. In Monagle, J. (ed.) Medical Ethics: A Guide for Health Professionals. Rockville, Md.: Aspen Publishers.

Kaplan, P., et al. 1991. Intellectual outcome in children with maple syrup urine disease. Journal of Pediatrics 119:46-50.

Kelsoe, J., et al. 1989. Reevaluation of the linkage relationship between chromosome 11p loci and the gene for bipolar affective disorder in the Old Order Amish. Nature 342:238-243.

Kevles, D. 1985. In the Name of Eugenics. Los Angeles: University of California Press.

Kevles, D. 1991. Presentation at the International Congress of Human Genetics, Washington, D.C., October.

King, R. 1992. In King, R., et al. (eds.) Genetic Basis of Common Diseases. New York: Oxford University Press.

Klinger, K. 1992 (published in 1994). New clinical and laboratory procedures: Fluorescence in situ hybridization. In Proceedings of the Committee on Assessing Genetic Risks. Washington, D.C.: National Academy Press.

Klinger K., et al. 1990. Prenatal detection of aneuploidy of 21, 18, 13, X or Y by interphase in situ hybridization. American Society of Human Genetics 47(3):A224.

Klinger K., et al. 1991. Interphase cytogenetics: Improved prenatal detection of aneuploidy in uncultured fetal cells: New results from a large blinded study. American Journal of Human Genetics 49(4):AIII.

Klinger, K., et al. 1992. Rapid detection of chromosome aneuploidies in uncultured amniocytes by using fluorescence in situ hybridization (FISH). American Journal of Human Genetics 51:55-65.

Knoppers, B., and LaBerge, C. (eds.). 1990. Genetic Screening: From Newborns to DNA Typing. New York: Excerpta Medica.

Kremer, E., et al. 1991. Mapping of DNA instability at the fragile X to a trinucleotide repeat sequence p(CGG)n. Science 252:1711-1714.

LaBerge, C., and Knoppers, B. 1992 (published in 1994). Newborn screening: Ethical and social considerations for the 1990s. In Fullarton, J. (ed.) Proceedings of the Committee on Assessing Genetic Risks. Washington, D.C.: National Academy Press.

Lancet. 1991. Chorionic villus sampling: Valuable addition or dangerous alternative? (editorial). Lancet 337:1513-1515.

Lancet. 1992. Screening for fetal abnormalities (editorial). Lancet 340:1006-1007.

Lappe, M., et al. 1972. Screening for genetic disease: Ethical and social issues in screening for genetic disease (statement from the Research Group on Ethical, Social and Legal Issues in Genetic Counseling and Genetic Engineering of the Hastings Institute). New England Journal of Medicine 286:1129-1132.

Laurence, K. 1990. Genetics and the prevention of neural tube defects and of "uncomplicated" hydrocephalus. Pp. 323-346 in Emery, A., et al. (eds.) Principles and Practice of Medical Genetics, Vol. I, 2nd Ed. Edinburgh: Churchill Livingstone.

Leahy, J., and Boyd, A. 1993. Diabetes genes in non-insulin-dependent diabetes mellitus. New England Journal of Medicine 328:56-57.

Li, F., et al. 1992. Recommendations on predictive testing for germ line p53 mutations among cancer-prone individuals. Journal of the National Cancer Institute 84(15):1156-1160.

Lichter, P., et al. 1988. Rapid detection of human chromosome 21 aberrations by in situ hybridization. Proceedings of the National Academy of Sciences USA 85:9664-9668.

Littlefield, J. 1970. The pregnancy at risk for a genetic disorder. New England Journal of Medicine 282:627-628.

Malkin, D., et al. 1990. Germ line p53 mutations in a familial syndrome of breast cancer, sarcomas and other neoplasms. Science 250:1233-1238.

Manchester, D., et al. 1988. Accuracy of ultrasound diagnoses in pregnancies complicated by suspected fetal abnormalities. Prenatal Diagnosis 8:109-117.

Marshall, E. 1993. Special report: The politics of breast cancer. Science 259:616-617.

Martin, J., and Gusella, J. 1986. Huntington's disease: Pathogenesis and management. New England Journal of Medicine 315:1267-1276.

Marx, J. 1992. Familial Alzheimer's linked to chromosome 14 gene. Science 258:550.

Matsubara, Y., et al. 1991. Prevalence of K329E mutation in medium-chain acyl-CoA dehydrogenase gene determined from Guthrie cards. Lancet 338:552-553.

McCabe, E. 1992 (published in 1994). Newborn screening: American Academy of Pediatrics policy statements and issues related to DNA and RNA microextraction from newborn screening blood spots. In Fullarton, J. (ed.) Proceedings of the Committee on Assessing Genetic Risks. Washington, D.C.: National Academy Press.

McKusick, V. 1992. Mendelian Inheritance in Man: Catalogs of Autosomal Dominant, Autosomal Recessive, and X-Linked Phenotypes (9th Ed.). Baltimore: Johns Hopkins University Press.

McLemore, T., et al. 1990. Expression of CYP1A1 gene in patients with lung cancer: Evidence for cigarette smoke-induced gene expression in normal lung tissue and for altered gene regulation in primary pulmonary carcinomas. Journal of the National Cancer Institute 82:1333-1339.

McPartlin, J., et al. 1993. Accelerated breakdown of folate in pregnancy. Lancet 341(8838):148-149.

Meaney, J. 1992 (published in 1994). Reports from the Networks for Genetic Services. In Fullarton, J. (ed.) Proceedings of the Committee on Assessing Genetic Risks. Washington, D.C.: National Academy Press.

Medical Research Council. 1991. Medical Research Council European trial of chorion villus sampling. Lancet 337:1491-1499.

Mennuti, M. 1989. Prenatal diagnosis—Advances bring new challenges. New England Journal of Medicine 230(10):661-663.

Merkatz, I., et al. 1984. An association between low maternal serum alpha-fetoprotein and fetal chromosomal abnormalities. American Journal of Obstetrics and Gynecology 148:886-894.

Milunsky, A. 1985. Prenatal diagnosis: New tools, new problems. In Milunsky, A., and Annas, G. (eds.) Genetics and Law III. New York: Plenum Press.

Modell, B. 1992. Current Trends in Early Prenatal Diagnosis. Hereditary Diseases Programme. World Health Organization Report. Geneva, May.

Motulsky, A. 1989. Genetic aspects of familial hypercholesterolemia and its diagnosis. Arteriosclerosis 9(S1):1-3 to 1-7.

Motulsky, A., and Brunzell, J. 1992. The genetics of coronary atherosclerosis. In King, R., et al. (eds.) The Genetic Basis of Common Diseases. New York: Oxford University Press.

Mueckler, M. 1993. Glucokinase, glucose sensing, and diabetes. Proceedings of the National Academy of Sciences 90(3):784-785.

National Academy of Sciences (NAS). 1975. Genetic Screening: Programs, Principles, and Research. Committee for the Study of Inborn Errors of Metabolism. Washington, D.C.: NAS.

National Institute of Child Health and Human Development (NICHD). 1979. Antenatal Diagnosis (Report of a Consensus Development Conference). NIH Publication No. 79-1973. U.S. Department of Health, Education and Welfare, Public Health Service, National Institutes of Health. Bethesda, Md.

National Institute of Child Health and Human Development (NICHD) National Registry for Amniocentesis Study Group. 1976. Midtrimester amniocentesis for prenatal diagnosis: Safety and accuracy. Journal of the American Medical Association 236:1471-1476.

National Institutes of Health (NIH). 1984. Diagnostic Ultrasound Imaging in Pregnancy. NIH Publication No. 84-667. Public Health Service. U.S. Department of Health and Human Services. Washington, D.C.: U.S. Government Printing Office.

National Institutes of Health Workshop on Population Screening for the Cystic Fibrosis Gene. 1990. New England Journal of Medicine 323:70-71.

National Institutes of Health (NIH) Workshop on Reproductive Genetic Testing. 1991. Reproductive Genetic Testing: Impact on Women. Bethesda, Md., November.

Nazar-Stewart, V., et al. 1993. The glutathione S-transferase Mu polymorphism as a marker for susceptibility to lung carcinoma. Cancer Research (in press).

New England Regional Genetics Group (NERGG). 1989. Combining maternal alpha-fetoprotein measurements and age to screen for Down syndrome in pregnant women under age 35: Report of New England Regional Genetics Group Prenatal Collaborative Study of Down Syndrome Screening. American Journal of Obstetrics and Gynecology 160:575-581.

Nicolaides, K., et al. 1992. Ultrasonographically detectable markers of fetal chromosomal abnormalities. Lancet 340:704-707.

Niederau, C., et al. 1985. Survival and causes of death in cirrhotic and in noncirrhotic patients with primary hemochromatosis. New England Journal of Medicine 313:1256-1262.

Niermeijer, M. 1988. Screening and counselling: Report of discussion group on genetic screening, counselling and intervention. In Bankowsky, Z., and Bryant, J. (ed.) Health Policy, Ethics and Human Values: European and North American Perspectives: Conference Highlights, Papers and Conclusions from the XXIst Council of International Organizations of Medical Science Conference, Geneva.

Nishisha, I. 1991. Mutations of chromosomes 5q21 genes in FAP and colorectal cancer patients. Science 253:665.

Oberle, I., et al. 1991. Instability of a 550-base pair DNA segment and abnormal methylation in fragile X syndrome. Science 252:1097-1102.

Office of Technology Assessment (OTA). 1992. Cystic Fibrosis and DNA Tests: Implications of Carrier Screening. OTA-BA-532. U.S. Congress. Washington, D.C.: U.S. Government Printing Office.

Oudet, C., et al. 1993. Linkage disequilibrium between the fragile X mutation and two closely linked CA repeats suggests that fragile X chromosomes are derived from a small number of founder chromosomes. American Journal of Human Genetics 52:298-304.

Parfrey, P., et al. 1990. The diagnosis and prognosis of autosomal dominant polycystic kidney disease. New England Journal of Medicine 323:1085-1090.

Platt, L., and Carlson, D. 1992. Prenatal diagnosis—When and how? New England Journal of Medicine 327:636-638.

President's Commission for the Study of the Ethical Problems in Medicine and Biomedical and Behavioral Research. 1983. Screening and Counseling for Genetic Conditions: The Ethical, Social, and Legal Implications of Genetic Screening, Counseling, and Education Programs. Washington, D.C.: Government Printing Office.

Press, N. and Browner, C. 1992 (published in 1994). Policy issues in maternal serum alpha-fetoprotein: The view from California. In Proceedings of the Committee on Assessing Genetic Risks. Washington, D.C.: National Academy Press.

Press, N., and Browner, C. 1993. Collective fictions: Similarities in the reasons for accepting MSAFP screening among women of diverse ethnic and social class backgrounds. Fetal Diagnosis and Therapy 8(Suppl. 1):97-106.

Privacy Commission of Canada. 1992. Genetic Testing and Privacy. Cat. No. IP34-3/1992. Ottawa: Minister of Supply and Services.

Propping, P. 1992. Alcoholism. Pp. 837-865 in King, R., et al. (eds.) The Genetic Basis of Common Diseases. New York: Oxford University Press.

Purkiss, S., et al. 1988. Surgical emergencies after prenatal treatment for intra-abdominal abnormality. Lancet 1:289-290.

Rapp, R. 1987. Moral pioneers: Women, men and fetuses on a frontier of reproductive technology. Women and Health 13:101-116.

Rapp, R. 1988a. Chromosomes and communication: The discourse of genetic counseling. Medical Anthropology Quarterly 2(2):143-157.

Rapp, R. 1988b. The power of "positive" diagnosis: Medical and maternal discourses on amniocentesis. In Michaelson, K. (ed.) Childbirth in America: Anthropological Perspectives. South Hadley, Mass.: Bergin & Garvey.

Rapp, R. 1991. Constructing amniocentesis: Maternal and medical discourses. In Ginsburg, F., and Tsing, A. (eds.) Negotiating Gender in American Culture. Boston: Beacon Press.

Ravine, D., et al. 1991. Treatable complications in undiagnosed cases of autosomal dominant polycystic kidney disease. Lancet 1:127-129.

Ravine, D., et al. 1992. Phenotype and genotype heterogeneity in autosomal dominant polycystic kidney disease. Lancet 340:1330-1333.

Rhoads, G., et al. 1989. The safety and efficacy of chorionic villus sampling for early prenatal diagnosis of cytogenetic abnormalities. New England Journal of Medicine 320(10):609-617.

Richards, R., et al. 1992. Evidence of founder chromosomes in fragile X syndrome. Nature Genetics 1:257-260.

Risch, N. 1992 (published in 1994). Genetic basis of mental disorders. In Fullarton, J. (ed.) Proceedings of the Committee on Assessing Genetic Risks. Washington, D.C.: National Academy Press.

Rothman, B. 1986. The Tentative Pregnancy: Prenatal Diagnosis and the Future of Motherhood. New York: Viking.

Rothman, B. 1992 (published in 1994). Early prenatal diagnosis: Unsolved problems. In Fullarton, J. (ed.) Proceedings of the Committee on Assessing Genetic Risks. Washington, D.C.: National Academy Press.

Rothman, B. 1993. The tentative pregnancy: Then and now. Fetal Diagnosis and Therapy 8(Suppl. 1):60-63.

Rotter, J., et al. 1992. Diabetes mellitus. Pp. 413-481 in King, R., et al. (eds.) The Genetic Basis of Common Diseases. New York: Oxford University Press.

Rousseau, F., et al. 1991. Direct diagnosis by DNA analysis of the fragile X syndrome of mental retardation. New England Journal of Medicine 325:1673-1681.

Schellenberg, G., et al. 1992. Genetic linkage evidence for a familial Alzheimer's disease locus on chromosome 14. Science 258:668-671.

Schimke, R. 1992. Cancers in families. In King, R., et al. (eds.) The Genetic Basis of Common Diseases. New York: Oxford University Press.

Scott, J., et al. 1991. Folic acid to prevent neural tube defects. Lancet 338:505.

Shapiro, L. 1991. The fragile X syndrome. New England Journal of Medicine 325:1736-1737.

Sherrington, R., et al. 1988. Localization of a susceptibility locus for schizophrenia on chromosome 5. Nature 336:164-167.

Simpson, J. and Carson, S. 1992. Editorial: Preimplantation genetic diagnosis. New England Journal of Medicine 327(13):951-953.

Singer, E. 1991. Public attitudes toward genetic testing. Population Research and Policy Review 10(3):235-255.

Society for Assisted Reproductive Technologies (SART). 1992. In vitro fertilization-embryo transfer (IVF-ET) in the United States: 1990 results from the IVF-ET Registry. Fertility Sterility 57:15-24.

Sorenson, J. 1976. From social movement to clinical medicine: The role of law and the medical profession in regulating applied genetics. Pp. 467-485 in Milunsky, A., and Annas, G. (eds.) Genetics and the Law. New York: Plenum.

St. George-Hyslop, P., et al. 1990. Genetic linkage studies suggest that Alzheimer's disease is not a single homogeneous disorder. Nature 347:194-197.

Steele, M., and Breg, W. 1966. Chromosome analysis of human amniotic fluid cells. Lancet 1:385.

Sujansky, E., et al. 1990. Attitudes of at risk and affected individuals regarding presymptomatic testing for autosomal dominant polycystic kidney disease. American Journal of Medical Genetics 35:510-515.

Sutherland, G., et al. 1991. Prenatal diagnosis of fragile X syndrome by direct detection of the unstable DNA sequence. New England Journal of Medicine 325:1720-1722.

Tabor, A., et al. 1986. Randomised controlled trial of genetic amniocentesis in 4606 low-risk women. Lancet 1:1287-1292.

Taussig, L., et al. 1983. Neonatal screening for cystic fibrosis. Pediatrics 72(6):741-744.

Therrell, B., et al. 1992. U.S. newborn screening system guidelines: Statement of the Council of Regional Networks for Genetic Services. Screening 1:135-147.

Tlucek, A., et al. 1990. Psychosocial impact of neonatal screening for cystic fibrosis on families with false-positive results. Journal of Developmental and Behavioral Pediatrics 13(3):181-196.

Townsend, R., et al. 1988. Factors affecting prenatal sonographic estimation of weight in extremely low birth-weight infants. Journal of Ultrasound in Medicine 7(4):183-187.

Tymstra, T. 1991. Prenatal diagnosis, prenatal screening, and the rise of the tentative pregnancy. International Journal of Technology Assessment 7(4):509-516.

Tymstra, T., et al. 1991. Women's opinions on the offer and use of prenatal diagnosis. Prenatal Diagnosis 11(12):893-898.

U.S. Preventive Services Task Force. 1989. Guide to Clinical Preventive Services: An Assessment of the Effectiveness of 169 Interventions. Baltimore: Williams & Wilkins.

Verkerk, A., et al. 1991. Identification of gene 9FMR-1 containing a CGG repeat coincident with a breakpoint cluster region exhibiting length variation in fragile X syndrome. Cell 65:905-914.

Verlinsky, Y., and Kuliev, I. (eds.). 1992. Pre-implantation Diagnosis of Genetic Diseases. New York: Liss.

Went, L. 1990. Ethical issues policy statement on Huntington's disease molecular genetics predictive test. Journal of Medical Genetics 27(1):34-38.

Wertz, D. 1992. Prenatal Diagnosis and Society. Royal Commission on New Reproductive Technologies, Ottawa, October.

Wertz, D., and Fletcher, J. 1988. Attitudes of genetic counselors: A multinational study. American Journal of Human Genetics 42:592-600.

Wertz, D., and Fletcher, J. 1989a. An international survey of attitudes of medical geneticists toward mass screening and access to results. Public Health Reports 104(1):35-44.

Wertz, D., and Fletcher, J. 1989b. Ethical problems in prenatal diagnosis: A cross-cultural survey of medical geneticists in 18 nations. Prenatal Diagnosis 9:145-158.

Wertz, D., et al. 1990. Medical geneticists confront ethical dilemmas: Cross-cultural comparisons among 18 nations. American Journal of Human Genetics 46:1200-1213.

Wexler, N. 1992. The Tiresias complex: Huntington's disease as a paradigm of testing for late-onset disorders. FASEB Journal 6:2820-2825.

Winchester, R. 1992. Genetic determination of susceptibility and severity in rheumatoid arthritis. Annals of Internal Medicine 117:869-871.

World Federation of Neurology Research Group on Huntington's Disease. 1990. Ethical issues policy statement on Huntington's disease molecular genetics predictive test. Journal of Medical Genetics 27:34-38.

World Health Organization (WHO). 1983. Report of a WHO Working Group on Fetal Diagnosis of Hereditary Diseases. Geneva: World Health Organization.

World Health Organization Expert Panel (WHO). 1992. Risk Evaluation of Chorionic Villus Sampling. Report of an Expert Panel. Copenhagen: World Health Organization.

Yu, S., et al. 1991. Fragile X genotype characterized by an unstable region of DNA. Science 252:1179-1181.

3

Laboratory Issues in
Human Genetics

The mapping of the human genome will lead to the identification of virtually all disease-causing genes and the development of tests to detect at least some of the mutations that are responsible for single-gene disorders and for susceptibility to many other common disorders. This proliferation of genetic tests will benefit those at risk of genetic and chromosomal disorders by permitting early treatment or, when treatment is not available, by providing prospective parents with options for avoiding the conception or birth of children affected with serious disorders. Consequently, errors in test performance and interpretation will detract from the benefit of genetic testing. Laboratory errors do occur. Errors have been documented in newborn screening (Holtzman et al., 1986; Hannon and Adam, 1991; Adam and Hannon, 1992), in biochemical genetic testing (Hommes et al., 1990), in karyotyping in cytogenetics* (Vockley et al., 1991), in linkage analysis, and in interpretation of results (P.M. Conneally, personal communication, February 1992).

Such errors in performance are likely to continue for the following reasons:

• many clinical laboratories are unfamiliar with the recombinant DNA techniques used in most new genetic tests;
• the use of very small samples with polymerase chain reaction (PCR) increases the chance of contamination with foreign DNA;
• the large volume of tests increases the chance of unintentional switching of samples;

Martinez v. Long Island Jewish Hillside Center, 512 N.E.2d. 535, New York; 1987.

- the vast majority of results will be in the normal range, a tendency that reduces the vigilance of those performing the test;
- the nature of genetic disorders increases the chance of errors in interpretation;
- tests at the DNA level may not detect all disease-causing or susceptibility-conferring mutations, resulting in false negative results; and
- a positive test result cannot always predict disease severity and, in some instances, may falsely predict the future occurrence of disease particularly in tests for predispositions to multifactorial disorders and disorders of variable expressivity.

This chapter reviews current programs and regulations for assessing the quality of laboratories providing genetic tests, including the interpretation of test results, and current provisions for assessing the safety and effectiveness of genetic test kits and their critical components. For purposes of the committee's definition, genetic tests are those that are used *primarily* for predicting the risk of genetic or gene-influenced disease either in the person being tested or in his or her descendants. Tests that are used primarily for other purposes, but may contribute to diagnosing a genetic disease (e.g., blood smears, certain serum chemistries), would not be covered by this definition.

Because the field of genetic testing is developing very rapidly, few systematic data are available on how many genetic tests are being done, who is doing them, or how well they are being done (Meaney, 1992). Some data are available on newborn screening (Holtzman et al., 1986; Hannon and Adam, 1991; Adam and Hannon, 1992; CORN, 1992). Similarly, few published data on genetic laboratory quality are available (Holtzman et al., 1986; Hommes et al., 1990; Hannon and Adam, 1991; Meaney, 1992). To assess the nature and extent of special laboratory issues in human genetics, therefore, the committee held an expert workshop to review existing voluntary, professional, and governmental regulatory efforts to ensure the quality of genetic laboratory testing (participants are listed in Appendix A of this report). Committee members also met with representatives of the Food and Drug Administration (FDA), the Health Care Financing Administration (HCFA), and the Centers for Disease Control and Prevention (CDC) to learn the agencies' current policies and plans for assessing the safety and effectiveness of genetic tests.

Identifying problems of the quality of genetic tests is complicated because of the ways in which they are provided. A few are sold as kits, primarily to clinical laboratories; these have to undergo scrutiny by the FDA. An increasing number of tests are being marketed as laboratory services by commercial laboratories and a few academic laboratories. Many more are being provided for clinical decision-making purposes by research laboratories in academic medical centers. Although the critical reagents (which usually are not part of FDA-approved kits) used for testing in commercial and research laboratories, and the laboratories themselves, are subject to new federal regulations, many laboratories and investigators are unaware of them. Part of the reason is the federal government's failure to apply current regulations to genetic tests on a systematic and thorough basis. Were it not for the availability of tests through research laboratories, many people at risk for rare diseases could be deprived of an opportunity to use these tests; they are of such limited commercial value that manufacturers of in vitro diagnostics have little interest in them. One regulatory challenge is to ensure quality without diminishing the availability of these tests. The committee is concerned that the regulatory burden not impede further development of tests or the provision of genetic testing services by laboratories that currently provide them.

PROGRAMS AND REGULATIONS FOR ASSESSING THE QUALITY OF LABORATORIES PROVIDING GENETIC TESTS

Assessment of the quality of laboratories providing genetic tests is currently conducted by a few states and by voluntary participation in the proficiency testing programs of private organizations. At present, only 10 states have some form of specific requirements for the licensing of clinical laboratories providing genetic tests (M. Watson, personal communication to Congressman Ted Weiss, 1992). Only New York State has specific legislation and regulations dealing with laboratories providing the full range of genetic tests, including DNA tests.

State Assessments of Laboratories Providing Genetic Tests

New York State began mandatory regulation of genetic testing when it established the first program assessment for cytogenetics laboratories in the United States in 1972, with cytogenetics proficiency testing beginning in 1974 (Willey, 1992). Since 1990, New York has been the only state that has specific mandatory standards and permits for DNA genetics laboratories performing tests on its citizens. It has a list of DNA tests approved for testing, including tests for sickle cell anemia, cystic fibrosis (CF), Duchenne and Becker muscular dystrophy, Tay-Sachs, and the thalassemias (A. Willey, Director, Laboratory of Human Genetics, New York State Department of Health, personal communication, January 1993). To be included on this list of approved DNA tests, the disorders must meet identified criteria (e.g., no form of the disorder that is undetectable because a mutation at another locus is known to exist; the method must identify 90 to 95 percent of cases; reagents and processes must be generally available in the laboratory community—or must be made available; if linkage analysis is required, the markers must be a specified map distance from the disease gene). To be approved to perform DNA tests from this list, the laboratories must demonstrate that they successfully perform the accepted test methodologies. New York developed a special training program for all inspectors who survey laboratories that perform genetic testing. New York has also developed standards for proficiency testing for

BOX 3-1 Congressional Oversight Hearing

To focus attention on the special issues in genetic laboratory testing, congressional hearings were held in July 1992 to highlight unresolved laboratory issues in human genetics (House Subcommittee on Human Resources and Intergovernmental Relations, 1992). The hearing included testimony from two patients who had had significant problems with genetic testing. One woman experienced long delays (more than seven months), high cost, and problems with her referring physician—all without receiving any results from the first physician and laboratory, when she sought presymptomatic diagnosis for Huntington disease. A pregnant woman testified about the anxiety caused by two positive reports from maternal serum alpha-fetoprotein (MSAFP) screening tests indicating a high risk for Down syndrome; only weeks later was it determined by amniocentesis that the fetus she carried did not have Down syndrome (Hoyt, 1992). Anxiety of this type is observed frequently while women are awaiting MSAFP results but usually abates when a negative result is reported (Holtzman et al., 1991).

The expert witnesses each presented cases of laboratory problems in various kinds of genetic diagnosis, testing, and screening. In one prominent medical center, the coordinator of the prenatal alpha-fetoprotein screening laboratory identified four significant problems over a two-month period, three involving commercial laboratories that provide MSAFP, and one problem of interpretation by a physician (Holtzman, 1992):

1. In one case, a laboratory reporting an abnormally low MSAFP result, failed to recognize that the woman's age of 36 (considered "advanced maternal age" for purposes of prenatal diagnosis) warranted proceeding directly to a definitive cytogenetic test. Waiting for the results of the tests it recommended could have delayed diagnosis and reduced the woman's options had the confirmatory test been positive.

2. In a second case, the laboratory director was uncertain whether the result had been adjusted for the patient's race and weight, key factors in interpreting test results.

3. In a third case, there was not enough information supplied on the request form to determine that the woman was further into her pregnancy than thought; the laboratory reported that her result was abnormal when, in fact, it was normal for her true stage of pregnancy.

4. In interpreting a woman's results, her physician correctly noted that she was not at increased risk for having a child with Down syndrome, but he failed to observe that she had an elevated MSAFP level and was, therefore, at increased risk for having a child with a neural tube defect.

NOTE: Witnesses at the July 23, 1992, hearing included three panels: (1) Heidi Hoyt, Washington, D.C., and "Kim" of Illinois (both patients reporting their experiences with genetic testing); (2) specialized genetics personnel: Elizabeth Gettig, M.S., Director of Genetic Counseling, West Penn Hospital, Pittsburgh, Pa.; Paul Billings, M.D., Chief, Division of Genetic Medicine, California Pacific Medical Center, Assistant Clinical Professor of Medicine, University of California, San Francisco, Calif.; Neil A. Holtzman, Professor of Pediatrics, Johns Hopkins School of Medicine, Baltimore, Md.; Patricia Murphy, Ph.D., Genica Pharmaceutical Corporation, Worcester, Mass.; and (3) representatives of U.S. Department of Health and Human Services agencies: William Toby, Acting Administrator of the Health Care Financing Administration (HCFA); Barbara Gagle, Acting Director, Health Standards and Quality Bureau, HCFA; Edward Baker, M.D., Director, Public Health Practice Program Office, Centers for Disease Control; Alan Anderson, M.D., Acting Director, Center for Devices and Radiological Health, Food and Drug Administration.

DNA tests, but these standards have not yet been implemented (Murphy, 1992a). The reach of the New York State program extends beyond the geographic borders of the state, since any laboratory wishing to perform a genetic test on a citizen of New York must be certified just as if it were located in New York; thus, most large commercial genetic testing laboratories who accept specimens from around the United States are licensed to meet New York DNA laboratory standards. Currently, no other state has developed as rigorous a program for the quality control of genetic testing as New York.

The California Department of Health Services contracts with private laboratories to provide newborn screening and maternal serum alpha-fetoprotein (MSAFP) testing. As part of the process it assesses the quality of the laboratories with whom it contracts. Since 1980, California has limited newborn screening to eight state-monitored laboratories, with centralized computer data collection, quality control, blind proficiency testing, and case follow-up. Fees for newborn screening are collected from the birth hospital or birth attendant. California also has centralized laboratory testing, quality control, and blind proficiency testing for its MSAFP screening program, which must be offered to every pregnant woman in California. California has developed draft regulations on DNA, cytogenetics, and microbiological testing, and for prenatal diagnosis centers and clinical centers; these draft regulations are awaiting public comment and public hearing (Cunningham, 1992).

Maryland has regulations requiring genetic testing and screening laboratories to demonstrate "continuing satisfactory performance" in external proficiency testing programs where they exist. The only approved laboratory for newborn screening in Maryland is the state laboratory, which participates in the U.S. Centers for Disease Control proficiency testing program for newborn screening (see below). Fourteen laboratories (including the state laboratory) are approved for MSAFP screening. Maryland regulations require laboratories doing Tay-Sachs testing to participate successfully in the proficiency testing program of the International Tay-Sachs Disease Quality Control Reference Standards and Data Collection Center (M. Kaback, personal communication, November 1992).

New Jersey requires its laboratories to comply with the New York system for genetic tests, and it now also recognizes College of American Pathology (CAP) proficiency testing for cytogenetics. Florida licenses cytogenetics laboratories using CAP guidelines and proficiency testing, but its legislation is now expiring. Iowa requires that MSAFP testing be done centrally in the state laboratory at the University of Iowa.

In addition, states in the Pacific Northwest Region (PacNoRGG) of the Council of Regional Networks for Genetic Services (CORN), including Washington, Oregon, Idaho, and Alaska, have adopted PacNoRGG proficiency testing standards as a condition for state laboratory license as a cytogenetics laboratory. The PacNoRGG cytogenetics proficiency test involves the provision of blind samples and requires the interpretation of clinical information on individuals and families.

Each round of proficiency testing gets more difficult as the proficiency of the participating laboratories improves.

Voluntary Quality Assurance and Proficiency Testing in Genetics

The Council of Regional Networks of Genetic Services, the College of American Pathologists, the Centers for Disease Control and Prevention, and several other organizations have developed specific genetic tests or tests for specific disorders. These include maternal serum alpha-fetoprotein, Tay-Sachs disease, and Huntington disease, for which the organizations have established voluntary proficiency tests (see Box 3-2). Other organizations interested in the quality of genetic tests include the Organization for Clinical Laboratory Genetics, the American Society for Histocompatibility and Immunogenetics, the American Association of Blood Banks, the Technical Working Group on DNA Analysis Methods (TWGDAM), the National Reference System for the Clinical Laboratory, the National Committee for Clinical Laboratory Standards (NCCLS), and the new American College of Medical Genetics (ACMG). Many of the voluntary quality assurance programs grew from the efforts of the American Society of Human Genetics (ASHG) (Punnett, 1992).

CORN was established in 1985 as a coordinating body for state genetic services programs organized in 10 regions. CORN is funded by the Genetic Services Program of the Maternal and Child Health Program, Health Resources and Services Administration (HRSA), U.S. Department of Health and Human Services (DHHS). Laboratory quality assurance quickly became and remains a high priority for CORN. CORN has a Quality Assurance Committee (for laboratory services), as well as other committees on quality assurance and proficiency testing, and education. CORN's national proficiency testing programs include alpha-fetoprotein, biochemical genetics, hemoglobinopathies and newborn screening, and most recently, DNA-based tests.

The College of American Pathologists developed guidelines, criteria, and methods for quality control and standards for clinical laboratories. CAP played a key role in the implementation of the Clinical Laboratory Improvement Act of 1967 (see below) when its quality assurance and proficiency testing standards and activities were recognized ("deemed") by the Secretary of Health and Human Services to fulfill the requirements of the law. Since 1967, CAP has worked to maintain itself and M.D.-pathologists as the appropriate professional group to judge the quality of clinical laboratories. CAP has voluntary proficiency testing programs for cytogenetics and MSAFP screening that are recognized by some states. With input from ASHG, CAP has spent two years developing guidelines for what it calls "molecular pathology." The ASHG role in setting standards for laboratory genetics will be assumed by the ACMG in 1993. ACMG laboratory standards for genetics are now under final revision and will be very important in quality assurance in genetic testing.

BOX 3-2   Voluntary Quality Assurance and Proficiency Testing Programs

New England Regional Genetics Group and the Foundation for Blood Research
The New England Regional Genetics Group (NERGG) sponsored the first proficiency testing program for MSAFP screening in pregnant women. Since 1983, the Foundation for Blood Research (FBR) in Maine has served as the national testing and training resource for the use of MSAFP. The foundation provides quality control and proficiency training programs that include (1) bimonthly quality assessment; (2) assessment of the ability of laboratories to measure MSAFP levels reliably; (3) assessment of the laboratories' ability to interpret the AFP result, adjust for critical variables, and make screening recommendations to referring laboratories; (4) assessment of the quality of commercial test kits as well as individual laboratory performance; and (5) telephone consultation on laboratory problems. In 1986, the College of American Pathologists also began to offer proficiency testing for MSAFP; since 1988, FBR and CAP have offered such proficiency testing jointly. In addition, FBR now offers proficiency testing for so-called triple-marker screening for Down syndrome; and this program is also offered jointly with CAP (Haddow and McKnight, 1992).

National Voluntary Biochemical Genetics Laboratory
Proficiency Testing Program
This voluntary program was established in 1985 by Frits Hommes and the Southeastern Region Genetics Group (SERGG) to provide quality standards and proficiency testing for biochemical genetic tests. It includes criteria for assessing adequate performance in (1) measuring inborn errors of metabolism of amino acids, organic acids, glycosaminoglycans, and oligosaccharides, as well as the assay of galactose-1-phosphate; (2) reporting analytical results; and (3) interpreting those results. A supervisory committee evaluates the results. Laboratories with unsatisfactory results are notified and offered a repeat test. Summary results of all participating laboratories are distributed after the supervisory committee has evaluated all the tests, including the repeat tests. Testing is performed twice a year, in February and September. Sixteen rounds of testing have been completed, with evidence of improved performance (Hommes, 1992).

International Tay-Sachs Disease Quality Control Reference Standards
and Data Collection Center
A voluntary, international laboratory quality assurance and proficiency testing program for Tay-Sachs disease has existed since 1973 (Kaback et al., 1977). Laboratories that make an error on the first round of proficiency testing on 25 unknown samples are not accredited but have an opportunity to be retested with 10 additional samples. If the laboratory achieves 100 percent accuracy in the second round, it can still be accredited; if there is an error on the second round, the laboratory is not accredited.

The list of accredited laboratories is widely disseminated to Jewish organizations by the National Tay-Sachs and Allied Diseases Association, Inc. Although the only leverage exerted is not to publish the names of laboratories that fail its proficiency programs, the system has effectively closed some laboratories, and has helped many others to improve their methodologies and quality in Tay-Sachs testing. The majority of laboratories doing Tay-Sachs identification have participated in this voluntary program, but new private laboratories can be started without meeting the requirements of this quality control program.

Huntington Disease Pilot Projects
The Huntington disease pilot projects also organized a voluntary laboratory quality assurance program. Early in the development of presymptomatic testing for Huntington disease, standards were developed for the original pilot studies to ensure the quality of the testing program, including rigorous laboratory standards.

Once funding for the pilots ceased, and other centers and laboratories began presymptomatic testing for Huntington disease, it was no longer possible to enforce the standards developed for the original pilot studies. Since this quality assurance program is voluntary, and involved only the laboratories participating in the Huntington pilot projects, it does not reach all laboratories performing marker analysis and identification of Huntington disease.

One recent study attempted to determine the accuracy of interpretation of complex linkage analysis for Huntington disease (Michael Conneally, personal communication, February, 1992). Selected family genetic linkage patterns (often called family "pedigrees") were distributed to a group of laboratories already performing complex linkage analysis for Huntington disease. Problems were found in the interpretation of inheritance patterns for Huntington disease by the responding laboratories.

Presymptomatic testing for Huntington disease—like many late-onset disorders—is extremely complex. The significance of the findings is so great that the standard for testing can tolerate no errors. Thus, prospects for the expansion of testing for Huntington disease without enforceable standards raise concerns about the quality of future testing for this disorder. The recent clarification of the basic mechanism of Huntington disease (Collaborative Research Group, 1993) now provides the possibility of direct DNA testing. Laboratory standards will be needed to ensure the quality of this new, more accurate testing method.

Although the Centers for Disease Control and Prevention attempted to establish its own cytogenetics proficiency testing program, it never progressed beyond a pilot program (Murphy, 1992a). CDC does run a voluntary proficiency testing program for newborn screening tests discussed below.

Costs, Benefits, and Limitations of State and Voluntary Quality Assurance Programs

In most state-run and voluntary programs, most of the costs of the quality control programs are paid by the participating laboratories. These costs could deter a research laboratory, or other small laboratory without cash reserves, from participating in the program. The costs of participation could be passed on to the consumer through higher laboratory prices, although the increases would not be a very large percentage of the current prices of most genetic tests. California now charges $40 for newborn screening and $55 for the MSAFP screening test, both of which include the cost of quality control and proficiency testing.

Rigorous state licensing provides protection to the citizens of that state, but continued reliance on the states will not afford equal protection to citizens of all states. Separate programs in each state could result in duplication of effort or in competing and, in some instances, conflicting laboratory standards. Many diagnostic laboratories do not now participate in voluntary quality assurance and proficiency testing in genetics. One incentive for such participation would be to publish the results of voluntary quality evaluations by laboratory name, as is now done by the National Tay-Sachs Disease and Allied Disorders Association, Inc., which publishes results of the quality assessment conducted by the International Tay-Sachs Disease Quality Control Reference Standards and Data Collection Center.

Federal Regulation of Clinical Laboratories

History

The Clinical Laboratory Improvement Act of 1967 (CLIA67) established federal control of laboratories providing more than 100 tests per year in interstate commerce for a profit. Only about 12,000 laboratories reimbursed by Medicare and Medicaid were covered. CLIA67 was originally administered by CDC, but authority was transferred to the Health Care Finance Administration in 1978. For laboratories under its purview, CLIA67 required the establishment of standards for laboratory directors and other laboratory personnel (CRS, 1990). The College of American Pathologists was recognized to set laboratory and personnel standards, and to develop a laboratory inspection system nationwide.

The Clinical Laboratory Improvement Amendments of 1988 (CLIA88) were enacted in response to rising concern over media reports of serious errors and variability in laboratory results, and inadequate training and supervision of personnel performing clinical laboratory tests. In particular, so-called Pap mills were found to have serious deficiencies in their cytology analysis of Papanicolaou tests, intended to detect cervical cancer. Public concern had also intensified about the quality of the increasing amount of unregulated laboratory services provided in physicians' office laboratories and other laboratories reimbursed by Medicare and Medicaid.

Laboratories Covered by CLIA88

With few exceptions, laboratories performing an "examination of materials derived from the human body for the purpose of providing information for the diagnosis, prevention, or treatment of any disease or impairment of, or the assessment of the health of, human beings" must obtain certification from HCFA under CLIA88 (Federal Register, 1992a). The exceptions are laboratories performing tests only for forensic purposes, research laboratories that do not report patient-specific results for the purposes defined above, and laboratories of federal agencies to the extent excepted by the Secretary of Health and Human Services (Federal Register, 1992a). How a laboratory derives its revenues, or even whether it charges for tests, is no longer a determinant of coverage under CLIA88. Thus, any laboratory that provided a genetic test result on which a clinical decision was based is subject to regulation.

More than 200,000 laboratories are estimated to be covered by CLIA88, over 100,000 of them in physicians' offices. Compliance with CLIA88, including CLIA certification is required for Medicare reimbursement of laboratory services, and many other third-party payers use Medicare certification as one criterion for reimbursement. However, HCFA may not know about laboratories that do not obtain certificates unless there is a complaint.

CLIA88 Regulations

In implementing CLIA88 the government sets standards for laboratories according to whether the tests they perform are of "moderate" or "high" complexity. The distinction between moderate and high complexity depends on a number of factors including knowledge needed to perform the test, characteristics of operational steps, judgment required, and interpretation of results. Thus far, CDC has classified 10,000 tests, approximately 25 percent as high complexity and 75 percent as moderate complexity (as of January 1993).

Laboratories performing tests of moderate or high complexity must conform to general quality control standards as well as those of the "specialty" under which the tests they perform are classified. (Some specialties are microbiology, chemistry, pathology, and hematology.) Laboratories must participate in proficiency testing programs for each specialty in which they perform tests and for which proficiency programs have been established. By 1995, a laboratory that fails a proficiency test two consecutive times or two out of three times will be subject to sanctions and may not continue to perform that test under its CLIA certificate. Nor will it be eligible for Medicare reimbursement for that test (CDC, 1992). HCFA had approved 12 of the 19 proficiency testing programs that had applied as of December 1992. None of these is in genetics (see below).

The absence of a complexity rating for a test does not exempt a laboratory performing only unrated tests from quality control. A laboratory test whose complexity has not been categorized "is considered to be a test of high complexity until PHS (Public Health Service), upon request, reviews the matter and notifies the applicant of its decision" (Federal Register, 1992b). In the meantime, "the laboratory must have a system for verifying the accuracy and reliability of its test results at least twice a year" (Federal Register, 1992c). Moreover, all laboratories filing a certificate of registration with HCFA will be inspected every two years, and the laboratory's quality control and internal proficiency test system will be assessed. HCFA has a training program for laboratory inspectors—many of whom are sent by states—provided by the Department of Laboratory Medicine of the Johns Hopkins University School of Medicine. HCFA may soon deem other organizations (CAP, Joint Committee on Accreditation of Health Organizations, specific states) as capable of conducting its surveys and accrediting laboratories. State accreditation can supplant HCFA accreditation when a state's program is deemed equivalent or more stringent than the federal program.

Quality control under CLIA88 is funded by fees charged to laboratories. Compliance fees vary substantially from hundreds to thousands of dollars depending on how many different types of tests the laboratory performs, their complexity, and the volume of testing.

Genetic Tests Under CLIA88

Very few genetic tests are on the list of tests whose complexity has been defined under CLIA88. Those that are listed have been classified as of moderate complexity including sweat chloride for CF, creatine kinase, and alpha-fetoprotein (AFP) for tumor marker (Federal Register, 1992d). A test subspecialty called "clinical cytogenetics" has been established, but there is no other genetic test subspecialty under CLIA88. Moreover, no proficiency testing for cytogenetic laboratories is required, although well-established programs (e.g., New York State and CAP) have been operating for years. Proficiency tests are not required for any other genetic tests, either.

Few laboratories performing genetic tests as their sole or principal activity are yet complying with the CLIA88 regulations. Based on the committee's workshops and other information, it appears that few genetics laboratories have applied for certification from HCFA even though they provide genetic test information for clinical use. Committee staff also surveyed the directors of 12 genetics laboratories in academic centers to ask if their laboratory had applied for certification, and only 1 laboratory indicated that it had.

Research Laboratories and Tests for Rare Disorders

Research laboratories are covered under CLIA88 if they also provide tests on which clinical decisions are based. Some of these laboratories provide genetic tests as clinical services that are not directly related to the research they perform, and they may have limited expertise in performing or interpreting such tests. In many large academic hospitals, the central laboratory is not even aware of all the laboratories that provide services. This situation could be rectified either by having these laboratories obtain their own certificates from HCFA or by having them (and the tests they perform) listed under the central laboratory's certificate. Although this would bring them under the purview of HCFA inspectors, it might not ensure quality. It is doubtful that external proficiency tests could be provided economically or efficiently for tests performed only occasionally by many laboratories or that occasional performance of a test can ensure high quality.

To ensure high quality in tests for rare disorders that are seldom performed, the genetics community, under CORN and the American College of Medical Genetics, could take the lead in fostering centralization of these tests. Once centralization occurs and the volume of specific tests performed by the central laboratory increases, a stronger argument can be made that external proficiency testing is economical and efficient. With the establishment of central laboratories, HCFA could consider setting a volume-of-test requirement necessary to ensure quality (as FDA has proposed for MSAFP testing). Laboratories not meeting that requirement would not pass inspection for that particular test. If challenged in court, however, such an arrangement might be considered a restraint of trade. Commercial laboratories, which are often subsidiaries of biotechnology companies, are expanding their range of services and contracting with hospitals, including some academic centers, to take over genetic testing functions.

Interpretation of Laboratory Test Results

For the reasons given earlier in this chapter, the misinterpretation of test results is more likely in genetic tests than in many other areas of clinical testing, and misinterpretation may have more serious consequences particularly in fetal diagnosis. The need for adequate interpretation is even greater when the health care providers ordering tests (1) are not expert in interpreting probabilistic clinical data (Holtzman, 1991); (2) are not expert in genetics; and (3) may not be aware of the implications of both positive and negative test results in genetics. As discussed further in Chapter 6, an increasing proportion of genetic tests will be ordered by primary care physicians, many of whom have limited knowledge of genetics (Hoffman, 1991; Holtzman et al., 1991; Hofman et al., 1993). Special concerns about interpretation also arise when tests may be provided by employers as part of fitness programs or by other organizations not skilled in genetics.

Interpretation can be very complex and can depend on the results of other family members. One way of ensuring that physicians who order tests understand the implications and limitations of results is to require that the laboratory performing the test provide adequate interpretation of the result in its report (Hommes, 1992), although all genetic testing laboratories may not be prepared to provide this service. With few exceptions the interpretation of a positive genetic test result should include the chance of future disease or the chance of having an affected child. In the latter case, the interpretation should note whether the chance is dependent on the carrier status of the mate of the person tested. If misattributed paternity might alter the interpretation, this should also be disclosed. The interpretation of test results should also indicate any confirmatory tests that are available and whether repeat or other follow-up testing is recommended. It might summarize the possible interventions. Interpretation of a negative test result should include the revised estimate of the chance of occurrence and make clear that the test result pertains only to a specific disorder, and within that disorder only to disease-causing mutations detectable by the test, which may not include all such mutations.

No matter how extensive or clear the laboratory's written interpretation, many individuals and couples with positive test results will benefit from genetic counseling as well. Some laboratories employ, or are affiliated with, genetic counselors or other personnel trained in genetics who can discuss test interpretation with referring physicians.

ENSURING THE SAFETY AND EFFECTIVENESS OF NEW GENETIC TESTS

FDA regulates medical devices under the Medical Devices Act of 1976 and the Safe Medical Device Amendments of 1990. This legislation gives FDA the authority to regulate an "in vitro reagent, or any other similar or related article, including any component, part or accessory, which is: intended for use in the diagnosis of disease or other conditions in man" (21 CFR 201(h)). Through classification of such "devices," FDA implements the legislation's intent to provide a "level of regulation necessary to afford reasonable assurance of safety and effectiveness of the device" (Tsakeris and Yoder, 1992, p. 2). Safety cannot be considered entirely separately from effectiveness. If a test cannot properly distinguish those at high risk of genetic disease from those at low risk, individuals who are mislabeled will suffer harm. False negatives will not be treated, while false positives may suffer from both unnecessary intervention and anxiety.

Only a small proportion of genetic tests in widespread use have been reviewed by FDA; these include tests for hypothyroidism, phenylketonuria (PKU), and MSAFP tests. The technologies used for the detection of most disease-related genotypes have not been submitted to FDA; these include biochemical reagents and DNA probes used in tests for CF, Huntington disease, muscular dystrophy, fragile X syndrome, and other disorders.

Premarket Approval of Medical Devices

Before a medical device can be legally marketed for in vitro diagnostic use, its sponsor (manufacturer, university, or individual scientist) must obtain premarket approval (PMA) or clearance (Tsakeris and Yoder, 1992). On receiving premarket notification from a sponsor, FDA will determine whether the device is "substantially equivalent" to a legally marketed "predicate" device. "Substantial equivalence means the new device must have the same intended use as the predicate device, the same technological characteristics (or, if different,) strong comparability of intended use and performance characteristics, and [not raise] new questions of safety and effectiveness" (Tsakeris and Yoder, 1992, p. 3). For the FDA to make a determination of substantial equivalence, the manufacturer has to demonstrate equivalent performance characteristics (as good as other legally marketed devices). If so, FDA will give the device either Class I or II designation, depending on the class of the predicate device. The safety and efficacy of Class I devices can be reasonably ensured if the manufacturer adheres to general controls that include good manufacturing practices in their production. Class II devices must meet not only general controls, but also special controls, in order to reasonably ensure safety and efficacy.

If FDA fails to find the device substantially equivalent, it will require full premarket approval, designating it a Class III device. This requires the manufacturer to present evidence of the device's safety and effectiveness. Genetic tests and devices placed in Class III include MSAFP kits (MSAFP is not approved by the FDA for use as a screening test for Down syndrome, although it is widely used for that purpose) and kits for the Philadelphia chromosome, tumor markers, and gene rearrangements. Class II tests include the sweat chloride test for CF, creatine kinase test for Duchenne muscular dystrophy, phenylalanine test for PKU, tests for coagulation defects (including detection of carriers of coagulation defects), and tests for sickle cell trait or disease. The copper test for Wilson disease is Class I (Tsakeris and Yoder, 1992).

The committee reviewed FDA's current definition of "substantial equivalence." Although the current definition (Tsakeris and Yoder, 1992) is reassuringly comprehensive, the FDA could interpret substantial equivalence too broadly, permitting a manufacturer to avoid the premarket approval process by claiming, for instance, that a DNA test marketed to detect sickle cell carriers was substantially equivalent to electrophoretic tests already on the market. Once marketed to detect carriers, the DNA test, unlike the electrophoretic test, could also be used for prenatal diagnosis. This would constitute an unapproved or "off-label" use of the device. Similarly, a DNA-based test for some CF mutations might be approved for the diagnosis of CF on the basis of substantial equivalence to the sweat chloride test, although only the DNA test could be used for carrier detection or prenatal diagnosis.

Despite the FDA's current definition of substantial equivalence, off-label use once a test is legally marketed remains an area of concern. Off-label use often goes undetected or unreported, although if manufacturers are aware of off-label use of a device, they must either withhold the product from the user (laboratory) or file a premarket notification of the new use. To prevent the problem of off-label use of genetic tests, FDA should require the manufacturer to indicate both intended and potential uses (which would include carrier screening, prenatal diagnosis, or presymptomatic testing, etc.). Increasing FDA's capability for postmarket surveillance would also reduce off-label use.

Collection of Data for Test Validation

The general principle that premarket data on test validity should be collected on subjects drawn from the same population as the intended targets of the test, after it is marketed, is often difficult to adhere to in the case of genetic tests. An underlying problem is that no confirmatory ("gold standard") test will be available. This will be the case for many direct tests that search for underlying disease-causing mutations. Only the appearance of the disease itself provides confirmation. With tests for rare diseases and diseases with a long time lag between the time of the test and the appearance of disease, it may not be feasible to determine sensitivity on subjects of the type in whom the test is intended to be used (e.g., asymptomatic, healthy subjects). Subjects with overt disease can be used to test sensitivity, and nonaffected subjects beyond the age at which the disease usually becomes manifest can be used to assess specificity. Because the age of such subjects will often be considerably older than those in whom such tests can be of value, the findings of such "shortcuts" may not be accurate predictors of sensitivity and specificity under conditions of intended use. Long-term follow-up is, therefore, a better means of assessing the validity of such tests. The assessment of the validity of tests for genetic predispositions will also require long, careful follow-up.

With tests intended for prenatal diagnosis in which only the fetal test result indicates the presence or absence of disease (i.e., there is no independent test or histopathological evidence to confirm the finding), validation will depend on test results in living subjects. In addition, when the parents elect to continue the pregnancy after a positive prenatal diagnostic test, the infant must be followed to determine whether the disease appears. Infants delivered after a prenatal diagnostic test was negative should also be followed, with a similar objective.

For tests for which a new treatment is being assessed in conjunction with test validation, a plan to withhold treatment from some subjects with positive test results is needed (e.g., randomized controlled trials). Otherwise it will be impossible to distinguish a person with a false positive result, who would never get sick, from a true positive in which the treatment was efficacious. When the false positive rate of a test is unknown, treating all people with positive results with an effective therapy will make it impossible to determine the specificity of the test unless the response to the therapy can distinguish true from false positives.

Humanitarian Exemptions

The Safe Medical Device Amendments of 1990 contains a "humanitarian device exemption" for conditions affecting less than 4,000 individuals in the United States. The safety of medical devices must be demonstrated prior to premarket approval, but demonstration of effectiveness can be postponed for 18 months. To qualify, no comparable devices to treat or diagnose the condition can be available and the probable benefit to health must outweigh the risk of illness or injury from its use. Such exempted devices may not be sold for more than the cost of research, development, fabrication, and distribution, and may only be used in institutions with local institutional review boards (IRBs), which approve the clinical use of the device and supervise its clinical testing. Proposed regulations were issued for this provision on December 21, 1992 (Federal Register, 1992e).

Although such an approach recognizes the difficulty of establishing the effectiveness of devices that will only be used occasionally (e.g., in diagnosing rare disorders), the 18-month delay will be insufficient to establish the effectiveness of many genetic tests for the reasons already noted. More importantly, manufacturers may be unwilling to go through premarket approval of tests for rare diseases because of their limited marketability. The Orphan Drug Act does not provide the incentives (including exclusivity for patents and tax credits) for development of medical devices that it does for drugs for orphan diseases. It does, however, offer grants for the development of devices, as well as for medical foods for rare diseases; $10 million is allocated for this purpose in fiscal year 1993 for grants of $100,000 to $200,000 per year for a period of two to three years for clinical tests of such products for rare diseases.

Investigational Use of New Devices

The collection of data to support PMA applications—that is, to determine safety and effectiveness—is the responsibility of the sponsor. To obtain these data the sponsor is allowed to use the device (including DNA probes and reagents) only for investigational purposes. Under FDA regulations, the device must be labeled for "investigational use only" and must be used in accord with a protocol (including specified period of study, number of sites, investigators, and patient samples) and must be approved by an IRB. Informed consent of participants in such studies may be required. This would always be the case if the participant was to be notified of the result or if a clinical decision was based on the result. Under "investigational use" exemptions, manufacturing costs can be recovered by charging for the device, but no profit can be made.

Under current FDA rules, an investigational "device and/or its results will not be used for diagnostic purposes without confirmation of the diagnosis by another, medically established diagnostic device or procedure" (R. Johnson, FDA, letter to device manufacturers, October 17, 1991, p. 3), unless an investigational device exemption has been approved by the FDA. The committee notes that, for many genetic tests involving direct determination of disease-causing mutations, the only confirmation that is possible is the clinical appearance of the disease, which may not happen until many years after the test is performed. In reply to the committee's inquiries, FDA wrote that obtaining an "approved Investigational Device Exemption (IDE) may be required for certain genetic products (e.g., *when there is no confirmatory test*) to assure the safe use of the device in collecting data to establish the performance characteristics of the device [emphasis added]" (Tsakeris and Yoder, 1992, p. 12).

Institutional Review Boards and Genetic Tests

The submission of protocols to IRBs for investigations covering such devices may overwhelm some IRBs. At some large academic centers, IRBs are appointing subcommittees to deal with new genetic investigations. Most IRBs will not have experts in genetics or individuals knowledgeable about ethical problems in genetic testing. The National Human Genome Research Center at the University of Iowa has created a unit to advise IRBs and other groups on ethical, legal, and social issues arising in genetics research.

Inappropriate Use of Investigational Devices

At some point in their development, genetic tests emerging from research laboratories in academic medical centers are offered as a clinical service. Research laboratories sometimes perform these tests at their convenience, with delays of months in reporting results (Hoffman, 1991; Klinger, 1992). If no manufacturers are interested in commercializing the tests as in vitro diagnostic devices, the research laboratory continues to provide them as a service. In many instances, academic research laboratories do not comply with investigational-use device requirements of FDA, despite the fact that performance of the test for clinical purposes requires them to do so.

FDA is aware of the problem of the use of medical devices that it has not reviewed for marketing and that are not in compliance with its regulations regarding investigational devices. One example is the use of the MSAFP test (which has FDA approval for detection of increased risk of fetal neural tube defects) for detection of increased risk of Down syndrome in the fetus (for which the test is not approved). FDA has proposed to deal with such problems by compiling an "accommodation list" of such tests that it believes to be essential to clinical care. Manufacturers or other sponsors of the tests on this list would be allowed an additional 30 months to collect data for premarket approval applications. Tests not on the list can no longer be legally provided unless they immediately comply with FDA requirements (FDA, 1992). ACMG has pointed out to FDA that the number of genetic tests in this category is very large and that the elimination of tests that are not listed will cause serious problems to patients with, or at risk for, genetic disorders (M. Watson and M. Cohen, letter to F. Yoder, FDA, August 18, 1992). Because many new genetic tests will be for rare diseases, the collection of adequate data to establish safety and effectiveness will take a long time, probably longer than the 30-month time limit given by FDA for devices on an accommodation list. For tests performed only occasionally, "provisional premarket approval" should be given (see below). Once granted, this will permit laboratories to charge a fair price for the test. This should serve as an incentive to accelerate data collection. Data collection can also be speeded by enabling investigators to collaborate, pooling their data. For very rare diseases, commercial sponsors of such collaboration are unlikely to be forthcoming. Support for collaborative studies will greatly speed the process of making these tests available to the public, and long-term support may be needed to conduct some of these studies.

NEWBORN AND OTHER GENETIC SCREENING PROGRAMS

An estimated 4 million screening blood specimens from heel-sticks of newborns are tested annually in the United States for at least one genetic disorder. Many of these tests are performed in state laboratories; some state laboratories subcontract work to commercial laboratories (Table 3-1). CDC provides the only proficiency testing program for newborn screening in the United States. For 39 state and territorial and 28 private laboratories participating in proficiency testing for newborn screening, CDC absorbs the cost of the testing program.

Participation in the program is voluntary; 115 organizations participate, including manufacturers and international laboratories, 39 state and territorial laboratories, and 28 private laboratories. Data on the quality of programs participating in CDC's voluntary program show substantial error rates, in excess of 5 percent false negatives (Holtzman et al., 1986; Adam and Hannon, 1992). CDC has consulted HCFA concerning approval of the CDC newborn screening proficiency testing program as a provider of proficiency testing under CLIA88; at present, CLIA88 regulations cover only one of the ten newborn screening tests, hypothyroidism (using thyroxine and thyroid stimulating hormone) (B. Adam, CDC, personal communication, January 1993).

Errors in screening for genetic disorders may also be greater than for other tests because it entails the testing of many people who will not have the condition being screened for. This is true in carrier and prenatal as well as newborn testing. When tests of high sensitivity and specificity are used in populations in which the condition being screened is of low prevalence, the predictive value of the result may be low. If, in addition, laboratory error adds substantially to the number of false negatives and false positives, the safety and benefit of screening come into question. This concern is all the more important because unlike many other medical procedures, it is usually not the patient who initiates the process but the health care provider or the state (in the case of newborn screening). This increases the possibility that the person being tested could misunderstand the objectives of testing and misinterpret the results. Errors in screening may also be greater than in other medical tests because many specimens are handled simultaneously and may be analyzed at a site far removed from where they were obtained. Thus the entire screening process, from informing the patient (or parent) through final disposition (giving the patient or parent the result or placing it on the patient's record), should be subject to quality control.

TABLE 3-1 Number and Types of Laboratories Providing Newborn Screening Tests

State	No. of Laboratories Operated by State	States Using Regional Laboratories	Private Laboratories Under State Regulations	Private Laboratories Without State Regulations	Total No. of Laboratories Doing Testing
Alabama	1				1
Alaska		Contracts with Oregon			0
Arizona		Contracts with Colorado			0
Arkansas	1				1
California	1[a]				8[a]
Colorado	1				1
Connecticut		Contracts with New York			0
Delaware		Contracts with Maryland			0
District of Columbia			1		1
Florida	1				1
Georgia	1				1
Hawaii			5		5
Idaho		Contracts with Oregon			0
Illinois	1				1
Indiana	1		3		3
Iowa	1				1
Kansas	1				1
Kentucky	1		3		4
Louisiana	1			3	4[b]
Maine		Contracts with Massachusetts			0
Maryland	1				1
Massachusetts	1				1[c]
Michigan	1				1
Minnesota	1				1
Mississippi		Contracts with Tennessee			0
Missouri	1				1
Montana	1				1

State						Total
Nebraska	1				16	17[d]
Nevada		Contracts with Oregon				0
New Hampshire		Contracts with Massachusetts				0
New Jersey	1					1
New Mexico	1					1
New York	1					1
North Carolina	1					1
North Dakota	1					1
Ohio	1					1
Oklahoma	1					1
Oregon	1					1
Pennsylvania	1[e]					3
Rhode Island	1[f]	Contracts with Massachusetts	1			1
South Carolina	1					1
South Dakota			8			8
Tennessee	1					1
Texas	1					1
Utah	1					1
Vermont		Contracts with Massachusetts				0
Virginia	1					1
Washington	1					1
West Virginia		Contracts with S. Carolina				0
Wisconsin	1					1
Wyoming		Contracts with Colorado				0
Puerto Rico	1					1
TOTAL	36	13	21	20	16	84

[a] Eight private laboratories under contract to California.
[b] 95% Central operated laboratory usage.
[c] One laboratory does tests for and provides services to other New England states.
[d] Plus some out of state laboratories.
[e] State laboratory does confirmatory and Q/A tests.
[f] Rhode Island state laboratory does some phenylketonuria tests.

SOURCE: CORN, 1992.

The regulation of laboratories under CLIA88 can only ensure that performance of the tests is as good as the intrinsic validity of the test. It does not address the inherent safety and effectiveness of the screening tests themselves. None of the current newborn screening tests has gone through the FDA's full premarket approval process. Tests for PKU and congenital hypothyroidism (for which all 50 states screen), sickle cell anemia (for which 42 states screen and 11 other states have limited screening or pilot studies), and galactosemia (for which 39 states screen) have been classified as Class II by FDA. It seems probable that the FDA has not even been notified of many of the "in vitro diagnostic devices" used in state laboratories for screening because they are not marketed outside that laboratory. It is also doubtful that in developing these devices, manufacturers (companies or individuals) have followed FDA requirements for investigational device exemption and use. Recently, mandatory newborn screening for CF has been undertaken in Colorado and Wyoming (Hammond et al., 1991). As far as the committee could determine, the immunoreactive trypsin assay used for CF screening by these states has not been submitted to FDA for premarket review for use in CF screening. An interesting policy dilemma arises if the organization performing the pilot study (e.g., a state laboratory) has no plans to market the test. It would then have no need to apply to FDA for premarket approval and could continue to handle the device as investigational even after screening becomes routine.

FINDINGS AND RECOMMENDATIONS

Ensuring the Quality of Laboratories

The safety and effectiveness of genetic tests must be established before these tests are used routinely and, once that comes to pass, great care must be taken in performance of the tests and interpretation of the results. Laboratory quality control falls into three areas:

• *The training and experience of the laboratory personnel:* **The nature of genetic tests and the implications of their interpretation suggest the need for special requirements for supervisory personnel (laboratory directors and technical supervisors) in laboratories involved in genetic testing.**

• *The structure and function of the laboratory itself:* **This requires inspectors with special training in assessing such laboratories.**

• *Proficiency testing:* **The most rigorous type should be conducted whenever possible, that is, external, blind proficiency testing in which an outside agency sends specimens to the laboratory under a fictitious patient's name.** The laboratory has no way of knowing that the specimen is for assessing laboratory quality. Other types of proficiency testing involve the sending of coded samples from a central source. **Proficiency testing should extend to all genetic laboratory tests and to the interpretation provided by the laboratory to referring physicians.**

Voluntary quality control programs have helped to establish criteria and standards for genetics laboratories and laboratory personnel. **The committee finds the current state of voluntary laboratory quality control programs in human genetics to be beneficial, but generally inadequate to address the special issues posed by genetic testing, because these programs lack essential enforcement authority.** The impact of these voluntary programs should be strengthened by the publication of the names of laboratories that have satisfied the proficiency and other requirements. Before names are withheld from a published list of "quality" laboratories, any laboratory not satisfying these requirements should be given an opportunity to rectify its deficiencies.

The clinical implications of commonly performed prenatal tests, particularly the abortion of presumably affected fetuses, warrant that laboratories performing them participate in proficiency testing programs.

The performance standard for genetic testing should be as *close to* **zero error as possible.** Laboratories with any error in proficiency testing should be placed on probation, with proficiency testing repeated using blinded methods. Unless the laboratory can attain the required standard in performing and interpreting any genetic test, its certification to perform that test should be removed.

The existing CLIA88 regulations could ensure the quality of genetic laboratory testing *were they to be fully implemented and applied to genetic testing.* Action by DHHS would help to ensure the quality of the most frequently performed genetic tests by (1) establishing genetics as a subspecialty under the CLIA88 regulations; (2) rating specific genetic tests for complexity; and (3) requiring proficiency testing for genetic tests.

The first step would be to require *all* laboratories providing any genetic test to obtain a certificate from HCFA. Next, would be development of a system for verifying the accuracy and reliability of the tests they perform. Third, laboratories performing genetic tests would be subject to inspection every two years. To make this approach meaningful, the laboratory inspectors would have to be well versed in the unique aspects of genetic tests, including the interpretation included in the report of results. A specific training unit on genetic testing should be included in HCFA's educational training program for inspectors, and the same training should be required of inspectors in agencies deemed by HCFA capable of performing inspections. In addition to these steps, HCFA could determine that existing proficiency programs for genetic tests satisfy its standards; HCFA could deem these proficiency testing programs to be required by laboratories providing those tests until such time as other programs are developed (see previous section on voluntary programs and Box 3-2 in this chapter). A laboratory that failed proficiency testing in a "deemed" program would be subject to HCFA sanctions even if that program was voluntary and did not itself impose sanctions.

It is doubtful that adequate quality control can be ensured with voluntary proficiency testing. This holds for newborn and other types of screening as well. **As with any genetic testing, participation in proficiency testing programs** should be required of laboratories providing newborn screening tests. This could be accomplished by designating genetic screening tests as moderate or high complexity under CLIA88. HCFA should examine the proficiency testing programs for genetic screening tests described earlier in this chapter and, if they meet its criteria, deem them acceptable.

The committee recommends that HCFA create a new specialty of clinical genetics into which it can incorporate the existing subspecialty of clinical cytogenetics, and also create new subspecialties of biochemical and molecular genetics. MSAFP testing and other methods of prenatal testing for birth defects should be incorporated into one of these three subspecialties. Most genetic tests should be classified as high complexity under CLIA88, primarily to ensure that supervisory personnel have adequate training in genetics. Although genetic tests might someday be simple enough to be feasible for home use, the difficulties of interpreting results would still render them of high complexity.

Within its existing authorities, HCFA can take steps to enhance the quality of tests for rare disorders, for which specific requirements may never be established. According to a HCFA representative, requirements for proficiency testing are unlikely to be established for low-volume tests unless their clinical or public health implications are high (J. Yost, HCFA, personal communication, January 1992). The establishment of such requirements could be costly both to HCFA and to laboratories that must participate.

The committee strongly recommends that the genetics community, under the leadership of its professional societies, designate a small number of laboratories as centralized facilities for tests for rare disorders. These organizations should establish and publicize a register of the tests performed by these central laboratories and encourage referral of specimens to them. The register should be easily accessible to a wide range of health care providers. It could also be included in the data bases of the National Library of Medicine. An external proficiency testing program should be established for the central laboratories. The genetics community should also study the possibility of setting a minimum volume of a genetic test that a laboratory must perform annually in order to obtain certification for that test and ensure the quality of test performance. With its informatics and data base capabilities, the National Library of Medicine should maintain a data base of centralized laboratories performing tests for rare disorders, genetic counseling centers, and support groups, which should be available to laboratories and providers at no charge.

HCFA and CDC should give high priority to requiring established proficiency programs for genetic tests. The New York State program can be considered a model for many genetic tests, although high priority should also be extended to setting specific requirements for other frequently performed prenatal tests. HCFA should incorporate standards and procedures for assessing genetic tests in its training programs for current and new laboratory inspectors.

Laboratories in academic health centers and elsewhere that conduct research, but that also perform genetic tests as a service (providing the results to referring laboratories or physicians, or directly to patients), should be subject to the same criteria, standards, and regulation as commercial genetic testing laboratories since they fall under the purview of CLIA88. The committee recommends that HCFA inform all hospitals of their legal responsibilities to register with HCFA every laboratory that provides results used in clinical decisions to physicians or patients.

The committee recommends that genetics laboratories provide reports in an easily understandable form for referring physicians who are not genetic specialists. These reports, including interpretation of the results, should be reviewed by HCFA as part of its inspection of laboratories performing genetic tests.

To ensure that physicians and patients receive consistent and accurate information, "package inserts" (information and instructions both for physicians and patients) should be provided by the manufacturer of genetic test kits through the laboratory from which the physician orders the test.

Ensuring the Safety of New Tests

Because genetic tests seldom will have perfect sensitivity or specificity, particularly when used for predictive purposes, because of the novelty of some genetic testing technologies, and because of the possibilities of misinterpretation of test results, full premarket approval is needed for all new genetic tests; that is, genetic tests should be in Class III. The concerns of the committee will be addressed only if FDA uses criteria for review that address these issues.

In its recent reply to the committee's inquiries, FDA indicated (Tsakeris and Yoder, 1992, p. 8) that a sponsor *may* be asked to provide information that includes when appropriate

- analytic sensitivity/limits of detection;
- analytic specificity/cross-reactivity/interference studies;
- accuracy studies;
- precision studies;
- reportable range;
- clinical sensitivity and specificity; and
- stability data.

The committee believes that data on all of these areas should be provided in premarket approval submissions for genetic tests. Specifically, sponsors should present evidence of sensitivity in terms not only of the ability of the test to detect specific mutations (*analytic sensitivity*) but of the proportion of people with clinically significant disease that are detected by the test (i.e., who have the specific mutation detected by the test; *clinical sensitivity*). One area of concern, for example, is the possibility of FDA approval of a (hypothetical) test kit for CF carriers that detects six mutations and might have 100 percent analytical sensitivity, but only 85 percent clinical sensitivity. The determination of an acceptable clinical sensitivity should be on a test-by-test basis, by taking into consideration not only the benefits of making correct predictions but the risks of making wrong ones.

The FDA should develop guidance to manufacturers for preparing premarket applications for genetic test devices. The application should include

• **the intended and potential use(s) of the test (e.g., presymptomatic diagnosis or prediction, carrier screening, prenatal diagnosis);**
• **for each intended use, data on the sensitivity and specificity of the test, with clinical manifestations serving as an end point in the absence of a "gold standard" test;**
• **procedures to be used by clinical laboratories to demonstrate their reliability (precision and accuracy) and proficiency in performance of the test; and**
• **description to be given to health care providers and to patients regarding the objectives of the test and the interpretations of negative or positive findings.**

For very rare diseases, it may take a long time to collect sufficient data on specificity and sensitivity. For diseases of late onset, a long lag will occur between the time of the test and the appearance of disease, and it will be difficult for applicants to provide adequate data on safety and effectiveness for subjects of the type in whom the test would be applied (e.g., presymptomatic individuals). It may also be impossible to assess the sensitivity and specificity of prenatal tests by independent tests or histopathological examination of aborted fetuses. **In all such cases, the committee recommends that data of the type described in the section "Collection of Data for Test Validation" be required. If these preliminary data suggest that the test is safe and effective for its intended use, the FDA should grant the applicant "provisional premarket approval" in order not to unduly delay submission for PMA.** Under this category, the test could be made more widely available, but the manufacturer would be responsible for obtaining and submitting additional periodic postmarket data of an adequate sample of subjects, until sufficient data are available to warrant full premarket approval. These data would be collected from patients' physicians either directly by the manufacturer or by the laboratories to whom it sells the device. The protocol used in the investigational phase (before provisional approval) would still apply, and informed consent would still be needed.

Once provisional premarket approval has been granted, however, the laboratories performing the test could charge a fair market price for the device or test kit. **The committee recommends that people receiving the test during this provisional period be informed that the safety and effectiveness of the test have not** been fully determined. **If the manufacturer is to contact physicians directly, testees must be informed if the manufacturer will have their names.** Once provisional premarket approval is granted, manufacturers should be allowed to charge a market price for the test. This process may require new legislation.

Provisional premarket approval, with periodic postmarket study for which the sponsor would be responsible, could also be used to cover the development of tests for rare conditions (which is the intent of the humanitarian device exemption). The committee therefore recommends that Congress consider the need for legislation in the spirit of the Orphan Drug Act that would give manufacturers the incentive to develop diagnostic medical devices for genetic tests of limited marketability.

The appearance of clinical disease is the only possible confirmation of many genetic tests, and that may not occur until many years after testing. **Investigators should be permitted to convey the results of investigational tests to subjects who are aware of the investigational nature of the test.** Thus, clinical decisions could be made on the basis of the results as long as the investigator has an approved investigational device exemption. FDA should make it clear that in such cases, with an approved IDE, results could be communicated to the patient or to his or her physician so that interventions can be instituted accordingly.

Since many IRBs are not experienced in the review of investigational genetic testing protocols, the committee recommends that the National Institutes of Health (NIH) Office for Protection from Research Risks (OPRR) and the National Center for Human Genome Research Ethical, Legal, and Social Implications (ELSI) Program coordinate efforts to assist IRBs in coping with this responsibility, and ELSI should consider supporting efforts to assist IRBs in this task. Other federal agencies (such as the FDA) and professional groups should also consider developing guidelines to help IRBs cope with this added responsibility (such as the informed consent guidelines for research involving genetic testing developed by the Alliance of Genetic Support Groups and the ASHG). The formation of a national advisory body on genetic testing could also be helpful in educating IRBs concerning research involving genetic testing (see Chapter 9). **IRBs used by commercial organizations should also have a broad, unbiased membership.**

Compliance with FDA requirements for premarket approval and approved investigational device exemption is essential to ensuring safe and effective use of a genetic test, just as compliance with CLIA88 is essential for any laboratory performing genetic tests for clinical purposes. The committee recommends that the FDA publicize widely to potential sponsors, including academic centers, that DNA probes and other reagents essential to the performance of genetic tests are medical devices. Consequently, whenever they are used for clinical purposes, genetic test devices (i.e., test kits, reagents, probes, etc.) either must be labeled "for investigational use only" (and must comply with FDA requirements for such use) or must have been approved or

or cleared for marketing by FDA. When genetic test devices are used investigationally for clinical purposes, manufacturers—including commercial or academically based laboratories preparing their own devices—should apply for FDA approval of an investigational device exemption, including an IRB-approved protocol, and periodic reports on the results of their investigations.

To speed the widespread availability of investigational devices of limited marketability, FDA should grant provisional premarket approval, as described earlier, when adequate preliminary evidence of safety and effectiveness has been collected. In addition, the NIH and private funding agencies should support meritorious studies designed to assess the safety and effectiveness of investigational genetic testing devices. To speed the collection of data on tests of limited marketability, national collaborative studies should be encouraged. Funding agencies should also support long-term studies on safety and effectiveness of genetic test devices (through the phase of provisional premarket approval) for diseases in which a long lag will occur between the time of the test and the clinical appearance of the disease.

The committee recommends that all genetic tests should either be designated as investigational devices—subject to IRB approval and FDA regulation—or be submitted to the FDA for premarket approval. FDA should clarify that when an approved IDE is obtained for a test for which no independent confirmatory test is available, the results may be given to the patient's health care provider or to the patient. When a device with an approved IDE is used to provide clinical information, the laboratory performing the test should be allowed to charge for the costs of testing, record keeping, and complying with reporting requirements. Because the investigational phase of new genetic tests may be prolonged, the laboratories performing these tests should be subject to external quality assessment. The committee recommends that HCFA inform every organization (e.g., academic health center or other hospital) that all laboratories in which investigational devices are being used for genetic testing are covered by CLIA88 and must register with HCFA to obtain CLIA88 certificates and be inspected.

The FDA has taken important first steps to increase the pool of advisors expert in genetics by inviting applications for service as FDA advisors ("special government employees") under its Clinical Chemistry and Toxicology Devices Panel of Experts. The agency should also consider developing workshops on critical aspects of genetic testing technology for manufacturers and clinical laboratories.

The committee is concerned that screening tests may become routine standard of care without adequate studies of their safety, effectiveness, or clinical utility. To ensure that adequate studies are conducted, the committee recommends that any new screening test should comply with FDA rules regarding investigational devices, including a protocol reviewed by an IRB. **The committee recommends that the decision to move from "pilot" or "investigational" use to rou-**

tine practice involve review of data collected in the pilot study and elsewhere by both FDA and a policy-making body, usually at the state level, that is independent of the organization directly responsible for conducting the pilot study. A national oversight body (see Chapter 9) could facilitate collection and dissemination of data from pilot "investigational" studies. An adequately conducted pilot study in one or a few states need not be repeated in others as long as the other state(s) can maintain the same standards of the pilot study in routine operation. The committee also recommends that some mechanism be found to resolve the dilemma posed by the need to demonstrate that the device is safe and effective for its intended use, whether or not it will be commercially marketed.

The preceding sections, as well as other chapters in this report, indicate that genetic tests for screening and other purposes differ in many respects from other laboratory tests. Some federal agencies, particularly FDA, have recognized this by planning special guidance for manufacturers of genetic tests and by inviting geneticists to participate on advisory groups. The committee welcomes such activity and encourages other agencies to do likewise. **In particular, the committee recommends a Genetic Device Advisory Panel to provide FDA with continuing and timely access to expert advice. In addition, the Clinical Laboratory Improvement Advisory Council should appoint a subcommittee on genetics to make recommendations on improving the quality of laboratories performing genetic tests under CLIA88.**

REFERENCES

Adam, B., and Hannon, W. 1992 (published in 1994). The Centers for Disease Control's infant screening quality assurance program: Overview, accomplishments, and initiatives. In Fullarton, J. (ed.) Proceedings of the Committee on Assessing Genetic Risks. Washington, D.C.: National Academy Press.

Benn, P., et al. 1992. A rapid (but wrong) prenatal diagnosis. New England Journal of Medicine 326(24):1638-1639.

Centers for Disease Control (CDC). 1992. Morbidity and Mortality Weekly Report 41 (RR-2), February 28.

Congressional Research Service (CRS). 1990. Clinical Laboratory Improvement Amendments of 1988. Washington, D.C.

Collaborative Research Group for Huntington's Disease. 1993. A novel gene containing a trinucleotide repeat that is expanded and unstable on Huntington's disease chromosomes. Cell 72:971-983.

Council of Regional Networks for Genetic Services (CORN). 1992. Newborn Screening Report: 1990 (Final report, February 1992).

Cunningham, G. 1992 (published in 1994). California newborn screening program. In Fullarton, J. (ed.) Proceedings of the Committee on Assessing Genetic Risks. Washington, D.C.: National Academy Press.

Federal Register. 1992a. 57 (40), February 28, 1992, Sec. 493.2, p. 7139; Sec. 493.3, p. 7140.

Federal Register. 1992b. 57 (40), February 28, 1992, Sec. 493.17{C}{4}, p. 7141.

Federal Register. 1992c. 57 (40), February 28, 1992, Sec. 493.1709, p. 7184).

Federal Register. 1992d. 57 (131), July 8, 1992.

Federal Register. 1992e. 57 (60491); 21 CFR 812, Docket 91N0404.

Food and Drug Administration (FDA). 1992. Draft "accommodation list" for device tests essential to clinical practice, but not approved by FDA for those uses. Washington, D.C. (personal communication of draft for comment, May 3, 1992).

Haddow J., and McKnight, G. 1992 (published in 1994). Quality of genetic laboratory procedures in the United States. In Fullarton, J. (ed.) Proceedings of the Committee on Assessing Genetic Risks. Washington, D.C.: National Academy Press.

Hammond, K., et al. 1991. Efficacy of statewide neonatal screening for cystic fibrosis by assay of trypsinogen concentrations. New England Journal of Medicine 325:769-774.

Hannon, W., and Adam, B. 1991. Identified problems found in the voluntary newborn screening proficiency testing program conducted by the Centers for Disease Control. In An overview of the national infant screening quality assurance program: Update and future directions. In Proceedings of the Eighth Annual Neonatal Screening Symposium, Saratoga Springs, N.Y., April.

Hoffman, E. 1991. Presentation at the Conference on Biotechnology and the Diagnosis of Genetic Disease: Forum on the Technical, Regulatory and Societal Issues. Program on Technology and Health Care, Department of Community and Family Medicine, Georgetown University Medical Center. Washington, D.C., April.

Hofman, K., et al. 1993. Physicians' Knowledge of Genetics and Genetic Tests. Academic Medicine 68(8):625-631.

Holtzman, C., et al. 1986. PKU newborn screening in descriptive epidemiology of missed cases of phenylketonuria and congenital hypothyroidism. Pediatrics 78(4):553-558.

Holtzman, N. 1991. The interpretation of laboratory results: The paradoxical effect of medical training. Journal of Clinical Ethics 2(4):1-2.

Holtzman, N. 1992. Testimony on genetic testing before the Subcommittee on Human Resources and Intergovernmental Relations, Committee on Government Operations, U.S. House of Representatives, July 23.

Holtzman, N., et al. 1991. Effect of education on physicians' knowledge of a new technology: The case of alpha-fetoprotein screening for neural tube defects. Journal of Clinical Ethics 2(4):1-5.

Hommes, F. 1992 (published in 1994). Laboratory quality assurance efforts in biochemical genetics. In Fullarton, J. (ed.) Proceedings of the Committee on Assessing Genetic Risks. Washington, D.C.: National Academy Press.

Hommes, F., et al. 1990. Documented errors and improvements in biochemical genetic testing. In Proficiency testing for biochemical genetics laboratories: The first ten rounds of testing. American Journal of Human Genetics 46:1001-1004.

House Subcommittee on Human Resources and Intergovernmental Relations. 1992. Committee on Government Operations, U.S. House of Representatives, hearing on genetic testing, July 23.

Hoyt, H. 1992. Testimony on genetic testing before the Subcommittee on Human Resources and Intergovernmental Relations, Committee on Government Operations, U.S. House of Representatives, July 23.

Kaback, M., et al. 1977. Tay-Sachs disease heterozygote detection: A quality control study. Tay-Sachs disease: Screening and prevention. In Kaback, M. (ed.) Progress in Clinical and Biological Research 18:267-277.

Klinger, K. 1992 (published in 1994). New developments in genetic testing. In Fullarton, J. (ed.) Proceedings of the Committee on Assessing Genetic Risks. Washington, D.C.: National Academy Press.

Meaney, J. 1992 (published in 1994). Council of Regional Networks for Genetic Services data on laboratory procedures. In Fullarton, J. (ed.) Proceedings of the Committee on Assessing Genetic Risks. Washington, D.C.: National Academy Press.

Murphy, P. 1992a (published in 1994). New York City DNA Laboratory Quality Assurance. In Fullarton, J. (ed.) Proceedings of the Committee on Assessing Genetic Risks. Washington, D.C.: National Academy Press.

Murphy, P. 1992b. Testimony on genetic testing before House Subcommittee on Human Resources and Intergovernmental Relations, Committee on Government Operations, U.S. House of Representatives, July 23.

Punnett, H. 1992 (published in 1994). Quality assurance efforts of the American Society of Human Genetics. In Fullarton, J. (ed.) Proceedings of the Committee on Assessing Genetic Risks. Washington, D.C.: National Academy Press.

Tsakeris, T., and Yoder, F. 1992 (published in 1994). FDA response to Institute of Medicine questions on regulation of human genetic devices. In Fullarton, J. (ed.)Proceedings of the Committee on Assessing Genetic Risks. Washington, D.C.: National Academy Press.

Vockley, J., et al. 1991. "Pseudomosaicism" for 4p– in amniotic fluid cell culture proven to be true mosaicism after birth. American Journal of Medical Genetics 39:81-83.

Ward, B., et al. 1992. Response. New England Journal of Medicine 326(24):1639-1640.

Willey, A. 1992 (published in 1994). New York State Genetic Quality Assurance Efforts. In Fullarton, J. (ed.) Proceedings of the Committee on Assessing Genetic Risks. Washington, D.C.: National Academy Press.

4

Issues in Genetic Counseling

It was a long and complex process. Blood samples from numerous members of my family had to be collected and analyzed. I underwent several months of genetic counseling to determine my ability to cope with any possible outcome. After a period of months, nothing remained but the nerve-racking wait for the results. . . . Finally, the wait was over: my test was negative. The DNA analysis has shown with 96 percent certainty (later increased to 99 percent, with refinement of the testing process) that I had not inherited the gene for Huntington's disease. When I learned the results I cried and laughed. It took months for the news to sink in. I am still adjusting. . . . The incomparable relief I felt at finally being free of the fear and uncertainty . . . was tempered by the painful knowledge that other family members had not been and would not be so lucky.

(Hayes, 1992)

It is but sorrow to be wise when wisdom profits not.

(Sophocles, *Oedipus Rex*)

Genetic testing raises a broad range of questions and issues for those considering testing and for those offering the test: How great are the risks of the test? How reliable is the test? What does this information mean for me, for my children, for my family, for future generations? What is the nature of the disorder? What is its severity? What options are available? How will we choose? What medical and support services will be needed? What resources are available? What does the future hold for health, longevity, quality of life? What does this informa-

146

tion mean for future insurability, employability, personal and social stigma, and discrimination? Along with their questions, people bring a wide variety of values and personal health beliefs about the central issues raised by genetic testing to the genetic testing and counseling experience.

Genetic counseling is the context for helping people address such issues. The communication of information and the process of counseling cannot be done in a vacuum; they are relevant only as they apply to each particular client's concerns and needs.

This chapter includes background information on the nature and basic components of genetic counseling in various settings (newborn screening, carrier detection, prenatal diagnosis, and screening for late-onset disorders). It also reviews critical issues facing genetic counseling today and for the future. Among these critical issues are nondirectiveness; informed consent; confidentiality; multiplex testing; recognizing social and cultural differences; and the need for a genetically literate public.

Many people who undergo genetic testing receive "good news" and reassurance with their genetic test results. They may learn definitively, or with a high probability, that neither they nor their children have a specific genetic disease. Many other people also learn that they and their children do not carry the gene(s) for that disorder. However, even favorable news and reassurance may affect people's concepts of themselves and their families, and may lead to what is called "survivor guilt" and a sense of ostracism from affected members of the family (Quaid, 1992; Wexler, 1992).

Other people who undergo genetic testing will be informed that a genetic disorder or genetic susceptibility has been identified in their fetus, their children, or themselves. Test results may be deeply troubling for those who receive a diagnosis of a genetic disorder or carrier status, raising fundamental questions of medical vulnerability, as well as personal and social image and identity. Individuals may perceive that they are "flawed," "imperfect," "defective," "inadequate," or "abnormal," or may have concerns that others will perceive them or their progeny in these terms (Kessler, 1979, 1981; Lipkin et al., 1986). The counselor acts as a resource in dealing with the sadness, loss, anger, guilt, or anxiety that genetic information can bring (Kessler et al., 1984).

In educating and counseling about genetics, the counselor must convey the varying nature of genetic risk and our varying ability to predict such risks. Our ability to predict genetic risk varies with mode of inheritance, severity of disorders, and other essential factors, such as environmental and/or combinations of genetic factors, that must be present before genetic susceptibility will be expressed as disease. The prediction of genetic risk also depends on the sensitivity and specificity of the test itself and the quality of laboratory procedures (see Chapter 3).

The immediacy of decision making is another key variable in genetic testing and counseling. The time pressure surrounding genetic testing varies by circumstances and disorders. For treatable disorders such as phenylketonuria (PKU), early identification of the disorder in newborns is critical so that dietary modification can be started early enough to prevent severe mental retardation. For many late-onset disorders and for preconceptional reproductive planning, genetic testing and counseling may occur in adulthood when the information will be of practical use; in these instances, the process of deciding whether to be tested need not be rushed. In other circumstances, it will be necessary to have information from genetic tests much more quickly so that decisions can be made. Although carrier testing is optimally performed before pregnancy, the most time-urgent of such decisions often surround reproduction, especially in prenatal diagnosis where safety dictates only a limited time during pregnancy in which to decide whether to be tested and to make decisions about whether to terminate or to carry to term a pregnancy if a genetic disorder is identified in the fetus.

There is tremendous variability in genetic counseling as provided today and envisioned for the future. As genetic testing expands with the growth of new genetic tests, genetic counseling and education will need to adapt to new modes and settings for the delivery of genetics services, *without sacrificing quality*. Health care providers will require an enhanced appreciation of the contribution of genetics to health, as well as an understanding of the complexities of genetic testing and decision making. This chapter reviews the basic tenets of genetic counseling as it has been defined and practiced in a variety of situations, and examines issues facing genetic counseling for the future.

BASIC COMPONENTS OF GENETIC COUNSELING

Genetic counseling is the process by which individuals and families come to learn and understand relevant aspects of genetics; it is also the process for obtaining assistance in clarifying options available for their decision making and coping with the significance of personal and family genetic knowledge in their lives. In 1975, the American Society of Human Genetics Ad Hoc Subcommittee on Genetic Counseling described genetic counseling (Epstein et al., 1975) as

> a communication process which deals with the human problems associated with the occurrence, or the risk of occurrence, of a genetic disorder in a family. This process involves an attempt by one or more appropriately trained persons to help the individual or family to (1) comprehend the medical facts, including the diagnosis, probable course of the disorder, and the available management; (2) appreciate the way heredity contributes to the disorder, and the risk of recurrence in specified relatives; (3) understand the alternatives for dealing with the risk of recurrence; (4) choose the course of action which seems to them appropriate in view of their risk, their family goals, and their ethical and religious standards, and to act in accordance with that decision; and (5) to make the best possible adjustment to the disorder in an affected family member and/or to the risk of recurrence of that disorder.

Others have applied clinical psychology theory and practice to the field of genetic counseling; this concept has been developed in the writings of Seymour Kessler (1979, 1981; Kessler and Jacopini, 1982; Kessler et al., 1984). Unquestionably, there are both educational and psychological support components to all levels of genetic counseling.

In the "classic" model of genetics services, genetic counseling is provided by a specialized team of professionals, including a clinical geneticist and genetic counselor, and is often provided in a genetics center (see Chapter 6 for discussion of personnel training and certification). The team might be much broader, particularly in specialty clinics where different disciplines are represented. For example, parents of children with cystic fibrosis (CF) often learn about recessive inheritance from pulmonologists, nurses, or social workers who provide care for their children in a CF clinic.

Increasingly, however, genetics services are being provided by primary care providers, who are not necessarily trained in human genetics. Primary care practitioners are also less likely to endorse an important principle of classical genetic counseling—that is, autonomous patient decision making (e.g., Geller et al., 1993; Stange et al., 1993); however, this more directive tradition in medical care is changing toward more autonomous decision making by patients, due in part to legal decisions on informed consent and the right to die (see Chapter 8).

The movement of genetics services into primary care is likely to increase as the number of genetic tests expands. Even if specialized genetics professionals are considered the best providers of genetic counseling services, there will simply be too few genetics professionals to meet the growing demand for services. However, traditional genetic counseling services, provided by specialized genetics professionals, are expected to remain a critical resource when test results reveal risks. Once genetic tests are judged to be "standard of care" for routine use, primary care practitioners are likely to be the ones to offer such testing and obtain informed consent. When risks are revealed, especially for nontreatable disorders including late-onset disorders and for those identified with carrier status, referral to specialized genetic counselors will usually be desirable because of the complexity of the issues in counseling for identified risk. Specialized genetics professionals will also increasingly need to train other personnel to provide genetic testing and counseling services as part of their professional activities.

In many genetic counseling situations, a client must decide whether to seek diagnosis and, if so, must then decide how to use the information resulting from the test. To date, genetic testing and genetic counseling lead to few opportunities for curative treatment of genetic conditions (see Chapter 2); thus, the primary emphasis in genetic counseling has been on facilitating autonomous decision making about receiving information on conditions for which treatment may not exist.

In a few conditions, accurate diagnosis can lead to medical interventions, such as newborn screening and follow-up treatment for PKU. For other conditions, carrier testing is available, permitting more options for reproductive planning, including avoiding conception. Prenatal diagnosis may provide reassurance as well as information for decisions on selective abortion if the fetus is determined to be at high risk for a diagnosable genetic disorder or in preparing for the birth of an affected child. Gene therapy has entered early clinical trials but is barely on the horizon for wide clinical use. This means that in many cases, the only intervention to be offered for a genetic disorder is communication about diagnosis, natural history, and information about available options, including a variety of reproductive options. In the absence of treatment, the psychological impact of this genetic information can be tremendous.

Awareness of the Impediments to Effective Genetic Counseling

Beyond the psychological consequences of receiving genetic testing information are the potential impacts on the family—not only the individual, but also the partner, parents, grandparents, siblings, and children of the individual being tested or screened. The diagnosis of a genetic condition or the results of a genetic test often have repercussions for future childbearing decisions as well, although this is only one of many components of genetic counseling. Social and psychological stress introduced by genetic diagnosis, as well as future financial and emotional burdens, can severely impact family functioning (Schild, 1979).

The provider of genetics services needs to be sensitive to the concept of the "teachable moment," that is, *the point(s) at which an individual, couple, or family is most able to comprehend and absorb the information being given*. The genetic counselor may not have the opportunity to counsel clients at more advantageous teachable moments—after some of the early shock and denial that often accompany genetic diagnosis have abated. Limited contact with the genetic counselor may often result from restrictions on insurance reimbursement (see Chapter 7) and other administrative impediments, such as the practice of scheduling counseling on the day of testing. These and other factors may help explain why certain studies show limited retention and understanding of the genetic information conveyed during counseling interactions (e.g., Childs et al., 1976; Sorenson et al., 1981; Chase et al., 1986; Wertz et al., 1986; Kessler, 1989). Potentially, one benefit of having primary care practitioners provide genetic counseling will be more continuity of care, since continuity of care provides more opportunities over time for *teachable moments*.

The psychological impact of a genetic diagnosis varies with its severity, treatability, and with the unique responses of different individuals and families (e.g., Kessler, 1979, 1980b; Kessler et al., 1984; Biesecker, 1992a; Wexler, 1992). Support, counseling, and follow-up can assist individuals and their families in coping with positive test results. The knowledge and skills of a properly trained counselor can help an individual understand the diagnosis, risk of recurrence, prognosis, and relevant preventive and therapeutic measures, and also aid in communicating important information to other family members.

There is general agreement that certain issues raised by testing should be discussed before an individual decides to be tested. Education and counseling include providing information and supportive counseling to people considering testing about what they need to know to decide whether to be tested—risk status, the benefits and burdens of testing, the limitations of available testing methods, and the implications of the test results, including the psychosocial consequences of such testing. Education and counseling are particularly important for genetic screening procedures, such as prenatal diagnosis for advanced maternal age or carrier screening for CF of an individual with no previous family history of the disease (see Chapter 2). In probabilistic terms, such individuals have a high likelihood of receiving good news—that their fetus is unaffected or that they are not carriers.[1] If conducted properly prior to testing, the groundwork for follow-up counseling will have been laid should test results come back indicating that a genetic condition is present.

Education and counseling following testing include interpretation of test results, discussion of the implications of that information, answering all questions (in a language and manner understandable to the person being counseled), providing supportive counseling, and offering information about community support groups and other follow-up resources. For some conditions, one visit might be sufficient to conduct posttest counseling, for example, after determination of Tay-Sachs carrier status in a nonpregnant female. Other disorders might require several visits or, rarely, long-term supportive care may be needed. The variability of genetic disorders and of their impact demands flexibility in the delivery of services, both diagnostic and psychological.

After genetic counseling, clients should have enough information at least to attempt to deal with the complex interaction among the risks and benefits of various courses of action and with their own values and personal choices (Quaid, 1992). Since genetic diagnosis can sometimes present more uncertainty than certainty, it is important to communicate both information and empathy, because information exchange may be taking place in an atmosphere that is filled with anxiety and unfamiliarity (Biesecker, 1992a). And while the content and nature of genetic counseling may vary, certain basic tenets will almost always apply: nondirectiveness, voluntariness, confidentiality, and respect for social and cultural differences.

Nondirectiveness

Carl Rogers, a clinical psychologist, coined the term *nondirectiveness* in 1942 to describe his psychotherapeutic approach of not advising, interpreting, or guiding his clients. Eventually, Rogers came to recognize that his very presence in a counseling relationship had directive components. By 1978, he had adopted the term *person centered* to describe his therapeutic approach, which is based on unconditional positive regard for the client as a self-actualizing person.

The early eugenics movement in the United States espoused improvement in the inborn characteristics of the human species by applying the rules of heredity to human reproduction (President's Commission, 1983; Kevles, 1985; Duster, 1990). Concern about early abuses in the eugenics movement helped to make the principle of nondirectiveness, and the corollary of respect for client autonomy, key concepts of genetic counseling today. Nevertheless, the issue of *nondirectiveness* in genetic counseling has led to controversy and confusion (Kessler, 1992; Biesecker, 1992a). The desirability as well as the practicability of nondirectiveness in genetic counseling has been challenged (e.g., Clarke, 1991; Morrison and Nevin, 1991; Kessler, 1992).

This controversy reflects an inherent tension in genetic counseling that arises from the complex functions of genetic counseling for different purposes in various settings. The continuum of genetic counseling includes, at a minimum, providing genetic information and education, as well as providing genetic counseling to explore the implications of the information; but it may also include providing specific medical *advice* for treatable conditions (e.g., Motulsky, 1989; Clarke, 1991; Harris and Hopkins, 1991; Pembrey, 1991; Super, 1991; Burke et al., 1993). Critics have challenged the ability of clinical geneticists and genetic counselors to practice nondirective counseling, and have raised concerns about the training and practice of primary care providers, which tends to encourage directive behavior (Epstein et al., 1975; Clarke, 1991; Stange et al., 1993). Primary care practitioners were found to be more directive in dealing with genetic situations than geneticists (Holmes-Seidle et al., 1987; Geller et al., 1993). Women who were counseled by a general obstetrician were more likely to terminate a pregnancy in which a sex chromosome abnormality had been diagnosed than if they were counseled by a geneticist (Holmes-Seidle et al., 1987).

Geneticists have recognized that their values often are not identical to those of their patients, thereby requiring that they respect patients' abilities to make decisions for themselves (Seller, 1982; Biesecker, 1992a; Kessler, 1992). The variation in approach among practitioners is part of the reason why patients must have the final decision about whether to be tested, even for disorders that are treatable. Biases are inherent to human nature and are often projected by health care providers in less than subtle ways. These biases may reflect the attitudes of health care providers about the nature and meaning of health and disease, the severity of genetic conditions and disorders, quality of life, the appropriateness of decisions related to genetic testing and counseling, acceptance of advice, and other issues of importance in genetics (Lin-Fu, 1981; Kessler, 1992; Uba, 1992). The use of language may be an important medium for the communication of values as well as facts in genetic counseling (see Box 4-1). Directiveness may also result from inadequate interviewing skills, including spending more time on or showing more enthusiasm for one option compared to another (Kessler, 1992).

BOX 4-1   Issues in the Use of Language in Genetics

Since a major component of genetic counseling deals with reproductive decision making, and since genetic counseling is necessarily so value laden and dependent on communication, it is natural that its language would be an important medium of transmitting values (Lin-Fu, 1981, 1987, 1989; Lippman, 1991, 1992a,b; Rapp, 1988a, 1991; Reinharz, 1988; Rothman, 1986, 1992, 1993; Wertz, 1992a-c). The meanings and implications of terminology commonly used in health may be altered in discussing genetics issues. The language of communicable disease and prevention takes on other connotations when applied to genetics, particularly the concept of "eradication" of genetic conditions (e.g., Hoffman, 1991; Cunningham, 1992). Much of the language used in genetics has connotations (or direct derivations) from the language of eugenics (Kevles, 1985; Duster, 1990; King, 1992; Lerman, 1992; Lippman, 1992a; Wertz, 1992b), with implications of perfectibility (Wertz, 1992a-c), which are far from the concepts of variation and kinship emphasized by current genetic counselors and underscored as a goal by this committee (see public education in genetics in Chapter 5). The enormous variability in our genetic makeup makes each of us unique, and we all are likely to carry several genes that contain a mutation having the potential to cause genetic disease in ourselves or in our descendants.

In becoming more self-conscious of their own language, geneticists have had insights that can benefit all of medicine in destigmatizing medical language. Use of terms such as *defect* rather than the more general and descriptive term *condition*, for example, tends to reflect more determinism about the immutability of genetic factors than may be appropriate in light of the importance of variability of genetic expression, and has harsh and negative connotations. In many other areas of medicine, the developing trend is away from the language of multiple morbidity and toward concepts of *functioning status* to reflect the variable severity and variable impact of disorders in human life. The language and concepts of genetic *defects* so common in genetics are especially problematic, raising deep personal concerns in individuals about being inherently flawed (Saxton, 1984, 1988; Asch, 1989; Waxman, 1992): the so-called defect or mutation in the gene is transferred to the person carrying it, rendering them "defective" or "mutant."

Calls for the eradication or prevention of genetic disease or of birth defects (e.g., Hoffman, 1991; Modell, 1991; Cunningham, 1992) use the language of infectious disease control but apply it to disorders such as muscular dystrophy and Huntington disease, which are largely untreatable today, where often the only intervention is to prevent the birth of affected fetuses. Such language and the concepts it reflects account for concerns of many persons in the disabilities community about genetic testing and the Human Genome Project. "You're not talking about eradicating disease; you're talking about eradicating me!" as a representative of a disability rights organization said recently (NIH Workshop, 1991). Similarly, language about reducing the incidence and burden of genetic disease to improve the health of society (Rowley et al., 1989; Modell, 1991; Caskey, 1993) employs the utilitarian language of cost-benefit and cost-effectiveness analysis. In the values and language of cost-benefit analysis, prenatal genetic testing programs in which fewer than 50 percent of parents chose to terminate a fetus diagnosed with a genetic disorder are considered to be a "failure" (OTA, 1992b).

continued

BOX 4-1—*Continued*

The language of medicine—and genetics as a subspecialty—may have a very different impact on the patients and clients who are faced with a diagnosis in themselves or in their fetus or child. For example, detection of a disorder is called a *positive* diagnosis by specialists—"positive for cancer or Huntington disease or Down syndrome—a matter that is anything but positive for the patient or family" (Rapp, 1988a). As discussed throughout this report, such diagnoses, particularly of genetic conditions, have conferred personal and social stigmatization (Duster, 1990; Lippman, 1991, 1992a; King, 1992), including loss of marriageability (Modell et al., 1980; Modell and Mouzouras, 1982; Modell and Petrou, 1988), as well as loss of insurability (Billings, 1991; Billings et al., 1992; see also testimony at the public forum of the Committee on Assessing Genetic Risks, Vol. 2, 1992) and employability (Gostin, 1990; Rothstein, 1992).

Terms describing utilization of genetic tests should be scrupulously value-neutral, particularly when no treatment is available. Stating merely that some "chose to be tested" or "chose not to be tested" avoids the value-laden connotations of "test acceptance or rejection," "uptake or declination" (terms that currently abound in the literature), with their positive and negative overtones.

Another example is the widespread use in genetics of the word *pedigree* for the pictorial family history chart that traces genetic characteristics and disorders in families. In normal parlance, "pedigree" more often brings to mind animal lineage in dogs or horses, for example; such language would be well replaced by the simpler language of "family chart." Given the deeply personal and value-laden nature of genetic information, it behooves everyone involved in any kind of genetic counseling to give careful and sensitive consideration not only to the impact of the language of genetics on clients, for whom the impact is the most immediate, but also to the implications of language on public understanding of the nature and meaning of genetics, and medicine in general should follow suit.

Nondirectiveness should not be mistaken for passivity, however. Some counselors, in their eagerness to be nondirective, may shrink from being interactive with clients, from fully exploring the personal implications to them of their alternatives and actions. Nondirective counseling is an active, engaging process built on psychodynamic understandings and concepts, not merely a neutral recital of facts.

The commitment to nondirectiveness in genetic counseling arises from respect for the patient's autonomy in decision making. In a multinational survey of geneticists conducted in 1985, nearly all of the respondents cited respect for patients' autonomy and support for their decisions as important goals of genetic counseling (Wertz and Fletcher, 1988). Most respondents did not consider more eugenic goals, such as improving the general health and vigor of the population, or reducing the number of carriers of genetic disorders in the population, as important. However, a significant number did *not* reject such goals as ones of secondary importance.

Genetic counseling is a highly value-laden endeavor, and it is essential that genetic counselors become aware of the values and biases they bring to their work (Lin-Fu, 1987; Wenger, 1991; Kessler, 1992). The experience and orientation of the genetics service provider influence descriptions and perceptions of disorders, variability, and especially, of severity; widely varying cultural, socioeconomic, educational, and ethical factors affect descriptions of genetic disorders and their possible outcomes (Lin-Fu, 1987; Biesecker, 1992a; Kessler, 1992). A more negative or more positive description of a disorder may result from the orientation of providers, as well as from their objective in providing genetic counseling (Kessler, 1992).

Individual values about genetic testing also vary. For example, since its limited availability in 1986, the number of people actually choosing to take a presymptomatic DNA linkage test for Huntington disease (a fatal, untreatable autosomal dominant disorder of late onset described in Chapter 2) has been lower (Craufurd et al., 1989; Quaid et al., 1989; Tyler and Craufurd, 1992; Wexler, 1992) than was predicted by earlier attitudinal studies (Meissen and Berchek, 1987). Of those who enter testing programs seeking to be tested, once they fully appreciate the ramifications of test information through pretest information and counseling, only 20 percent continue the process to have the test; fully 80 percent choose not to utilize the genetic test. Among the members of the Dutch Huntington's Disease Association who decided not to undergo testing, a large proportion assumed negative consequences even if the Huntington disease gene was shown *not* to be present, for example, so-called survivor guilt, depression, and ostracism from their family (Huggins et al., 1992; Tibben et al., 1992). The test for Huntington disease has only been given in a few centers familiar with the disease. Now that a test for the gene is possible, great caution must be taken. Serious harms (i.e., unexpected impacts of not considering all the implications of deciding whether to be tested) could emerge from an existing trend to reduce the amount of counseling below the level recommended in the international guidelines and the U.S. protocol on presymptomatic testing for Huntington disease (Quaid, 1992; Wexler, 1992).

In the future, tensions surrounding the ethics of genetic counseling will become increasingly evident as more effective treatment becomes available for some genetic disorders, and even more tests are provided in primary care settings. Treatability poses additional dilemmas in deciding whether to give advice to patients to undergo testing beyond providing nondirective genetic counseling. The availability of effective treatment tends to shift the nature of the interaction closer to the model for provision of medical advice and guidance within the context of the ordinary practice of medicine; treatment may be aimed directly at the underlying disease or, in the case of cancer susceptibility, the intervention may involve frequent monitoring for early signs of tumor development.

The preservation of autonomous reproductive decision making may also come in direct conflict with traditional public health perspectives, which emphasize choices for societal good in terms of improved health by reducing the overall burden of disease or decreasing social and health care costs. Some clients will choose not to reproduce or to selectively abort affected fetuses, and their decisions will coincide with public health objectives. The weighing of risks and harms is complicated since *general benefits to society* from reducing the societal burden of disease may compete with the *particular harms to the individual* of losing autonomy and self-determination in areas as deeply personal and defining as genetics and reproduction. As a society, we have decided that such a health trade-off is socially acceptable for certain infectious diseases that pose an imminent threat to health, often to large numbers of people. However, as a society, we have also reached a consensus that such a trade-off is *not* appropriate for genetic disorders; thus, most compulsory sterilization laws enacted earlier in the twentieth century were subsequently repealed (Andrews, 1987).

Informed Consent

Principles of informed consent in the provision of genetic testing services, whether experimental or routine, include (1) fair explanation of the procedures to be followed and their purposes, including identification of any that are experimental; (2) description of risks and benefits to be reasonably expected, including the risks and benefits of future treatment; (3) disclosure of appropriate alternative procedures that might be advantageous to the participant; (4) information on what future decisions participants might be asked to make, including the possibility of abortion; (5) offer to answer inquiries; (6) instruction that the participant may refuse the test; and (7) documentation of the consent (see further discussion in Chapter 8).

In theory, informed consent has been accepted as an essential component of the doctor-patient relationship, but in general medical practice, physicians frequently fail to communicate elements essential for informed participation by patients (Wu and Pearlman, 1992). Few health care providers have been trained in the psychosocial skills needed to work effectively with patients in the informed consent process (Johnson et al., 1992), which may be associated with a historical reluctance by practicing physicians to factor patients' goals and values into decisions regarding their health care (Hollander, 1992).

In 1975, the National Academy of Sciences emphasized the need for obtaining consent by pointing to the nature of the hazards that have been experienced in genetic screening programs, including stigmatization, loss of employment or insurance, and family discord (NAS, 1975). In addition, the 1975 committee stressed that persons being screened or tested should be made fully aware of the limitations of the particular test, such as the risk of false positive or false negative findings and what can be done to minimize that risk. These concerns will become especially relevant as more tests are offered that have lowered sensitivity or specificity, such as those for non-Mendelian multifactorial diseases. The Alliance of Genetic Support Groups (1993) worked with a variety of professional and consumer organizations to develop informed consent guidelines for research involving genetic testing; these have now been released by the Alliance.[2] This joint development process involving professional bodies and consumers exemplifies the overall principles of this report.

To support this effort, there is a need for the development of balanced educational and counseling materials that describe genetic disorders. Such materials would help all providers of genetic testing and counseling to offer accurate and reliable education to their clients, and could help to reduce areas of bias or directiveness in genetic counseling. Balanced materials should be of special help to primary care practitioners who have to advise patients about a range of newly developing genetic tests. Since genetic tests are being developed so rapidly, there will also be a need to ensure that this kind of information reflects the latest scientific knowledge.

Because much of current genetic testing and related counseling now occurs in a research setting, there are important issues related to informed consent and other aspects of the protection of research subjects in large family research studies in genetics, often called genetic *pedigree studies*. The Ethical, Legal, and Social Implications (ELSI) Program at the National Institutes of Health (NIH) supported a 1992 American Association for the Advancement of Science workshop on these issues; more recently, ELSI, in cooperation with the NIH Office for Protection from Research Risks, convened a working group to consider additional guidelines for large family studies in genetics, and developed a special section on human genetic research for the *IRB Guidebook* (OPPR, 1993). The committee commends this first assessment and policy development process related to special issues in research involving genetic testing and counseling.

Confidentiality

Because confidentiality is so essential in preserving client autonomy, its role in genetic diagnosis and testing is sometimes more complicated than in other medical tests or research protocols. Potential effects on other family members, are greater, as is the possibility for discrimination in employment or insurance, for example, where test results may only indicate an increased susceptibility to illness in an otherwise healthy person. The National Society of Genetic Counselors (NSGC, 1991) developed *Guiding Principles* that include a policy statement on the confidentiality of test results:

> The NSGC supports individual confidentiality regarding results of genetic testing. It is the right and responsibility of the individual to determine who shall have access to medical information, particularly results of testing for genetic conditions.

Communicating Risks and Dealing with Uncertainty

One of the goals of genetic counseling is to calculate and communicate risks (Holtzman, 1989). Risk communication, however, entails far more than just accurately determining the numerical risk and transmitting that information to a client.

Clients come to the counseling session with experiential, emotional, religious, and situational concerns that will influence not only their perception and interpretation of risk but also the manner in which they receive the information presented to them. Communicating, understanding, interpreting, and using information on genetic risk involve a "series of complex, multidimensional processes with major rational and nonrational components" (Kessler, 1979).

Risk interpretation is usually associated with acceptability of the risk, that is, the willingness of an individual to deal with the outcome (Wertz et al., 1986). For example, when confronted with the risk of genetic disease in their offspring and when making reproductive decisions, people are likely to place greater weight on their ability to cope with a disabled or fatally ill child than on precise numerical risks (Lippman-Hand and Fraser, 1979d). Risk perception is also influenced by a number of additional subjective interpretations, such as preexisting notions about the degree of risk, whether the risk is under the individual's control (Slovic et al., 1984), whether it is reversible or treatable, whether it is visible, and whether one knows an individual with the disorder (Kahneman and Tversky, 1982; Evers-Kiebooms and van den Berghe, 1987; Hodgkinson et al., 1990). In addition, cultural differences can have a profound effect on the interpretation of risk (Lin-Fu, 1981, 1987, 1988, 1989; Miller, 1992; Uba, 1992) (see below). Finally, interpretation and understanding of risk may be affected by a limited understanding of risk in arithmetic terms, particularly probability (Kessler, 1979); for example, in a Maryland study of 190 predominantly Caucasian, middle-class women, more than one-fifth thought that "1 out of 1,000" meant 10 percent, and 6 percent thought it meant greater than 10 percent (Chase et al., 1986).

Furthermore, the manner in which risks are posed can influence a client's choices. The provider—as well as the presentation—may have a profound effect on perception of risk (Biesecker, 1992a; Kessler, 1992). Most counselors attempt to present risks numerically and avoid expressions of risk such as "high" or "unlikely" (Shiloh and Sagi, 1989). Deciding to have a genetic test can be different if the risk is presented as a 25 percent chance of having an affected child rather than a 75 percent chance of having an unaffected child (Holtzman, 1989). Interpretation of risk also varies according to whether it is presented as a single figure or in comparison with a variety of genetic and other risks (Shiloh and Sagi, 1989).

For the young adult child of a person with Huntington disease with a 50 percent risk of inheriting the disorder, is the risk of being tested for the disease worth the potential employment or insurance discrimination he or she might face? For a 35-year-old pregnant woman, is a 1 in 250 chance of having a child with Down syndrome worth the risk of miscarriage of an unaffected fetus due to the prenatal diagnosis procedure? In these situations, choices can be made among various courses of action, based on the values and beliefs of those making the choices (Juengst, 1988). In prenatal counseling, regardless of actual risk, parents might perceive the chance of occurrence in a binary manner, it either will or will not happen. By processing risks in this way, individuals simplify probabilistic information and shift their focus to the implications of being at risk and the potential impact of what could occur. As Lippman-Hand and Fraser (1979a) point out, "the 'one' in the numerator never disappears no matter the size of the denominator, and the 'one' could be the counselee's child." Risk presentation and interpretation, therefore, are important in the decision-making process and are important components of the genetic counseling process.

These and other factors can also influence the results of studies of retention of risk information. In a study of 190 individuals from 100 families in which there is at least one person with autosomal dominant polycystic kidney disease (PKD), most tested poorly on questions reflecting their knowledge of the genetics of PKD (Hodgkinson et al., 1990). An analysis of nine studies on counseling published since 1970 concluded that "many parents of children with a genetic disorder have an inadequate understanding of the genetic implications of the disease, even after one or more genetic counseling sessions" (Evers-Kiebooms and van den Berghe, 1987). In one study, most (87 percent) who came for counseling with inaccurate knowledge of risk still had inaccurate knowledge after counseling, and some of those who came with accurate knowledge, had inaccurate knowledge after counseling (Sorenson et al., 1981). As described above, a number of factors undoubtedly influence understanding of risk and ability to report risk accurately. In the future, with an increase in the number of tests available to predict genetic disease and pressure to streamline the counseling process, those providing genetic counseling will find themselves facing even greater challenges in communicating risk.

Recognizing Social and Cultural Differences

Combined, the minority groups of Asian and Pacific Islanders, African-Americans, Hispanics, and Native Americans comprise nearly one-fourth of the U.S. population, increasing at a rate more than three times that of the total U.S. population (U.S. Bureau of the Census, 1988; U.S. Immigration and Naturalization Service, 1989). Projections for the year 2000 indicate that a majority of the U.S. population will be people of color (King, 1992); thus people who now comprise racial or ethnic minorities are sometimes referred to as the "emerging majority." The issue of cultural and racial variation in the receipt of genetic information poses additional challenges for those providing genetic counseling.

The sickle cell and Tay-Sachs carrier screening programs of the past provide valuable information on the importance of understanding the culture and values of the population being screened, and providing education and counseling tailored to that population, and of optimizing the settings in which screening occurs (see Chapters 1 and 2). Persons from different cultures, socioeconomic classes, and educational backgrounds may interpret and value the information provided through genetic testing and screening differently. This variability may be due to differences in people's views on reproduction and abortion, the role of children in the society, the significance of genetic disorders and diagnoses in terms of overall

---

**BOX 4-2   Ethnic and Cultural Perspectives
on Genetic Information**

Studies that examine cultural issues in genetics among Asian-Americans are illustrative of the types of issues counselors should be sensitive to in providing pretest and posttest education and counseling to an ethnic minority (Muecke, 1983; Hoang and Erickson, 1985; Lin-Fu, 1987-1989; Uba, 1992). For many Asian-Americans, health means the absence of symptoms; thus, the concept of pre-symptomatic identification implicit in carrier screening or prenatal diagnosis can be unfamiliar and confusing (Muecke, 1983; Hoang and Erickson, 1985). Among some Asian-Americans, particularly recent immigrants, the cause of illness may be attributed to supernatural forces, such as demons and evil spirits, or accepted as fate or punishment for wrongdoing (even of one's ancestors). Shame about illness as punishment plays an important role in some Asian cultures, and denial may be common; thus, some Asian-Americans may not reveal stillbirths or the birth of a child with a congenital malformation in reporting their family history. For persons whose religious values stem from Taoism or Naturalism, disruption of the natural harmony of the body through amniocentesis or other invasive procedures (even blood sampling) is seen as highly undesirable; others do not wish to interfere with their fate (Harwood, 1981; Muecke, 1983). Prenatal counseling is often not de-sired by those who believe that the mere mention of diseases during pregnancy may result in a bad outcome to the pregnancy, and Asian-American women, par-ticularly new immigrants, generally are held responsible by their spouses and in-laws for any poor outcome of a pregnancy, including the birth of a baby with a genetic disorder. In contrast to the high value placed on individual independence in the dominant American culture, Asian cultures are highly family oriented and give greater importance to family reputation than to individual happiness; thus, medical decisions, including those surrounding reproduction and genetic counsel-ing, often involve parents and in-laws as well as spouses (Lin-Fu, 1989).

---

health, concepts of responsibility, blame and social stigma, labeling of genetic conditions in pejorative terms, and the relative importance and interaction of indi-viduals, families, and the larger society. The social and cultural meaning of class, race, ethnicity, and religion all impact on genetic testing and reproductive deci-sion making (Rapp, 1988a,b, 1991, 1993). Although genetics services providers may believe that they are providing vital information essential to autonomous decision making, those receiving it might have no context or practical use for understanding the information being provided. Furthermore, the information may challenge their basic individual and cultural values, thereby increasing their con-fusion and anxiety (see Box 4-2).

Some common diagnosable genetic disorders in the United States have a higher prevalence in minority and immigrant populations and their descendants, including sickle cell anemia, thalassemia, and Tay-Sachs disease. For thalas-semia, for example, the U.S. population at risk includes persons who originated from Italy, Greece, the Middle East, the Indian subcontinent, South China, Southeast Asia, and Africa (Lin-Fu, 1981). Many of those at high risk for thalassemia are recent immigrants and refugees for whom ethnocultural barriers are a serious deterrent to genetics and other health services. To break down ethnocultural barriers, geneticists and other health professionals must not only become aware of their own cultural values, but also understand, appreciate, and respect the cultures of those to whom service is offered, which may be very different from their own (Lin-Fu, 1981, 1989; Uba, 1992). Ethnocultural factors play a key role not only in communications (which encompasses far more than the simple use of language), but also in the perception and acceptance of risk, and in beliefs about health and genetic disorders in general (Wenger, 1991).

Differences in perception and use of genetics services may also be a function of socioeconomic status. In the United States and the United Kingdom, studies have shown that women of upper socioeconomic groups were more likely to use prenatal diagnostic procedures (Wertz and Fletcher, 1988; Wertz, 1992a-c). Acceptance of Tay-Sachs and sickle cell screening by adults, as well as retention of information presented by counselors and doctors, correlated with education and social status (NAS, 1975). Similarly, a study of families at high risk for X-linked diseases found that those with higher incomes and greater education were more likely to utilize prenatal diagnosis in an attempt to ensure that their offspring would be healthy (Beeson and Golbus, 1985).

Consequently, a general assessment of the client's education, family structure, family decision making, degree of acculturation, concept of and approaches to disease, and expectations of the service provider may represent an important first step in genetic counseling. Differences in language and culture can be important barriers in informed consent and in genetic counseling. For example, a recent survey of genetic counselors and nurses in genetics revealed that only 14 percent were fluent in a language other than English (OTA, 1992a). In addition, the vast majority of genetic counselors are Caucasian (more than 90 percent), although 25 percent of genetics services clients are estimated to be from racial and ethnic groups that are not Caucasian (CORN, 1992; OTA, 1992a). In some settings, individuals of the same background as the clients have been trained to assist genetic counselors in overcoming cultural, linguistic, geographic, or economic barriers (see Chapter 6). In one demonstration of delivery of prenatal genetics services for hemoglobinopathy screening, key features were distinguishing the different ethnic groups and providing a distinctive approach to medical care of each, providing interpreter service, and meeting with leaders of each ethnic group to obtain their support (Rowley et al., 1987).

THE CONTEXTS OF GENETIC COUNSELING

Genetic counseling takes place in many contexts and settings: it can take place following the birth of a child, during childhood or adolescence, as a part of reproductive planning, and in pregnancy and adulthood. At each stage in the life process, different concerns and questions will arise based on the need to make a decision or the need to cope with troubling information. Genetic counseling takes place surrounding the process of genetic screening or genetic testing or following referral by physicians based on signs and symptoms. Although each context for genetic counseling described below requires adherence to the basic principles described above—respect for autonomy, informed consent, balanced and accurate presentation of risks, and respect for privacy—each context presents some particular challenges to client-centered counseling for the genetic counselor. Some of these challenges are also discussed in Chapters 1, 2, and 8.

Newborn Screening

Newborns may now be screened for more than 11 genetic and metabolic disorders, but screening programs vary significantly by state. As discussed in Chapter 2, broad population screening such as newborn screening inevitably results in a high rate of false positive test results in the initial stages of newborn screening; this necessitates accurate and timely confirmatory diagnosis as well as follow-up counseling for families whose newborn has initial positive tests results.

Newborn screening is not a trivial intervention and may raise important health and social issues. For example, detection of an affected child can disrupt the relationship between the parents and the newborn. Parents often experience guilt at having passed a genetic disorder to their child. In addition, there may be social stigma, and such stigma may be increased if a reliable carrier screening test was available *before* pregnancy or birth (although such a test is *not* available for PKU or hypothyroidism). In all cases, the parents of an affected child should be informed about the availability of carrier testing for their relatives. The counselor should be sensitive to the possibility, however, that this information might not be desired by the parents, and the wishes of the parents should be respected.

There have been suggestions that newborn screening could also serve as a strategy for providing carrier screening (Cunningham, 1992). These suggestions have been based on reasons of convenience, since most babies are born in hospitals where genetic screening programs are available. However, there are practical as well as social and ethical problems with obtaining and using information on carrier status obtained from newborns. First, as a practical matter, newborns determined to be carriers would have to be followed until their reproductive years to ensure that they are aware of their carrier status when they may choose to know the information. Second, the detection of carrier status in newborns might raise the anxiety level of parents without providing necessary resources to address such concerns, and may create personal and social stigma for the newborn child. Third, newborn screening is an inefficient way of detecting carriers, and other approaches to carrier screening in young adulthood give more options to people identified as carriers (see below). Further, the information may become lost to the individuals before they are old enough to use it, or it may be unwelcome information. In some newborn screening tests, such as the test for sickle cell anemia, the same test reveals both the carrier status and the disease status of the newborn simultaneously. The test for sickle cell anemia indicates if the newborn is a carrier of one copy of the gene or two copies and is affected with the disease. Questions arise about whether genetic information on the carrier status of the newborn should be revealed to the parents. One advantage of telling the parents is to give them information relevant to their own future reproductive plans.

An additional dilemma that arises in newborn screening—if a newborn is diagnosed with an autosomal recessive disease and the parents are subsequently tested—is that genetic information may reveal misattributed paternity. The President's Commission (1983) recommended that misattributed paternity be disclosed, suggesting that counselors counsel the mother separately. The committee takes the view that such information should not be volunteered to the woman's partner.

Determining Carrier Status

Individuals or couples generally request a genetic test to determine carrier status in order to make their reproductive plans. Most people seeking carrier testing have already learned that they are related to an affected individual or someone who is known to be a carrier or that they are at higher risk because of ethnic or racial status (e.g., Tay-Sachs disease, sickle cell anemia, thalassemia, cystic fibrosis). They request carrier tests for reassurance or for the opportunity for information that may be used in prevention (which may take many forms) or both. Prevention may include avoiding marriage to (or reproduction with) another carrier, reproductive planning through prenatal diagnosis and selective abortion, artificial sperm insemination by donor, ova or embryo donation, adoption, surrogacy, or experimental procedures for preimplantation diagnosis.

At present, most carrier screening takes place in the context of reproductive planning and often is conducted during pregnancy. Current debate surrounding CF carrier screening, for example, focuses on whether the goals are best accomplished by screening preconceptional adults or pregnant women (OTA, 1992a). These approaches can be complementary; the question revolves around when the information is best assimilated. Many feel that it would be better for individuals to know their risks before getting pregnant; they suggest screening earlier before pregnancy is likely to occur, when more options are available (Lipkin et al., 1986). Others argue that individuals not facing a pregnancy are not motivated to seek or use information on their carrier status; they will not value this information until they are either planning a family or starting a family (Brock, 1984). The committee favors giving pertinent information prior to conception when options are greater.

Past carrier screening programs have demonstrated the benefits of appropriate community education prior to screening people with no previous family history of the condition for which they are being screened (see Chapter 1). These programs include Tay-Sachs screening programs in the United States (Kaback, 1977; Githens et al., 1990; Scriver and Clow, 1990) and thalassemia screening programs in North America (Fisher et al., 1981; Scriver et al., 1984; Rowley et al., 1991), Sardinia (Cao et al., 1989), Canada (Scriver et al., 1984), Cyprus (Angastiniotis, 1991), and among Cypriots in London (Modell and Mouzouras, 1982; Modell and Petrou, 1988). In the 1970s, the woeful lack of appropriate public education at every level—from government officials to health professionals to the general community—about sickle cell disease and particularly about carrier status—is thought to have contributed to early problems in sickle cell testing and screening programs. More public awareness about genetic diseases and tests will undoubtedly help individual counseling.

Carrier screening provides a good example of the need for education and counseling both before and after testing. Education and counseling are needed before a person decides to undergo carrier testing to inform about the test and the meaning of acquiring this information to the individual. If an individual is tested and found to be a carrier, counseling after the test is also essential. However, if an individual is not found to be a carrier, counseling might not be necessary following the test as long as participants truly understand the results. Some general genetics education and counseling can be provided by informed primary health care providers. Before providing analysis for carrier status, it is important to discuss the client's a priori risk—that is, the individual's risk prior to any test result. At the present time, with a negative family history for a variety of autosomal recessive disorders, an individual's ethnic background is most important in defining a priori risk (e.g., CF in Caucasians, sickle cell in African-Americans). In the future, however, racial and ethnic status may not be as important a risk predictor; this has already happened in Tay-Sachs disease, where more births of infants with Tay-Sachs disease now occur in non-Jews than among Jews.

The complexity of genetic counseling for CF carrier screening serves as an example of the challenges posed by carrier detection. Cystic fibrosis is highly variable in its severity, and severity cannot be predicted by genetic testing. Median life span is increasing, conventional treatment of CF is improving, and prospects for effective gene therapy are growing. Any education and counseling before screening for carrier status should, therefore, include information about the individual's risk, the limits of existing tests to identify all carriers, the potentially limited availability of definitive prenatal diagnosis for at-risk couples, the variable nature of the disease, and prospects for the current and future of treatment of CF. In the case of a negative screening result, individuals must clearly be informed that there is still a chance that they could be carriers. Research is needed to evaluate simple and innovative alternative methods of conveying such information, for example, in pamphlets written in easily understood language.

Although genetic counseling should be flexible and tailored to the particular situation, follow-up counseling and support are needed when carrier status is identified. Usually clients need supportive counseling immediately. Some may want genetic education and counseling right away; others might learn more if genetic education and counseling were delayed. News of carrier status can be accompanied by feelings that impede the person's ability to receive information on both emotional and practical levels. People's perceptions of their own health may worsen, which occurred for some when they were made aware of their carrier status for Tay-Sachs disease (Marteau, 1989, 1990); such anxiety can be prolonged (Zeesman et al., 1984). Knowledge of carrier status can also have an impact on reproductive intentions or behavior, including decisions relating to marriage or choice of marriage partner (Modell et al., 1980; Sujansky et al., 1990).

The moment at which a person is identified as a carrier of a recessive genetic trait may not always be the "teachable moment" at which the person is most able to comprehend the full significance of the information. More teachable moments might come later after the initial information has been absorbed and the person has formulated questions related to the significance of the genetic information, particularly for future reproductive decision making. Thus, education and counseling for persons identified as carriers might well come in two stages, supportive counseling first with the initial detection of carrier status and, later, more detailed genetic education and counseling, when the person has had an opportunity to evaluate the significance of the new information.

In genetic counseling for carrier status, the person being tested, (the *proband*) is routinely advised of risks to other family members. If, for example, an individual is found to be a carrier for an autosomal recessive disorder such as CF or Tay-Sachs disease, the genetic counselor informs the individual that siblings also each have a 50 percent chance of being carriers. In most cases, the suggestion is made that the individual contact his or her siblings and that they consult with their personal physician or attend a genetics clinic for counseling. The genetic counselor does not typically confirm that the proband has informed relevant family members due to limits on time, access, and legal requirements for confidentiality in the counselor-client relationship. Often the family member requests the genetic counselor to assist by seeing other relatives or by guiding the disclosure process. Most people do inform their relatives of genetic information relevant to their health. However, the nature of some family relationships may impede full disclosure to the family by the patient.

Breaching confidentiality to disclose medical information to relatives raises legal and ethical issues, as well as psychosocial ones. Some argue that genetics providers should be legally permitted to disclose such relevant information to relatives at risk (Wertz and Fletcher, 1988). Not all relatives want genetic information (Quaid, 1992; Wexler, 1992). Sharing highly personal medical information that involves reproductive and health futures can raise many emotional and practical issues for family members and can lead to withholding relevant health information from other family members, and thereby not providing them the option to seek testing. The committee believes that clients should be encouraged to inform relatives about pertinent genetic information, but that only rare circumstances would warrant disclosure of genetic information without the consent of the client (see Chapter 8),

Prenatal Diagnosis

Some of the most difficult issues today in genetic diagnosis, testing, and screening surround prenatal diagnosis. The ability to diagnose genetic disorders far exceeds any ability to treat or cure them, and this situation is likely to prevail for a substantial period into the future. Since few diagnosable disorders are now treatable or preventable, few options yet exist for the use of genetics knowledge. Reproductive planning and decision making constitute one of the principal uses of such genetic knowledge, including evaluation of reproductive risk, decisions about whether to selectively abort fetuses identified as affected or highly likely to be affected by diagnosable genetic disorders, or preparing for the birth of an affected child. To compound the difficulties and uncertainties of such decision making, many of the genetic disorders that can now be diagnosed are highly variable in their expressivity, yet information about severity is rarely available through prenatal diagnosis. Prenatal diagnostic decisions are among the most personal in anyone's life and involve difficult psychological, ethical, legal, and social issues for anyone faced with them.

Some prenatal tests are screening tests (e.g., maternal serum alpha-fetoprotein), and other techniques permit diagnosis of certain genetic disorders. Again, the education and counseling needs will differ depending on the nature of the disorder for which the test is being done and the indication for the procedure. The majority of prenatal diagnoses are conducted for advanced maternal age, which increases the risk of a chromosomal abnormality, such as Down syndrome, in the fetus. In general, prenatal diagnosis for advanced maternal age is considered a genetic screening procedure because, although the risk of a chromosomal abnormality increases with age, it does so uniformly across the population (i.e., women of the same age carry the same risk). The majority of obstetrician-gynecologists now routinely offer prenatal diagnosis to women aged 35 and older. These physicians could conduct pretest education and counseling, and/or nurses appropriately trained in prenatal genetics could also provide pretest education and counseling. In the event a fetus is identified to have or be at high risk for a genetic disorder, however, posttest counseling should be conducted by a trained genetics professional in collaboration with the primary care physician.

The educational component of prenatal diagnosis includes information about the testing procedure, as well as the risks of the procedure for both mother and fetus in relation to the chances of detecting an abnormality. All of the options available when an abnormality is detected should then be discussed with the client, including the option of terminating the pregnancy. Psychosocial counseling becomes most important when clients have been provided basic information and are making their own, independent decision whether to undergo testing. The counselor encourages patients to discuss the meaning the information has for them, including the patients' feelings about potential sources of support should they choose to raise a child with a disability, what they might perceive as intolerable disability, the option of terminating the pregnancy, family reactions and values, and previous experiences (Biesecker, 1992b). Counselors should take into consideration the cultural and social differences described above and integrate into their counseling a recognition of how different backgrounds might shape the values and expectations of the counselees (Lin-Fu, 1981, 1987; Kessler, 1992).

A substantial body of literature has been written about the complexity of decisions surrounding prenatal diagnosis, including whether to have the test and what to do about the information it produces (Evers-Kiebooms and van den Berghe, 1987; Sissine et al., 1981; Saxton, 1984, 1988; Beeson and Golbus, 1985; Faden et al, 1987). Some of these studies focus on rational decision making (Pauker and Pauker, 1979), while other concentrate on socially determined responses (Lippman-Hand and Fraser, 1979a-d; Cote, 1983; Wertz et al., 1991). Much of this literature presents an idealized model about how such decisions should be made (Beeson and Golbus, 1985). Some studies have raised concerns that the process of prenatal diagnosis interrupts the formation of the maternal-infant bonding, a process than has been called the "tentative pregnancy" (Rothman, 1986, 1992; Tymstra, 1991).

In one study, interviews with 53 mothers or couples led them to conclude that decision making regarding prenatal diagnosis and the uncertainties related to reproductive decisions were most often dealt with by envisioning the various outcomes and speculating as to how others will view the decision, rather than by "rational decision making" (Lippman-Hand and Fraser, 1979a-d; Lippman, 1992a). Probabilities were not particularly useful as a basis for parental decision making; the predominant perception of parents was a binary one—that a particular outcome will or will not happen. Parents then made a decision based on minimizing potential losses (Lippman-Hand and Fraser, 1979a-d).

Recent data from a large number of studies of families with a prior history of diagnosable genetic disorders indicate that even the most knowledgeable and experienced people employ somewhat differing values about selective abortion (Kaback et al., 1984, 1986; Faden et al., 1987; Wertz et al., 1991; Kaback, 1992; Wertz, 1992a-c). Parents considering prenatal diagnosis often saw only one tenable course of action, and thus did not see themselves as engaged in decision making. More than half of them had made clear decisions about their willingness to risk bearing an affected child before genetic counseling, reflecting attitudes they held long before the current pregnancy; parents viewed counseling as a source of information on carrier status and available options to implement prior decisions. The woman's religion was a key factor in decision making; lower educational attainment and income were associated with more willingness to have an affected child; but the most important variable was a previously affected child—those with a severely affected child were less likely to risk the birth of another child with a potentially severe disorder (Beeson and Golbus, 1985). However, persons from families with personal experience of the disorder also often have ambivalent feelings about selective abortion, regarding it as a rejection of their affected relative (Hodgkinson et al., 1990; Wertz et al., 1991; Wertz, 1992a-c).

Increasingly, prenatal diagnostic services are being provided not in genetic centers, but in private hospitals and clinics, and or in the offices of obstetricians and family physicians. There is little standardization in how services are provided, and the majority of women undergoing prenatal testing may receive only a subset of the counseling previously described. Some receive group counseling with or without individual assessment and counseling, some receive written information, and some receive information over the telephone prior to testing. Procedures for informed consent also vary widely (Biesecker, 1992b).

The institutionalization of prenatal screening and diagnosis, and the provision of these services en masse, may not provide appropriate attention to the individual concerns and needs of pregnant women. For example, maternal serum alpha-fetoprotein (MSAFP) screening during pregnancy has become widespread (see description of MSAFP screening test in Chapter 2). California has a program requiring that all providers of obstetrical services in California inform their patients of the availability of the MSAFP screening test (Cunningham, 1992). Press and Browner (1992, 1993) studied the understanding of women participating in the MSAFP program in California; despite the brochure given to each pregnant woman and the opportunity for her to consent or refuse testing, the majority of women studied reported that they believed they had been told to have the test rather than informed about the existence of the test, and many did not understand that the test was a *screening* test to predict increased risk rather than a *diagnostic* test capable of identifying genetic disorders in a fetus. Some physicians may have problems in the mathematics required for correct interpretation of laboratory test results (Holtzman, 1992) (see Chapters 2 and 3). There are also reports of considerable anxiety associated with MSAFP findings of increased risk of neural tube defects or Down syndrome in the developing fetus (Hoyt, 1992).

Screening for Late-Onset Disorders

Diagnosing the predisposition or susceptibility to future disease through genetic analyses will be troublesome for a society accustomed to medical tests that remove uncertainty. Such tests are likely to modify or reduce some uncertainties, but are not likely to remove them; indeed, these tests are likely to add new uncertainties. As predisposing genes are identified, genetic counselors and primary care providers will be faced with the task of helping at-risk individuals to understand the meaning of genetic predisposition and cope with the ambiguity. The late age of onset of these disorders makes test results particularly problematic, in that individuals may have to wait many years before finding out whether or not they will be affected by the disease. Late onset and difficulty in arriving at a specific diagnosis—because of and combined with variable gene penetrance, gene-gene interaction, variable disease severity, and environmental influences—create a complex of ambiguities that present an increasing challenge to genetic counseling now and in the future.

What are persons identified as being at risk to do about marriage, reproduction, and other life decisions, as well as about changing behaviors that may contribute to prevention of the disorder? The severity of a disease and its amenability to treatment or prevention will play a major role in both the presentation and the reception of genetic information. The most unacceptable psychological impact of facing the uncertainties of untreatable illness may be the feeling of being the passive victim of a totally random event (Wexler, 1992). In addition, for many conditions, questions arise about their prospects for insurability, employability, and other critical aspects of their lives. This kind of uncertainty is very difficult for even the most well-trained and dedicated counselors to convey even to relatively well-educated and well-informed people.

What does a counselor tell someone who has been identified as a carrier of a predisposing gene, especially when a gene has incomplete penetrance? Of necessity, counseling will be supportive rather than prescriptive. In counseling for non-Mendelian disorders, it is unlikely that individuals will be grouped easily into two distinct categories—those at no (or very low) risk and those at high risk (Risch, 1992). The proper model for counseling may include a very large number of categories, with the risk ranging from low to high depending on the particular constellation of genes at many loci. It is also critical to discuss the availability of effective presymptomatic interventions for those conditions where they are available. For example, avoidance of potentially health impairing habits, such as smoking, could be offered as a plan of action to individuals found to be at risk for lung cancer or coronary heart disease. Individuals identified at high risk for colon cancer could be counseled to have periodic medical examinations. Such interventions are not harmful and are warranted based on genetic predisposition alone. Little is known about the extent to which knowing genetic predisposition will affect the acceptance of genetic testing or compliance with medical interventions. Earlier research showed that knowing the increased risk of carrying the Tay-Sachs disease gene among young people of Ashkenazi Jewish descent did not increase acceptance of genetic screening (Clow and Scriver, 1977).

In the case of late-onset autosomal dominant disorders such as Huntington disease, adults face a double dilemma. Before the availability of predictive tests, individuals who knew of their risk status could forgo childbearing as the only way of avoiding passing on the trait. Now that presymptomatic tests are becoming available for some disorders, and those at risk can find out whether they will most likely develop the disease, they are presented with new options. If not at risk, they can reproduce without the burden of passing the gene to their children. If found to be carriers of the gene, they can elect to have prenatal diagnosis to determine whether their offspring will also inherit the fatal gene.

Multiplex Testing

In the future, genetic testing is likely to be provided in groups of tests (see discussion of such "multiplexing" of tests in Chapters 1, 2, and 8). The prospect of multiplex testing will undoubtedly create new challenges for the genetic counselor, once tests are available that can detect multiple genetic traits in an individual at one time. If the multiplex testing is to be used for carrier screening, then the individual must understand that multiple tests assessing the risk for different disorders will be available.

NEED FOR A MORE GENETICALLY LITERATE PUBLIC

The public is generally not well prepared to face the increasing number and complexity of personal and public policy decisions likely to emerge from advances in human genetics. In the genetic counseling setting, individuals and families may be confronting genetic diagnoses and information in a state of crisis, characterized by shock, perceived threat, anxiety, or disbelief. The challenge to genetic counseling is to convey, during a stressful time, complex information about often rare genetic disorders and the probabilistic nature of the information, and to explore the meaning and significance of this information for the person, the family, and their future. Increasingly, the responsibility of preparing individuals to deal effectively with their own genetic health care must also fall to the public education system, a key enabler of scientific literacy. Every client brings some knowledge of genetics, whether accurate or sufficient or not, to the genetic counseling session; well-informed clients are better prepared to consider the issues in genetic testing and counseling and to make informed decisions appropriate to their own values. Chapter 5 addresses the need for improved public genetics education to increase the understanding of genetics, including variation, kinship, and diversity so that citizens can make informed decisions about genetic testing and participate in public debate about the scientific, ethical, legal, and social issues related to genetics.

CONCLUSIONS AND RECOMMENDATIONS

Components of Genetic Counseling

The committee believes that genetic counseling and education must be an integral part of genetic testing; anyone who is offering, or referring for, genetic testing must provide—or refer for—appropriate genetic counseling and education prior to testing and follow-up after testing. If effective treatment can prevent serious disease or symptomatology, the committee believes that patients at risk for treatable illnesses should be informed of the potential bene-fits—as well as potential medical, social, and economic harms—of genetic testing and about possible treatment interventions. Nondirectiveness should remain the standard of care for reproductive planning and reproductive decisions surround-ing prenatal diagnosis, as well as counseling concerning untreatable disorders. Full informed consent before genetic testing based on consideration of all the available options will continue to be essential whether or not the condition is treatable (see Chapter 8). Even when diseases are treatable and physicians offer medical advice about genetic testing and follow-up treatment, it will still be im-portant for physicians to balance their medical advice with concern for their pa-tient's right to make an informed decision different from the one recommended by the physician. This is especially crucial in genetic testing, since genetic informa-tion carries more personal, family, and social risks and burdens than many other kinds of medical information. Research to demonstrate high specificity and sen-sitivity will be especially critical before genetic tests for treatable disorders should be recommended by physicians or other health professionals. Where treatment or prevention is only partially effective, detailed counseling will be needed to de-scribe the outcomes of various treatment options within the context of the natural history of the disorder. Patients need knowledgeable advisors to provide the latest information on possible outcomes to serve as the basis for informed decision making. Considerations of quality of life also need to be discussed when therapy is only partially effective. The committee believes that genetic counseling, if truly person centered, should be inherently flexible and variable. A standard of care should be based on the objectives of genetic counseling: to support the client in making voluntary informed decisions and help the client to cope with the emo-tional suffering related to genetic conditions. **A goal of reducing the incidence of genetic conditions is not acceptable, since this aim is explicitly eugenic. Also, professionals should not harbor implicitly eugenic goals of preventing births or otherwise influencing reproductive or other decisions. The princi-ple of autonomous decision making requires that providers not present any reproductive decisions as "correct" or advantageous for a person or society.** Since couples at risk for genetic diseases in their offspring may differ in their reproductive choices, the decisions about whether to reproduce or to abort an affected fetus are individual choices that should be left to each couple. Similarly, a decision about whether to test for the presence of genes or gene complexes that predict the likely development of future disease that cannot be treated should be an individual decision, and will often require extensive genetic counseling to con-sider the benefits and burdens of such a choice; in these circumstances, some persons will choose testing and others will not. Even when treatment becomes possible, some of these decisions may be still be painful, costly, and uncertain, and still require extensive genetic counseling.

The committee believes that informed consent is essential to ensure indi-vidual autonomy in decision making. The committee therefore recommends

that informed consent be obtained before any genetic testing (see Chapter 8). The committee also endorses the use of the guidelines developed under the auspices of the Alliance of Genetic Support Groups (AGSG) and American Society of Human Genetics (ASHG). More research is needed about what clients need to know in order to make an informed decision concerning genetic testing and about the most effective manner in which to educate patients in a nonbiased way, and about what standards should be set to ensure that all testing and screening programs meet requirements for informed consent.

The committee recommends the development of balanced descriptions of genetic disorders in culturally appropriate language that is respectful of persons with the disorder(s) and avoids the use of pejorative terms and language. Appropriate genetics professional groups should undertake the development of balanced descriptions of particular disorders, perhaps starting with more common disorders, such as neural tube defects, Down syndrome, and sickle cell disease for which screening is already widespread. Cystic fibrosis would also be a useful example for the development of such balanced descriptions, because the circumstances surrounding CF are changing, such as (1) rapid increases in the identification of additional alleles; (2) improvements in median life expectancy; (3) advances in conventional therapies; and (4) early trials of genetic therapies. Balanced materials should be developed with the participation of individuals and families affected by the disorder as well as by specialized genetics personnel. Such materials should also be tested before use and evaluated to determine their effectiveness and possible sources of bias in communicating information both about the particular disorder and about the potential risks and harms of tests available for the disorder. Any such materials developed and tested in this painstaking way should be shared widely. Dissemination should be carried out through professional societies and voluntary health organizations.

The committee endorses the National Society of Genetic Counselors (NSGC) policy statement on confidentiality. The genetic counselor, as the messenger of potentially devastating or discriminatory information, must honor the patient's desire for confidentiality except under rare special circumstances (discussed in Chapter 8) where breach of confidentiality is necessary to avert serious harm. These special circumstances may involve the potential effects of genetic information on other family members or the potential harm to others if the information is not disclosed. Should a counselor feel a professional or personal need to disclose genetic information to a party other than the patient with whom he or she is consulting, then the potential for that disclosure should be addressed before any diagnostic services are rendered.

Providing Genetic Counseling

As more genetic tests are administered, what is ultimately more important is not who provides such services, but that genetic counseling is provided

and provided appropriately. To ensure that adequate genetic counseling is provided to all those seeking genetics services, a cadre of individuals trained in medical genetics and counseling will be needed. Primary care practitioners and allied health professionals will need a minimal basic understanding of medical genetics and counseling (see Chapter 6), and efforts must be made to ensure that the public is sufficiently educated to be informed consumers of genetics services (see Chapter 5). Despite the variety in the substantive information and the nature of genetic counseling, certain basic tenets should apply regardless of who is conducting the counseling and where it is being done. They include respect for the autonomy and privacy of the individual, the need for informed consent, and sensitivity to the tendency of the genetic counselor toward directiveness and paternalism (see Chapters 1 and 8). Research will clearly be needed to test methods for adapting genetic counseling to various providers and settings and to evaluate the impact of such changes.

Since genetics education and counseling are likely to be provided increasingly by primary care practitioners, the committee recommends that training programs be developed for these practitioners to help them perform these educational and counseling functions appropriately and to know when to refer patients to specialized genetics personnel. Innovative educational devices should be developed and evaluated (e.g., video, interactive computer systems, and on-line data bases), along with other resources to support genetics education and counseling in primary care settings. The adequacy of genetics education and counseling in primary care settings should also be evaluated, including behavior related to nondirectiveness in situations involving untreatable disorders or reproductive decision making. Genetics education and counseling tasks should be analyzed to determine what level of complexity can appropriately be delivered by various kinds of practitioners and in various settings, as well as to determine what degree of complexity will require the training and experience of specialized genetics personnel. The committee believes that the more complex and significant the implications and decisions to be made—including reproductive decision making and testing for untreatable late-onset disorders—the more training will be needed to provide appropriate genetics education and counseling.

The committee recommends additional research on issues in directiveness as genetic testing expands (see Chapter 9). The committee also recommends pilot studies on alternative approaches to genetic counseling, especially for untreatable, fatal, late-onset disorders such as Huntington disease. Such research should include adequate evaluation of aspects of directiveness, as well as the effects of differing levels of intensity of counseling and education both before testing and after testing (see Chapter 9).

More research is also needed to understand clients' risk interpretation and assimilation, particularly to determine factors influencing the timing of genetic counseling interventions to take advantage of the teachable moment(s) for genetic counseling. The committee recommends that research on the best ways to provide essential genetics education and counseling—by a variety of providers in a variety of settings—precede efforts to streamline genetic counseling (some approaches to these issues are discussed in Chapter 6). However, the committee believes that understanding and recalling numerical risks are too limited as measures of the success of or need for counseling. Beyond mere comprehension of numerical risk, genetic counseling must assist individuals in determining their own acceptable risk. Since risk perceptions vary among individuals and among counselees and counselors, there is no one right way to present or interpret risk information; information must be balanced, with all the options given, and the process must be tailored to the client.

The committee also believes that ethnocultural sensitivity is essential in genetic counseling. The committee therefore recommends that genetic counseling should be tailored to the cultural perspective of the client, with special attention to differing cultural perspectives on the role of persons in authority. The committee recommends research to determine how best to provide genetic counseling in ways that are sensitive and appropriate to a variety of cultures and language. Such research should be planned, conducted, and evaluated with the participation of persons from the cultures being studied. Once developed, the results of this research should be widely disseminated not only throughout the professional genetics community, but among health care professionals generally. The committee also recommends that training in culturally appropriate language and delivery of genetics services be included in the preparation of all health and genetics professionals who are likely to provide genetic testing and counseling in the future. As one step in this process, genetic counseling and other genetics training programs should actively seek to increase the number of minority practitioners prepared to provide a variety of genetic counseling roles in a variety of settings (see Chapter 6).

The Contexts of Genetic Counseling

Newborn Screening

Newborn screening programs should ʋe conducted for one purpose only—the identification of treatable disease and benefit to the newborn child (see Chapters 1, 2, and 8). In general, newborn screening should not be conducted if no therapeutic intervention is available (except for carefully defined peer-reviewed research studies). Thus, the committee recommends that newborns not be screened for the purpose of determining the carrier status of the newborn (see Chapters 1 and 8). In the event that a genetic disease is confirmed in a newborn, the parents should be counseled by a knowledgeable pediatrician, genetic counselor, or nurse, not only about the prognosis and treatment options for the newborn, but also about the significance of the findings should the parents choose to have additional children.

There have been suggestions that newborn screening could also serve as a strategy for providing carrier screening (Cunningham, 1992). These suggestions have been based on reasons of convenience, since most babies are born in hospitals where genetic screening programs are available. However, there are practical as well as social and ethical problems with obtaining and using information on carrier status obtained from newborns. First, as a practical matter, newborns determined to be carriers would have to be followed until their reproductive years to ensure that they are aware of their carrier status when they may choose to know the information. Second, the detection of carrier status in newborns might raise the anxiety level of parents without providing necessary resources to address such concerns, and may create personal and social stigma for the newborn child, including impact on insurability or other negative repercussions. Third, newborn screening is an inefficient way of detecting carriers, and other approaches to carrier screening in young adulthood give more options to people identified as carriers.

The committee believes that newborn screening is not the optimal way to determine genetic carrier status of the parents. If carrier status in the newborn or other children is revealed through genetic testing for treatable disease, parents should be informed prior to the screening of the newborn (1) of the possible availability of the information; and (2) the benefits and harms of knowing the carrier status of their children, including that the information has no relevance to the health of the newborn. Because of the risk of possible stigma affecting the development of the child, such information is best provided in the context of genetic counseling; the decisions of the parents about whether to receive such information should always be respected.

Finally, genetic services should not be disruptive to families. In general, the committee recommends that misattributed paternity detected through follow-up to newborn screening should only be revealed to the mother and should not be volunteered to the social father (see Chapters 2 and 8). This extremely sensitive issue is likely to become increasingly problematic as genetic testing expands, and the committee recommends research and evaluation of current policies and practices in genetic testing and screening related to identification of misattributed paternity.

Determining Carrier Status

The committee believes that, ideally, carrier screening should be conducted before a pregnancy occurs, thereby offering individuals more options should they find they are at risk for disease in their future offspring. The committee recognizes that carrier screening often takes place during pregnancy, but recommends the development of innovative methods for practical carrier screening of adults before pregnancy. Better public and provider education may increase preconceptional carrier testing. Research is needed to evaluate simple and innovative alternative methods of conveying such information, for example, in pamphlets written in easily understood language.

Research is needed to determine how well primary care practitioners are prepared for genetic counseling tasks and what education and training will be required to prepare them for expanded genetic testing and counseling (see Chapter 6). Counseling about identified carrier status may require referral for specialized genetic counseling, for example, in complex or untreatable disorders. In addition, when the sensitivity or specificity of the carrier test is less than optimal and there are social concerns about confidentiality and discrimination; under these circumstances, specialized genetic counseling may also be needed before any genetic test to help clients make a decision about whether to pursue carrier testing.

The committee believes that patients should disclose to relatives genetic information relevant to the health of those relatives. However, the committee recommends that confidentiality be breached only in rare circumstances to prevent serious avoidable harm under conditions described in Chapter 8. If there is a possibility that confidentiality may be breached, those circumstances should be fully disclosed in the informed consent process before carrier screening or any other type of genetic service. Under those rare circumstances where unauthorized disclosure of genetic information is deemed warranted, the genetic counselor should first try to obtain the permission of the person to release the information. To facilitate the disclosure of relevant genetic information to family members, accurate and balanced materials should be developed to assist individuals in informing their families and in providing access to further information, as well as access to testing if relatives should choose to be tested.

Prenatal Diagnosis

The committee is concerned that not enough genetic pretest education and counseling is now given surrounding prenatal diagnosis, and the committee recommends education and counseling both before and after prenatal diagnosis. In most cases, this education and counseling should be provided by a trained genetics professional or a primary care practitioner with special training in genetics. Special training in genetics is needed by anyone offering prenatal or other reproductive genetic testing (see Chapter 6). Prenatal diagnosis may also be offered for high-risk pregnancies, where there was a previously affected child or family member, both parents are carriers of an autosomal recessive disorder, or one parent carries a dominant trait.

Pretest genetic education and counseling should help people determine whether they wish to undertake prenatal testing. All of the options available when an abnormality is detected should then be discussed with the client before the test is given. The education and counseling process before prenatal diagnosis entails assessment of family, medical, and pregnancy history; information regarding testing and its implications; and supported decision making. In this process, certain ethical principles should be maintained: (1) testing will be voluntary; (2) confidentiality will be maintained; and (3) parental options will be protected and respected.

The committee recommends that additional research be conducted in two areas related to genetic counseling in prenatal diagnosis:

- A variety of approaches to counseling and informing of results should be evaluated in terms of (1) what the client has learned; (2) whether the client has been offered the opportunity to explore his/her feelings and reactions to the information; and (3) general satisfaction with the way counseling was provided and information reported.

- Additional research is needed on the impact of prenatal diagnosis, particularly its immediate and long-term impact on women. Such research should include the psychosocial implications—both at the time of pregnancy and later in life—of decision making about selective abortion of a fetus diagnosed with a genetic disorder that may develop early in life. The committee believes that such research will provide important information for the design and evaluation of genetic counseling for prenatal diagnosis for the future both in primary care and in specialized genetics settings.

Screening for Late-Onset Disorders

In general, neither physicians nor genetic counselors are yet well prepared to deal with the complexities of counseling for late-onset disorders. Therefore, the committee believes that such counseling initially should be provided in a specialized genetics center familiar with the genetics and psychosocial aspects of the disorder in the context of pilot studies. The committee recognizes that—once direct DNA testing can be performed in an individual for the single-gene defects predisposing to breast and colon cancer—there are not enough trained personnel to carry out the recommended counseling. The committee recommends research on genetic testing for breast and colon cancer, including psychosocial impacts, the impact of knowledge about susceptibility genes on the willingness to be tested, and compliance with recommended medical regimens. This research should include caregivers other than geneticists, since it is likely that much testing of this kind will be carried out by nongeneticists in the future.

Multiplex Testing

The committee recommends the development of innovative methods for multiplex testing, with the grouping of tests by related types of disorders that raise similar issues in terms of the significance of their implications (including the availability of effective treatment and how soon treatment needs to be

instituted), to allow appropriate education, informed consent, and genetic counseling. This will be a critical issue for the future of genetic testing and genetic counseling. Tests should not be grouped together just because it is technically feasible or economically advantageous; for example, a test for PKU that is treatable should not grouped together with a test for Huntington disease that is not treatable. Tests should be grouped with other tests that have the same implications and issues for genetic education and counseling so that people can make informed decisions about genetic testing; tests should not be grouped according to marketplace exigencies. Research will be required to develop and evaluate innovative methods for the grouping of genetic tests in a way that will make it possible for multiplex testing to embody the committee's basic principles on informed consent and the need for genetics education and counseling (see Chapters 2 and 8).

NOTES

1. It is important to distinguish between the terms "positive result" and "negative result" in both lay and medical terminology. While a physician would describe test results that reveal the presence of a fetal abnormality as "positive" in terms of detecting the condition for which the test was defined, a lay person would be most likely to describe this result as "negative" in social, emotional, or psychological terms (see discussion of language of genetics, Box 4-1).

2. These guidelines are available from the Alliance of Genetic Support Groups, 35 Wisconsin Circle, Suite 440, Chevy Chase, MD 20815, 301-652-5553.

REFERENCES

Alliance of Genetic Support Groups. 1993. Informed Consent: Participation in Genetic Research Studies. Chevy Chase, Md.

Andrews, L. 1987. Medical Genetics: A Legal Frontier. Chicago: American Bar Foundation.

Angastiniotis, M. 1991. Development of Genetics Services from Disease Oriented National Genetics Programs (Cypress Thalassemia Centre, Archbishop Makarios III Hospital, Nicosia, Cyprus). Presentation at the 8th International Congress of Human Genetics, Washington, D.C., October.

Asch, A. 1989. Reproductive technology and disability. In Cohen, S., and Taub, N. (eds.) Reproductive Laws for the 1990s. Clifton, N.J.: Humana Press.

Beeson, D., and Golbus, M. 1985. Decision making: Whether or not to have prenatal diagnosis and abortion for X-linked conditions. American Journal of Medical Genetics 20:107-114.

Biesecker. B. 1992a (published in 1994). Genetic counseling: Settings, providers and goals, current and future. In Fullarton, J. (ed.) Proceedings of the Committee on Assessing Genetic Risks. Washington, D.C.: National Academy Press.

Biesecker, B. 1992b (published in 1994). Issues in genetic counseling for prenatal diagnosis. In Fullarton, J. (ed.) Proceedings of the Committee on Assessing Genetic Risks. Washington, D.C.: National Academy Press.

Billings, P. 1991. Causes of discrimination in health insurance. Genewatch 7(6):2-3.

Billings, P., et al. 1992. Genetic discrimination in insurance. American Journal of Human Genetics 50:476-482.

Brock, D. 1984. Cystic fibrosis. In Wald, N. (ed.) Antenatal and Neonatal Screening. New York: Oxford University Press.

Burke, W., et al. 1993. Clinical implications of genetic susceptibility testing: Nondirective counseling vs. medical advice (submitted for publication in the Journal of the American Medical Association).

Capron, A. 1979. Tort liability in genetic counseling. Columbia Law Review 79:619, 680.

Cao, A., et al. 1989. The prevention of thalassemia in Sardinia. Clinical Genetics 36:277-285.

Caskey, C. 1993. Molecular medicine: A spin-off from the helix. Journal of the American Medical Association 269(15):1986-1992.

Chase, G., et al. 1986. Assessment of risk by pregnant women: Implications for genetic counseling and education. Social Biology 33:57-64.

Childs, B., et al. 1976. Tay-Sachs screening: Motives for participating and knowledge of genetics and probability. American Journal of Human Genetics 28:537-49.

Clarke, A. 1991. Is Non-Directive Genetic Counselling Possible. Lancet 338:998-1001.

Clow, C., and Scriver, C. 1977. The adolescent copes with genetic screening: A study of Tay-Sachs screening among high school students. In Kaback, M. (ed.) Tay-Sachs Disease: Screening and Prevention. New York: Alan Liss.

Collins, F. 1992. Cystic fibrosis: Molecular biology and therapeutic implications. Science 256(5058): 774-779.

Committee on Assessing Genetic Risks. 1992. Vol. 2: Proceedings. Washington, D.C.: National Academy Press.

Cote, G. 1983. Reproductive drive and genetic counseling. Clinical Genetics 23:359-362.

Council of Regional Networks for Genetic Services (CORN). 1992. Presentation by Ilana Mittman at the January 24, 1993, meeting of the Joint Working Group on the Ethical, Legal and Social Implications of the Human Genome Project, Bethesda, Md.

Craufurd, D., et al. 1989. Uptake of presymptomatic predictive testing for Huntington's disease. Lancet ii:603-605.

Cunningham, G. 1992 (published in 1994). Maternal serum alpha-fetoprotein screening in California. In Fullarton, J. (ed.) Proceedings of the Committee on Assessing Genetic Risks. Washington, D.C.: National Academy Press.

Duster, Troy. 1990. Backdoor to Eugenics. New York: Routledge.

Epstein, C., et al. 1975. Genetic counseling (statement of the American Society of Human Genetics Ad Hoc Committee on Genetic Counseling). American Journal of Human Genetics 27:240-242.

Evers-Kiebooms, G., and van den Berghe, H. 1987. Impact of genetic counseling: A review of published follow-up studies. Clinical Genetics 15:465-474.

Faden, R., et al. 1987. Prenatal screening and pregnant women's attitudes toward the abortion of defective fetuses. American Journal of Public Health 77:288-290.

Fisher, L., et al. 1981. Genetic counseling for β-thalassemia trait following health screening in a health maintenance organization: Comparison of programmed and conventional counseling. American Journal of Human Genetics 33:987-994.

Gabow, P. 1992 (published in 1994). Autosomal dominant polycystic kidney disease. In Fullarton, J. (ed.) Proceedings of the Committee on Assessing Genetic Risks. Washington, D.C.: National Academy Press.

Geller, A., et al. 1993. How will primary care physicians incorporate genetic testing? Directiveness in counseling. Medical Care 31:989-1001.

Githens, J., et al. 1990. Newborn screening for hemoglobinopathies in Colorado: The first 10 years. American Journal of Diseases of Children 144:466-470.

Gostin, L. 1990. Genetic discrimination: The use of genetically based diagnostic and prognostic tests by employers and insurers. American Journal of Law and Medicine 17(1&2):109-144.

Harris, R., and Hopkins, A. 1991. Non-directive genetic counseling. Lancet 38:1267-1268.

Harwood, A. (ed). 1981. Ethnicity and Medical Care. Cambridge, Mass.: Harvard University Press.

Hayes, C. 1992. Genetic testing for Huntington's disease—A family issue. New England Journal of Medicine 327(20):1449-1451.

Hoang, G., and Erickson, R. 1985. Cultural barriers to effective medical care among Indochinese patients. Annual Review of Medicine 36:229-239.

Hodgkinson, K., et al. 1990. Adult polycystic kidney disease: Knowledge, experience, and attitudes to prenatal diagnosis. Journal of Medical Genetics 27:552-558.

Hoffman, E. 1991. Presentation at the Conference on Biotechnology and the Diagnosis of Genetic Disease: Forum on the Technical, Regulatory and Societal Issues. Program on Technology and Health Care, Department of Community and Family Medicine, Georgetown University Medical Center. Washington, D.C., April.

Hofman, K., et al. 1993. Physicians' knowledge of genetics and genetic tests. Academic Medicine 68(8):625-631.

Hollander, R. 1992. In Johnson, S., et al. Teaching the process of obtaining informed consent to medical students. Academic Medicine 67(9):598-600.

Holmes-Seidle, M., et al. 1987. Parental decisions regarding termination of pregnancy following prenatal detection of sex chromosome abnormality. Prenatal Diagnosis 7:239-244.

Holtzman, N. 1989. Proceed with Caution: Predicting Genetic Risks in the Recombinant DNA Era. Baltimore, Md.: The Johns Hopkins University Press.

Holtzman, N. 1990. Prenatal screening: When and for whom? Journal of General Internal Medicine 5(S):542-546.

Holtzman, N. 1992. The interpretation of laboratory results: The paradoxical effect of medical training. Journal of Clinical Ethics 2(4):1-2.

Hoyt, Heidi. 1992. Testimony before the Human Resources and Intergovernmental Relations Subcommittee of the Committee on Government Operations. U.S. Congress, House of Representatives. Washington, D.C., July 23.

Huggins, M., et al. 1992. Predictive testing for Huntington disease in Canada: Adverse effects and unexpected results in those receiving a decreased risk. American Journal of Medical Genetics 42:508-515.

Johnson, S., et al. 1992. Teaching the process of obtaining informed consent to medical students. Academic Medicine 67(9):598-600.

Juengst, E. 1988. Prenatal diagnosis and the ethics of uncertainty. In Monagle, J. (ed.) Medical Ethics: A Guide for Health Professionals. Rockville, Md.: Aspen Publishers.

Kaback, M. 1977. Tay-Sachs disease: From clinical description to prospective control. In Kaback, M. (ed.) Tay-Sachs Disease: Screening and Prevention. Progress in Clinical and Biological Research 18:1-7.

Kaback, M. 1992 (published in 1994). Genetic knowledge and attitudes: A multi-ethnic study. In Fullarton, J. (ed.) Proceedings of the Committee on Assessing Genetic Risks. Washington, D.C.: National Academy Press.

Kaback, M., et al. 1984. Attitudes toward prenatal diagnosis of cystic fibrosis among parents of affected children. Pp. 15-28 in Lawson, D. (ed.) Cystic Fibrosis Horizons. Proceedings of the 9th International Cystic Fibrosis Congress. Chichester, N.Y.: Wiley.

Kaback, M., et al. 1986. Genetic knowledge and attitudes: A multiethnic study. National Technical Information Service. PB87162947/AS. Washington, D.C.: U.S. Department of Commerce.

Kahneman, D., and Tversky, A. 1982. The psychology of preference. Scientific American 246:160-171.

Kenen, R., and Schmidt, R. 1978. Stigmatization of carrier status: Social implications of heterozygote genetic screening programs. American Journal of Public Health 68:1116-1120.

Kessler, S. (ed.). 1979. Genetic Counseling: Psychological Dimensions. New York: Academic Press.

Kessler, S. 1980a. Genetic associates/counselors in genetic services. American Journal of Human Genetics 7:323-334.

Kessler, S. 1980b. A psychological paradigm shift in genetic counseling. Social Biology 27(3):153-167.

Kessler, S. 1981. Psychological aspects of genetic counseling: Analysis of a transcript. American Journal of Medical Genetics 8:137-153.

Kessler, S. 1989. Psychological aspects of genetic counseling. VI: A critical review of the literature dealing with education and reproduction. American Journal of Medical Genetics 34:340-353.

Kessler, S. 1992. Psychological aspects of genetic counseling. VII: Thoughts on directiveness. Journal of Clinical Counseling 1(1):9-17.

Kessler, S., and Jacopini, A. 1982. Psychological aspects of genetic counseling. II: Quantitative analysis of a transcript of a genetic counseling session. American Journal of Medical Genetics 12:421-435.

Kessler, S., et al. 1984. Psychological aspects of genetic counseling. III: Management of guilt and shame. American Journal of Medical Genetics 17:673-697.

Kevles, D. 1985. In the Name of Eugenics. Los Angeles, Calif.: University of California Press.

King, P. 1992. The past as prologue: Race, class, and gene discrimination. In Annas, G., and Elias, S. (eds.) Gene Mapping: Using Law and Ethics as Guides. New York: Oxford University Press.

Lerman, R. 1992. Final Solutions: Biology, Prejudice, and Genocide. University Park: Pennsylvania State University Press.

Levi-Pearl, Sue. 1992 (published in 1994). From a consumer's point of view (statement at the public forum). In Fullarton, J. (ed.) Proceedings of the Committee on Assessing Genetic Risks. Washington, D.C.: National Academy Press.

Lin-Fu, J. 1981. Cooley's Anemia: A Medical Review. Publication No. (HSA) 81-5125. Rockville, Md.: U.S. Department of Health and Human Services.

Lin-Fu, J. 1987. Meeting the needs of Southeast Asian refugees in maternal and child health and primary care programs. Maternal and Child Health Technical Information Series 2-11. Rockville, Md.: Maternal and Child Health Bureau, Department of Health and Human Services.

Lin-Fu, J. 1988. Population characteristics and health care needs of Asian Pacific Americans. Public Health Reports 103:18-28.

Lin-Fu, J. 1989. Ethnocultural factors in genetic counseling: The Asian-Americans as a model. Presentation at the Conference on the Thalassemias: Diagnosis, Management, Future Perspective for Therapy, New York Hospital-Cornell Medical Center, New York, May 15.

Lipkin, M., et al. 1986. Genetic counseling of asymptomatic carriers in a primary care setting. Annals of Internal Medicine 105:115-123.

Lippman, A. 1991. Prenatal genetic testing and screening: Constructing needs and reinforcing inequities. American Journal of Law and Medicine 17:15-50.

Lippman, A. 1992a (published in 1994). The goals and purposes of genetics: Language, policy, and the construction of inequities. In Fullarton, J. (ed.) Proceedings of the Committee on Assessing Genetic Risks. Washington, D.C.: National Academy Press.

Lippman, A. 1992b. Geneticization and the Construction of Health: Biomedicine as Biopolitics. Address to the Royal Society of Medicine. London, October.

Lippman-Hand, A., and Fraser, F. 1979a. Genetic counseling—Parents' responses to uncertainty. Birth Defects: Original Article Series 15:325-339.

Lippman-Hand, A., and Fraser, F. 1979b. Genetic counseling: Provision and perception of information. American Journal of Medical Genetics 3:113-127.

Lippman-Hand, A., and Fraser, F. 1979c. Genetic counseling—The postcounseling period. I: Parents' perceptions of uncertainty. American Journal of Medical Genetics 4:51-71.

Lippman-Hand, A., and Fraser, F. 1979d. Genetic counseling—The postcounseling period. II: Making reproductive choices. American Journal of Medical Genetics 4:73-87.

Loader, S., et al. 1991. Prenatal screening for hemoglobinopathies. II. Evaluation of counseling. American Journal of Human Genetics 48:447-451.

March of Dimes. 1990. Symposium on Genetic Services for Underserved Populations (May 1988). Birth Defects: Original Article Series.

Marteau, T. 1989. The impact of prenatal screening and diagnostic testing upon the cognitions, emotions, and behaviour of pregnant women. Journal of Psychosomatic Research 33:7-16.

Marteau, T. 1990. Reducing the psychological costs. British Medical Journal 301:26-28.

Meissen, G., and Berchek, R. 1987. Intended use of predictive testing by those at risk for Huntington's disease. American Journal of Human Genetics 26:283-293.

Miller, J. 1992. The Public Understanding of Science and Technology in the United States, 1990. Report to the National Science Foundation. Washington, D.C.

Modell, B. 1991. Genetic fitness. Presentation at the International Congress on Human Genetics. Washington, D.C., October.

Modell, B., and Mouzouras, M. 1982. Social consequences of introducing antenatal diagnosis for thalassemia. In Cao, A., et al. (eds.) Thalassemia: Recent Advances in Detection and Treatment. Birth Defects 19(7):285-291.

Modell, B., and Petrou, M. 1988. Review of control programs and future trends in the United Kingdom. Birth Defects: Original Article Series 23(5B):433-442.

Modell, B., et al. 1980. Effect of introducing antenatal diagnosis on reproductive behaviour of families at risk for thalassemia major. British Medical Journal 280:1347-1350.

Morrison, P., and Nevin, N. 1991. Non-directive genetic counseling. Lancet 38:1267.

Motulsky, A. 1989. Societal problems in human and medical genetics. Genome 31:870-875.

Muecke, M. 1983. In search of healers: Southeast Asian refugees in the American health care system. Western Journal of Medicine 139:835-840.

National Academy of Sciences (NAS). 1975. Genetic Screening: Programs, Principles, and Research. Report of the Committee for the Study of Inborn Errors of Metabolism. Washington, D.C.: NAS.

National Institutes of Health (NIH) Workshop on Reproductive Genetic Testing: Impact on Women. 1991. Bethesda, Md., November 21-22.

National Society of Genetic Counselors (NSGC). 1991. Guiding principles and resolutions. Perspectives in Genetic Counseling 14(1):3.

Office of Protection from Research Risks (OPPR). 1993. Human genetic research. Protecting Human Research Subjects: IRB Guidebook. National Institutes of Health. Bethesda, Md.

Office of Technology Assessment (OTA). 1992a. Genetic Counseling and Cystic Fibrosis Carrier Screening: Results of a Survey. OTA-BP-BA-97. U.S. Congress. Washington, D.C.: U.S. Government Printing Office.

Office of Technology Assessment (OTA). 1992b. Panel on Genetic Counseling and Cystic Fibrosis Carrier Screening. U.S. Congress. Washington, D.C., March 10-12.

Pauker, S., and Pauker, S. 1979. The amniocentesis decision: An explicit guide for parents. Birth Defects: Original Article Series 15:289-324.

Pembrey, M. 1991. Non-directive genetic counseling. Lancet 38:1267.

President's Commission for the Study of Ethical Problems in Medicine and Biomedical and Behavioral Research. 1983. Screening and Counseling for Genetic Conditions. Washington, D.C.: U.S. Government Printing Office.

Press, N., and Browner, C. 1992 (published in 1994). Policy issues in maternal serum alpha-fetoprotein: The view from California. In Fullarton, J. (ed.) Proceedings of the Committee on Assessing Genetic Risks. Washington, D.C.: National Academy Press.

Press, N., and Browner, C. 1993. Collective fictions: Similarities in the reasons for accepting MSAFP screening among women of diverse ethnic and social class backgrounds. Fetal Diagnosis and Therapy 8(Suppl. 1):97-106.

Quaid, K. 1992 (published in 1994). Streamlining genetic counseling for broader application. In Fullarton, J. (ed.) Proceedings of the Committee on Assessing Genetic Risks. Washington, D.C.: National Academy Press.

Quaid, K., et al. 1989. Knowledge, attitude, and the decision to be tested for Huntington's disease. Clinical Genetics 36:431-438.

Rapp, R. 1988a. Chromosomes and communication: The discourse of genetic counseling. Medical Anthropology Quarterly 2(2):143-157.

Rapp, R. 1988b. The power of "positive" diagnosis: Medical and maternal discourses and amniocentesis. In Michaelson, K. (ed.) Childbirth in America: Anthropological Perspectives. South Hadley, Mass.: Bergin & Garvey.

Rapp, R. 1991. Constructing amniocentesis: Maternal and medical discourses. In Ginsburg, F., and Tsing, A. (eds.) Negotiating Gender in American Culture. Boston: Beacon Press.

Rapp, R. 1993. Sociocultural differences in the impact of amniocentesis: An anthropological research report. Fetal Diagnosis and Therapy 8:S1:90-96.

Reinharz, S. 1988. Controlling women's lives: A cross-cultural interpretation of miscarriage accounts. Pp. 3-37 in Research in the Sociology of Health Care. New York: JAI Press, Inc.

Risch, N. 1992 (published in 1994). Genetic testing and mental illness. In Fullarton, J. (ed.) Proceedings of the Committee on Assessing Genetic Risks. Washington, D.C.: National Academy Press.

Rothman, B. 1986. The Tentative Pregnancy: Prenatal Diagnosis and the Future of Motherhood. New York: Viking.

Rothman, B. 1992 (published in 1994). Early prenatal diagnosis: Unsolved problems. In Fullarton, J. (ed.) Proceedings of the Committee on Assessing Genetic Risks. Washington, D.C.: National Academy Press.

Rothman, B. 1993. The tentative pregnancy: Then and now. Fetal Diagnosis and Therapy 8(Suppl. 1):60-63.

Rothstein, M. 1992. Genetic discrimination in employment and the Americans with Disabilities Act. Houston Law Review 29(1):23-84.

Rowley, P., et al. 1984. Screening and genetic counseling for β-thalassemia in a population unselected for interest: Effects on knowledge and mood. American Journal of Human Genetics 31:718-730.

Rowley, P., et al. 1987. Prenatal hemoglobinopathy screening: Receptivity of Southeast Asian refugees. American Journal of Preventive Medicine 3:317-327.

Rowley, P., et al. 1989. Do pregnant women benefit from hemoglobinopathy carrier detection? Annals of the New York Academy of Sciences 565:152-160.

Rowley, P., et al. 1991. Prenatal screening for hemoglobinopathies. I. A prospective regional trial. American Journal of Human Genetics 48:439-446.

Saxton, M. 1984. Born and unborn: The implications of reproductive technologies for people with disabilities. Pp. 298-312 in Arditt, R., et al. (eds.) Test-Tube Women: What Future for Motherhood? Boston: Pandora Press.

Saxton, M. 1988. Prenatal screening and discriminatory attitudes about disability. In Baruch, E., et al. (eds.) Embryos, Ethics, and Women's Rights: Exploring the New Reproductive Technologies. New York: Harrington Park Press.

Schild, S. 1979. Psychological issues in genetic counseling of phenylketonuria. In Kessler, S. (ed.) Genetic Counseling: Psychological Dimensions. New York: Academic Press.

Scriver, C., et al. 1984. β-thalassemia disease prevention: Genetic medicine applied. American Journal of Human Genetics 36:1024-1038.

Scriver, C., and Clow, C. 1990. Carrier screening for Tay-Sachs disease. Lancet 336:191.

Seller, M. 1982. Ethical aspects of genetic counseling. Journal of Medical Ethics 8:185-188.

Shiloh, S., and Sagi, M. 1989. Effect of framing on the perception of genetic recurrence risks. American Journal of Medical Genetics 33:130-135.

Sissine, F., et al. 1981. Statistical analysis of genetic counseling impacts: A multi-method approach to retrospective data. Evaluation Reviews 5:745-757.

Slovic, P., et al. 1984. Characterizing perceived risk. Pp. 91-124 in Kates, R. et al. (eds.) Perilous Progress: Managing the Hazards of Technology. Boulder, Colo.: Westview Press.

Sokal, D., et al. 1980. Prenatal chromosome analysis: Social and geographic variation for older women in Georgia. Journal of the American Medical Association 244(13):1355-1357.

Sorenson, J., et al. 1981. Reproductive Pasts, Reproductive Futures: Genetic Counseling and Its Effectiveness. New York: Liss.

Sorenson, J., et al. 1984. Parental response to repeat testing of infants with 'false-positive' results in a newborn screening program. Pediatrics 73:183-187.

Stange, K., et al. 1993. Physician agreement with U.S. Preventive Services Task Force recommendations. Journal of Family Practice 34:409-416.

Sujansky, E., et al. 1990. Attitudes of at risk and affected individuals regarding presymptomatic testing for autosomal dominant polycystic kidney disease. American Journal of Medical Genetics 35:510-515.

Super, M. 1991. Non-directive genetic counseling. Lancet 338:1266.

Thiederman, S. 1986. Ethnocentrism: A barrier to effective health care. The Nurse Practitioner (January).

Tibben, A., et al. 1992. DNA testing for Huntington's disease in the Netherlands: A retrospective study on psychosocial effects. American Journal of Medical Genetics 44(1):94-99.

Tyler, A., and Craufurd, D. 1992. Presymptomatic testing for Huntington's disease in the United Kingdom. British Medical Journal 304:1593-1596.

Tymstra, T. 1991. Prenatal diagnosis, prenatal screening, and the rise of the tentative pregnancy. International Journal of Technology Assessment 7(4):509-516.

Uba, L. 1992. Cultural barriers to health care for Southeast Asian refugees. Public Health Reports 107:544-548.

U.S. Bureau of the Census. 1988. United States Population Estimates by Age, Sex, and Race: 1980 to 1987. Washington, D.C.

U.S. Immigration and Naturalization Service, Statistical Analysis Branch. 1989. Immigrants Admitted by Country or Region of Birth, FY 81 to FY 88. Washington, D.C.

Waxman, B. 1992 (published in 1994). Human Genome Program: A disability perspective. In Fullarton, J. (ed.) Proceedings of the Committee on Assessing Genetic Risks. Washington, D.C.: National Academy Press.

Wenger, F. 1991. Knowing yourself culturally: Influence on clinical practice. Paper presented at the conference on Ethnocultural Diversity in the 90s. Florida Department of Health and Rehabilitative Services, Orlando, Fla., October 29.

Wertz, D. 1992a. How parents of affected children view selective abortion. In Holmes, H. (ed.) Issues in Reproductive Technology. Garland Press.

Wertz, D. 1992b (published in 1994). Issues in prenatal diagnosis: Policy implications of my research. In Fullarton, J. (ed.) Proceedings of the Committee on Assessing Genetic Risks. Washington, D.C.: National Academy Press.

Wertz, D. 1992c. Prenatal diagnosis and society. Royal Commission on New Reproductive Technologies. Ottawa, October.

Wertz, D., and Fletcher, J. 1988. Attitudes of genetic counselors: A multinational survey. American Journal of Human Genetics 42:592-600.

Wertz, D., et al. 1986. Clients' interpretation of risks provided in genetic counseling. American Journal of Human Genetics 39:253-264.

Wertz, D., et al. 1988. Communication in health professional-lay encounters: How often does each party know what the other wants to discuss? In Ruben, B. (ed.) Information and Behavior, vol. 2. New Brunswick, N.J.: Transaction Books.

Wertz, D., et al. 1991. Attitudes toward abortion among parents of children with cystic fibrosis. American Journal of Public Health 81:992-996.

Wexler, N. 1992. The Tiresias complex: Huntington's disease as a paradigm of testing for late-onset disorders. FASEB Journal 6:2820-2825.

Wiggins, S., et al. 1992. The psychological consequences of predictive testing for Huntington's disease. New England Journal of Medicine 327(20):1401-1405.

Wu, W., and Pearlman, R. 1992. Consent in medical decision making: The role of communication. In Johnson, S., et al. (eds.) Teaching the process of obtaining informed consent to medical students. Academic Medicine 67(9):598-600.

Zeesman, S., et al. 1984. A private view of heterozygosity: Eight year follow-up study on carriers of the Tay-Sachs gene detected by high school screening in Montreal. American Journal of Medical Genetics 18:769-778.

5

Public Education in Genetics

There is a growing recognition that scientific literacy generally, and genetic literacy in particular, are essential to informed public decision making:

> There is the need to have an enlightened citizenry, people who are aware of the nature of science, who use the scientific approach in their decision-making.
>
> (Ebert, 1993)

Scientific literacy encompasses an appreciation of scientific information, but it also requires application of knowledge to personal and societal problems, as well as a recognition of the ethical, economic, political, and legal implications of scientific progress (Hurd, 1985; Bybee, 1986; McInerney, 1987a; Rutherford and Ahlgren, 1988). In addition, scientific literacy must include an understanding of the scientific process. The public is often confused about conflicting scientific information in the popular media. An understanding that information is often incomplete and imperfect in issues of public health would help the public appreciate that conflict and controversy are part of an open process of scientific discovery, investigation, and debate. In addition, mistakes are made in science; scientists need to exercise reasonable caution in reporting results, but the public and the media must also be better able to evaluate scientific claims (Levi-Pearl, 1992).

The Human Genome Project also has recognized an educational imperative in the development of its programs (USDHHS and DOE, 1990, 1991). This imperative is intended to develop a genetically literate public that understands basic biological research, understands elements of the personal and health implications of genetics, and participates effectively in public policy issues involving genetic information. This imperative also is intended to develop an understanding of the widely varying personal values and cultural perspectives in our society about complex issues related to genetics.

Genetics professionals and qualified educators must assume responsibility for identifying the essential components of genetic literacy. What do we want people to know, value, and do about genetic information? For example, ideally members of the public should know that DNA is the information molecule; they should value the variation and diversity that is expressed from that molecule; and they should be able to participate in public debate about the use of genetic information (J. McInerney, personal communication, 1993). However, the public also needs to understand the interaction and interdependence of genes, the individual, and the environment. Perhaps the most important contribution of new knowledge about genetics is its ability to document a major biological basis for human variation. The old argument about nature versus nurture is outdated; as discussed throughout this report, both nature (genes) and nurture (environment) are important to human health. Broad public understanding of the potential and limits of genetics is essential to avoid genetic reductionism (Holtzman, 1989; Keller, 1992). This is a "tall" order indeed; even many well-educated people lack understanding of these concepts. Nevertheless, the increasing impact of genetic decision making in health and disease makes it important to educate the public in these matters.

Much of the responsibility for genetics education must fall to two components of the public education system: formal education, which takes place in the schools; and informal education, which includes educational interventions outside of school. Public education has long been viewed as a key enabler of democratic pluralism, providing individuals with access to elements of cultural, political, and scientific literacy. Understanding the basis of genetics—variability and evolution—reinforces this democratic pluralism with values of personal autonomy, kinship, and respect for variation, thereby helping to decrease artificial social divisions.

This conclusion has been echoed twice in the last two decades. In 1975 the National Academy of Sciences (NAS) Committee on Inborn Errors of Metabolism recommended (NAS, 1975):

> It is essential to begin the study of human biology, including genetics and probability, in primary school, continuing with a more health-related program in secondary school. . . . Sufficient knowledge of genetics, probability, and medicine leading to appropriate perceptions of susceptibility to and seriousness of genetic disease and of carrier status cannot be acquired as a consequence of incidental, accidental, or haphazard learning. . . .

These health education precepts (including media coverage and personal counseling) have been utilized with some success in other areas of mass public health education such as cardiac risk reduction (Farquhar, 1992). In 1983, the President's Commission for the Study of Ethical Problems in Medicine and Biomedical and Behavioral Research reaffirmed the importance of public education about genetics (President's Commission, 1983):

Efforts to develop genetics curricula [at all levels] and to work with educators to incorporate appropriate materials into the classroom . . . should be furthered. The knowledge imparted is not only important in itself but also promotes values of personal autonomy and informed public participation.

BARRIERS TO OVERCOME

The world's supply of information increases daily, and nowhere is the flood greater than in science. Much of the news of science has to do with human biology, genetics, and medicine—subjects bearing on individual health and well-being. Because of this avalanche of new information, however, scientific literacy among most members of the public lags far behind the technological trends and innovations.

If the public is to have a sufficient knowledge of topics such as human diversity, human development, and genetics, the educational process must begin early in life when children's flexibility and scientific interest are at a maximum. Children must understand the nature and methods of science in general, as well as the broad principles of genetics. In addition, the applications of genetics tend to be driven by technology; children therefore need to understand and appreciate the science behind this technology. Students should understand that technology may have unintended consequences and that it may be fallible (AAAS, 1989a). For example, technology helps scientists to identify certain genes in an individual, but it also may reveal much more information about that individual, including information about families. Similarly, the technology for genetic testing has technical limitations (Chapters 2 and 3). Such knowledge can influence the physical, intellectual, and cultural development of patients, parents, and informed citizens.

Educational interventions should encourage open minds and intellectual flexibility, which allow receptivity to new ideas in order to appreciate diversity and variability. This perspective can help people overcome the perception that they have lost control to a medical enterprise that itself has difficulty keeping up with new facts and concepts.

WHAT DO PEOPLE KNOW?[1]

Periodic studies sponsored by the National Science Foundation (NSF) and conducted since 1979 show that general scientific illiteracy is a persistent problem in the United States. A 1990 NSF study suggests that only about 7 percent of Americans can be considered scientifically literate (i.e., having minimal understanding of scientific terms, concepts, methods, and their societal impact). Only 24 percent understand DNA's relationship to inheritance. However, Americans maintain a lively interest in medical news, appear to understand the rudiments of human genetics, and have already formed opinions about important issues in genetic testing. Seven out of ten Americans are very interested in issues about new medical discoveries, and 52 percent are able to understand a simple problem dealing with the inheritance of a genetic illness (Miller, 1992).

Recent national surveys paint a conflicting picture of the state of public consciousness of genetic disease and the issues surrounding genetic testing. In recent U.S. surveys, more than one-third (37 percent) of respondents report having an immediate family member who has had, is at risk for, or is a carrier of a genetic disease (OTA, 1987). However, it appears that most people harbor a simplistic concept of genetic disease focused on physical deformities and mental retardation, which may not be genetic in origin (NORC, 1990). And although 85 percent of those surveyed claimed to have heard or read little or nothing about genetic screening per se (NORC, 1991), they nevertheless have opinions about genetic testing and appear to sense its potential for misuse: 72 percent believe that the benefits of science generally outweigh any harmful effects (Miller, 1992), and only 48 percent think genetic screening will do more good than harm (NORC, 1991). More than 8 of 10 respondents believed that (1) employers should not have the right to require that prospective employees take genetic screening tests or to use screening results in hiring decisions (ABC, 1990; NORC, 1991); (2) employers should be required to provide a workplace free of carcinogens, rather than exclude workers with an inherited susceptibility to cancer (NORC, 1990); and (3) insurance companies are not justified in refusing to insure a person based on test indications of his or her future susceptibility to serious disease (ABC, 1990).

Although initial reporting of an October 1992 survey commissioned by the March of Dimes indicated that a majority of the respondents reported believing that someone else had a right to an individual's genetic information (March of Dimes, 1992a), less than 20 percent of the total respondents thought that an employer had a right to genetic information (19 percent of the total) (March of Dimes, 1992b). This survey also confirmed that a majority of the respondents knew little or nothing about genetic testing or gene therapy (68 and 87 percent, respectively). The results of these polls and surveys indicate public confusion and concern about genetics and genetic testing, as well as ambivalence about the complex social and ethical implications of genetic testing discussed throughout this report.

WHAT IS GENETICS EDUCATION?

There is a wide spectrum of public education interventions in genetics. Beginning with broadly based fundamental scientific literacy and appreciation for human diversity and variability, which are acquired mostly in school, educational interventions then should focus more narrowly on the general public awareness of human genetics, genetic disorders, genetic services (such as newborn screening), and prevention. Finally, the focus of genetics educational interventions narrows to specific disorders that may affect an individual, leading to a range of complex, individualized genetic counseling services (see Chapter 4).

Formal Genetics Education

There is a growing awareness among educators that a basic understanding of genetics, disease risk, and health choices is an essential element of cultural literacy—as important in the education of a developing child as a basic understanding of hygiene and nutrition. For example, high school biology teachers who participated in training workshops sponsored by Cold Spring Harbor Laboratory rated genetics and ecology as the biology topics "most important in preparing students for adult life" (Micklos and Kruper, 1991).

Systematic genetics education in the context of broader scientific and biological literacy should begin in elementary school with principles of human variability and diversity in the context of the total environment, and then progress through middle school and into high school. This effort should (1) inculcate basic tenets of genetic literacy that are essential for all students as they assume management of personal and family health care as adults; (2) help some students prepare for their future roles as opinion leaders in government, industry, education, medicine, and law; and (3) maintain and broaden the interest of the approximately 15 percent of science-interested students who are focusing on biology or health-related majors (Astin et al., 1991), as well as stimulate this interest in other motivated students. This educational imperative has been unchanged since an educational needs assessment by the Biological Sciences Curriculum Study (1978) and the March of Dimes recommended the following:

> Education in human genetics should begin in elementary school and continue throughout adult life in settings outside the formal classroom. The orientation should be interdisciplinary, combining factual material in basic genetics with content from the behavioral and social sciences.

Genetics education offers an almost unparalleled opportunity to integrate concepts from several sciences, as well as the personal and social implications of new technologies. Public policy issues in genetics must be broadened to include discussions of personal autonomy; the allocation of public resources; and guarantees of equity for women, minorities, and persons with disabilities. This is consistent with the innovative approaches of "whole learning," "across curricula," and "science-technology-society" that synthesize information from various disciplines and relate learning to the student's personal life and culture (Walker et al., 1980; Bybee, 1986; AAAS, 1989b).

Therefore, the basis of scientific and genetic literacy must be a fundamental grasp by elementary school students of the abundant diversity available to them in their own physical and cultural environments, as well as in nature (via nature walks, zoos, and museums of natural history). Comparisons between themselves and other species can stimulate their sense of biological variety and kinship. Students will also see comparisons within their own group, as well as between and within classes at school, or between and within families. The understanding of *variety and kinship in the context of environment* is well within the grasp of elementary school children; this broad foundation will prepare them for formal study of biology and genetics, including variations that may take the form of disease. This kind of knowledge will help enable them as adults to interpret the scientific information that appears in the media, as well as prepare them for medical problems that may befall them or those they care for.

Genetics Education for the Future

It is not likely that there will be enough specialized genetics personnel in the United States to perform the essential health education that will be required as genetic testing or screening becomes more widespread. In addition, data from large-scale testing programs suggest that a clinic or a doctor's office is not the best context for a first exposure to genetic testing information, and that public education campaigns and counseling, generally, have a greater impact on individuals with some previous exposure to genetic concepts (Reilly, 1989; Yager, 1991; Saunders, 1992). Decisions about genetic testing and its potential personal impact ultimately must be tied to preexisting knowledge and value systems. Without such knowledge, individuals are more likely to make uninformed decisions or to cede all decisions about genetic testing to their doctors. To prepare citizens for informed personal and societal decision making, school children will have to be taught the basics of the relevant science and technology, and the ethical, legal, and social issues stemming from that science and technology will have to be integrated into the science instruction. Several formal programs warrant further study.[2]

DNA Learning Center

One such program is the DNA Learning Center (DNALC) at Cold Spring Harbor Laboratory, which extends that institution's traditional postgraduate research and education mission to the college, precollege, and public levels. The "human genome education center" includes a hands-on student laboratory, student multimedia computing laboratory, and research laboratory. Through a number of grant-supported activities and programs, the DNALC (1) develops new instructional technologies to make genetics accessible to the public, and especially to young people; (2) trains educators for laboratory-based teaching in genetics; (3) provides an interactive learning environment for students, teachers, and nonscientists; (4) extends enrichment activities to underserved populations including minorities, the disabled, the economically disadvantaged, and those living in nonurban areas; (5) provides a forum for public discussion of the personal, social, and ethical implications of genetic technology; and (6) serves as a national clearinghouse for information on genetics, genetic medicine, molecular biology, and biotechnology.[3]

Biological Sciences Curriculum Study

Another model program is the Biological Sciences Curriculum Studies (BSCS) program in Colorado. Under a 16-month grant from the U.S. Department of Energy, the BSCS has developed an educational module for the high school biology classroom titled *Mapping and Sequencing the Human Genome: Science, Ethics, and Public Policy.* This module was distributed free of charge to more than 50,000 high school biology teachers and educators nationwide in mid-October 1992. The module contains two units of background information for the teacher—the first unit deals with the science of the Human Genome Project, and the second discusses ethics and public policy and how to teach these topics to students. BSCS collaborated with the American Medical Association in developing these materials; the American Society of Human Genetics, National Society of Genetic Counselors, Council of Regional Networks for Genetic Services, and other professionals have provided independent reviews. Each activity has been field-tested in classrooms nationwide.[4]

Project Genethics

Project Genethics consists of a series of model workshops on human genetics and bioethical decision making conducted by the staff of the Human Genetics and Bioethics Laboratory at Ball State University in Indiana. The workshops are taught by teams of outstanding secondary school biology teachers who have completed an intensive four-week summer component (at Ball State University), an academic year follow-up, and mentor teacher training. The objectives of the two-week workshops are designed to meet human genetics/bioethics educational needs of teachers. Among other things, each participant will be able to apply an understanding of Mendelian inheritance and human pedigree analysis procedures to assessing problems related to genetic screening and genetic counseling. These skills are then used to analyze the social, ethical, legal, psychological, or philosophical problems that can arise as a result of practices such as genetic screening programs, genetics education, amniocentesis, chorionic villus sampling, artificial insemination by donor (AID), and DNA-based paternity identification.[5]

University of Kansas Medical Center

Another Human Genome Project-funded program at the University of Kansas supports a series of workshops for middle and secondary science teachers to address the lack of public information on the ethical, legal, and social issues of the Human Genome Project. Teachers are selected for a four-phase national program to prepare them to become "resource" teachers. Teachers are recruited from public, parochial, private, and special schools (e.g., schools for the visually or hearing impaired). Resource teachers are chosen for their knowledge, experience, and links with existing teacher organizations. Workshops are conducted to update and expand the use of human genetics materials in school curricula.[6]

Informal Educational Interventions

Public concerns about genetics and genetic testing are an appropriate focus of informal educational interventions, which should facilitate dialogue about the scientific, ethical, legal, and social issues in genetics such as the following:

• *Knowledge of Genetics for Understanding Personal and Family Health.* Focusing on the concepts of genetic variability and diversity will avoid simplistic explanations of genetics concepts and risk as either categorically good news— that an individual has essentially zero risk for a particular disease—or categorically bad news—that he or she is virtually certain to develop it. Many genetic disorders are of variable and often unpredictable severity, and much genetic risk assessment is of an inherently probabilistic nature. Since many genetic tests are developed long before effective treatment, the availability of the test should not be considered a technological imperative, as may often be the case in prenatal diagnosis (Lippman, 1992; Press and Browner, 1992; Rothman, 1992). Understanding these complexities will be essential for informed personal and family health decision making in the future.

• *Implicit Goals and Possible Outcomes of Genetic Testing.* A variety of implicit goals and outcomes have been identified for genetic testing in different contexts and settings (see Chapter 4). In the case of prenatal diagnosis and population screening, these goals include contributing to family planning, preparing individuals and/or family members to deal psychologically and emotionally with a genetic condition, and providing time to initiate life-style changes or therapies that may mitigate the severity of symptoms. Other, more controversial goals and outcomes of genetic testing, which may be implicit or explicit, include eliminating disease genes from the population by identifying carriers or by encouraging termination of affected pregnancies (Press and Browner, 1992).

• *Concept of Eugenics.* The potential for manipulation or direction of human reproduction is also implicit in genetic testing. The public needs to understand that testing for genetic conditions raises value judgments about what is normal versus what is abnormal—and that the social and legal acceptance of such judgments can create a pressure for genetic conformity. The concept of genetic conformity may not only result in disease prevention, but also produce an intolerance of ethnic or racial populations. The eugenics movement in the United States and Europe during the first four decades of the twentieth century attempted to promote "genetic hygiene" to reduce disease; more recently, "ethnic cleansing" in the former Yugoslavia and elsewhere has renewed debate about the possible return of organized policies for social eugenics (see discussion of autonomy in Chapter 8).

• *Relationship Between Genetic Testing and Abortion.* Rational discussion of this sensitive issue is critical and must be based on facts and options, and not merely on values or opinions. In recent years, there has been a pervasive trend to separate abortion from the discussion of genetic testing. For example, all direct reference to abortion was deleted just prior to publication of educational materials for participants in the California maternal serum alpha-fetoprotein (MSAFP) screening (Cunningham, 1992). Avoiding discussion of abortion makes it impossible to consider the full implications of prenatal genetic testing and the range of choices available to parents. Discussion of abortion—as with other sensitive matters related to reproduction—often arouses strong reactions in local schools and communities. Nevertheless, awareness of the possibility of abortion among the considerations that follow genetic testing is an essential part of informed consent for any such testing (see Chapters 4 and 8).

• *Sensitivity to Genetic Disadvantage.* James Watson (1992), co-discoverer of the structure of DNA and founding director of the National Center for Human Genome Research, offered this analysis of genetic disadvantage:

> Some people get a bad start in life because they are born into poverty, and some people get a bad start in life because they are born with a bad set of genes. The function of a compassionate society is to deal with both kinds of inequality.

Formal biology education typically emphasizes gene states, using terms such as "mutant" and "abnormal" to describe the genes involved in disease conditions. Sensitivity to the challenges and problems of genetic disorders includes care in the use of language (Lippman, 1992) and the avoidance of dehumanizing terms. This is the context in which basic concepts of variety and kinship can help to reduce the stigma associated with genetic disorders.

• *Genetics of Complex Disorders.* In addition to understanding variety and kinship, the public will need to develop an understanding of the role of both genetic and environmental factors in complex disorders such as heart disease and some cancers. Although genetic factors are being identified in many common diseases of late onset, they often require environmental interaction to produce disease. This additional public perspective on genetics is essential to help dispel concepts of determinism that overemphasize the role of genetics in health behavior.

The Human Genome Project's Ethical, Legal, and Social Implications Program has funded the development of two television series intended to contribute to this public dialogue. One project, coordinated by the WGBH Educational Foundation in Boston, produced eight one-hour programs for release in 1993 through the Public Broadcasting System. These programs are designed to prepare viewers for informed participation in public debate; it will try to make molecular biology intelligible, moving beyond sensational headlines to illustrate the molecular revolution in biology and medicine, and explore the social issues raised by advances in molecular biology. A second project by WNET in New York aired one segment on genetics as part of a 10-part series also on public television in 1993. Public television may only reach a small percentage of the American public, but these programs can also be used in schools and a variety of other settings to educate the public. It will be important to study their use and effectiveness as educational tools in various settings.

PUBLIC HEALTH EDUCATION

The goal of health education interventions is to prevent disease and promote health. A traditional public health model is to define a problem, identify risk factors, develop and test interventions, implement these interventions, evaluate prevention effectiveness, and develop a national program (Rosenburg, 1992). This model could prove effective in addressing those genetic disorders that are treatable and for which testing is available. However, it could also mistakenly encourage the public to believe that screening or genetics knowledge will make the outcome of every pregnancy a perfectly healthy baby, eliminate all disease, or make everyone "normal" (NAS, 1975).

Health educators traditionally equate healthy behaviors with "good" decision making. However, it is impossible to apply this measure of decision making when examining the genetic testing process (Lippman-Hand and Fraser, 1979). The confounding issue in this model, as it applies to genetic disorders, is that many times the disorders cannot yet be prevented because there is no cure; what has been prevented is the births of babies with these diseases. For example, a public health educator may be tempted to use the prevailing public health model in analyzing muscular dystrophy: define the health problem as muscular dystrophy, identify the risk factor in being a member of a family in which it appears, develop and test interventions such as a prenatal DNA diagnostic test, implement such interventions by advising obstetricians of the DNA test as the standard of care, evaluate effectiveness by measuring the number of births with muscular dystrophy, and develop a national program that might mandate prenatal DNA diagnostic testing for muscular dystrophy. Health educators need to recognize the limitations of the traditional model in the context of genetics.

The 1975 NAS Committee on Inborn Errors of Metabolism recommended the utilization of theories and precepts developed by the health education community:

> Screening authorities could improve the effectiveness of public education by studying and employing methods devised and tested by professional students of health behavior and health education. The use of the mass communication media and other techniques to change attitudes and behavior has not been particularly successful, partly because of failure to follow the appropriate precepts.

The "health belief model" hypothesizes that health-related action depends upon three factors: (1) sufficient motivation (or health concern) to make health issues salient or relevant, (2) perceived threat of a serious health problem, and (3) the belief that following a particular health recommendation would be beneficial in reducing the perceived threat at an acceptable cost (Rosenstock et al., 1988). Some studies have shown that this model has only a very limited value in predicting behavior following genetics-related education (Kaback, 1992).

The social cognitive learning theory (Bandura, 1986) says that behavior is determined by expectancies and incentives (Rosenstock et al., 1988). *Expectancies* include beliefs about how events are connected, opinions about how one's own behavior is likely to influence outcomes, and the ability to influence outcomes. *Incentives* include the value of a particular object or outcome (which may be health status, physical appearance, or other consequences as interpreted by the individual).

BENEFITS AND BURDENS OF GENETICS KNOWLEDGE

Understanding of genetics enhances cultural literacy, engenders understanding of the variety and diversity in ourselves and others, and holds the promise of improved treatment and even possible prevention of some diseases (see Chapter 2). Some experts downplay concerns about the emergence of a "new eugenics" (Motulsky and Murray, 1983; Kevles and Hood, 1992; Motulsky, 1992). However, media attention and recent survey data indicate increasing public concern about these burdens, particularly about discrimination (Miller, 1992). Such burdens include the possible misuse of genetic information (e.g., on particular physical traits[7] such as stature[8] or from behavioral genetics[9]), and possible social stigma or discrimination in personal and family relationships, as well as in insurance, employment, and education.

An informed public is the best societal protection from possible abuses of genetic technology and information in the future. The task, therefore, is to educate the public so that each individual is capable of making an informed decision about seeking or accepting genetic testing and considering personal courses of action. In addition, the public and policy makers must be educated to help them develop appropriate public policy regarding genetic testing and screening. Genetic counseling will ultimately be made more effective by a better-educated public.

FINDINGS AND RECOMMENDATIONS

With the explosion of genetic information over the coming decade, the committee believes that there is both the need and the opportunity to increase public literacy about genetics and genetic testing. Genetic testing is not an end in itself. This educational imperative is intended to develop a genetically literate public that understands basic biological research, understands elements of the personal and health implications of genetics, and participates effectively in public policy issues involving genetic information. This imperative is also intended to develop an understanding of the widely varying personal values and cultural perspectives in our society about complex issues related to genetics.

The committee believes that genetic literacy is essential to individual and public empowerment—for understanding not only ourselves, but our relationships to our families, our communities, and the world.

In contrast to most health behavior strategies, the committee recommends that the goal of genetics health education *not* be to elicit any particular behavioral change, but rather to produce informed decision makers by providing genetics knowledge to increase options, help people make informed choices, and promote an appreciation and acceptance of human variation and differences. The committee recommends more analysis of the implications of applying concepts of public health education to genetics, including analysis of what has been learned from the concepts of the health belief model and the social cognitive theory in relation to health-related decision making in genetics.

The committee therefore recommends that specific funding be devoted to ensuring that all school children receive sufficient education in genetics to enable them to make informed decisions as adults. The committee recommends that systematic genetics education begin in elementary school and be continued throughout formal education. Model programs like those described in this chapter can help to provide the foundation for a genetically informed public, and will be enhanced by the inclusion of ethical, legal, and social issues in genetics. With a solid foundation in school-based education, the public will be better prepared to respond to both scientific and social issues arising from genetics technologies. However, the committee is concerned about the rate of adoption of information imparted by these programs. Further assessment is needed of the impact of these programs and the utilization of the knowledge gained. Evaluation should also include identification of the barriers to integrating genetics—including the social implications—into school curricula, and methods for reducing such barriers.

Variation and kinship in the context of the environment should be the fundamental concepts of genetics education for the public. The committee recommends that genetics education include ethical, legal, and social issues stemming from science and technology. To ensure quality, programs will need the continuing advice of genetics experts to keep them current; this will be a considerable challenge given the rapid rate of knowledge development in genetics.

There is no prospect of having enough specialized professional genetics personnel in the United States to provide the essential education required to prepare the public for personal and public policy decisions as genetic testing becomes more widespread. Nevertheless, the committee recommends that genetics professionals and qualified educators assume responsibility for identifying the essential components of genetic literacy to serve as the basis for expanded public genetics education. This approach to public education about genetics will not be a small or an easy task.

The committee recommends that the Human Genome Project's Ethical, Legal, and Social Implications (ELSI) Program at the National Institutes of Health and the Department of Energy coordinate a public education initiative in genetics and expand its support for such efforts. It will be necessary to bring leaders from education and other professions, other federal agencies, support groups, foundations, and consumers to formulate appropriate goals and strategies. Among the important strategies to be considered are (1) to ensure that appropriate educational messages about genetic tests and their implications reach the public; (2) to incorporate principles, concepts, and skills training that supports informed decision making about genetic testing into all levels of schooling—kindergarten through college; (3) to enhance consumers' knowledge and ability to make informed decisions in either seeking or accepting genetic tests; (4) to establish systems for designing, implementing, and maintaining community-based interventions for the improvement of genetics education among population groups at higher risk of particular genetic disorders (e.g., increased risk related to race or ethnicity); and (5) to enlist the mass media to help decrease consumer confusion and increase the knowledge and skills that will equip consumers to make the most appropriate decisions for themselves.

The National Science Foundation should (1) expand its programs that support model educational initiatives in science for precollege and college programs in molecular biology; (2) collaborate with the ELSI program of the Human Genome Project to encourage such programs to focus the attention of students on the health, social, legal, and ethical issues raised by genetic testing and screening as well as on science; and (3) require evaluation of educational interventions.

Broad public participation will be required to develop educational approaches that respect the widely varying personal and cultural perspectives on issues of genetics, and are tolerant of individuals with genetic disorders of all kinds. Particular effort will be needed to include the perspectives of women, minorities, and persons with disabilities, who may feel especially affected by developing genetics technologies. There is much to be learned from those who are particularly affected by genetic testing technologies, and from those affected by genetic disorders, including persons with disabilities and their families and support groups.

Strategies for enhanced public education could include:

(a) meetings of representatives of national groups of clinical geneticists, counselors, educators, laboratories, foundations, public health officials, genetic support groups, and consumers to explore common interests and develop a common educational initiative;

(b) support for the review of current genetics educational materials prepared by various groups, to foster balance in the presentation of information (including balanced information on the nature of genetic disorders, as well as the benefits and harms of genetic testing), and to ensure that the information is understandable and appropriate to the intended audience;

(c) development and evaluation of existing teacher-tested lessons on genetics for use in a variety of classroom settings at different grade levels;

(d) design of model curricula for teaching and evaluating genetics, as well as the ethical and societal implications of genetic testing and screening, from kindergarten through grade 12—including concepts of respect for genetic diversity (differences) and kinship that can be understood by children of all ages, and treatment of sensitive issues related to reproduction;

(e) recommendation to state boards of education to mandate inclusion of at least one human genetics course in requirements for teacher preparation;

(f) development of a "Consumer's Guide to Genetic Testing" on genetic services, various genetic tests, and the implications of the tests so as to provide balanced, reliable, readily understandable, and available sources of needed information;

(g) support for the development of community-based programs, that focus on the particular needs of special populations who may be at high risk for particular genetic disorders as a consequence of race or ethnicity, and involve appropriate community leaders, centers, churches, and synagogues; and

(h) support for a working group on the role of the media in increasing consumer knowledge about genetics and its application, and considering approaches to decreasing consumer confusion resulting from media reporting of genetics, particularly the impact of exaggeration or sensationalism on public understanding of genetics, as well as on individuals and families affected by genetic disorders.

NOTES

1. In developing its recommendations for the educational interventions for the future, the committee had the benefit of a background paper on current public knowledge and attitudes about genetics prepared by David A. Micklos. Director, DNA Learning Center at Cold Spring Harbor Laboratory (Micklos, 1992).

2. There are a few model programs in addition to those mentioned in this chapter; the North Carolina Biotechnology Center in Research Triangle Park is developing instructional materials and conducting workshops for teachers. The demand for continuing education may increase as teachers are required to prove subject competence and remain conversant with developments in their respective fields (see McInerney, 1987a); testing for human genetic disorders using recombinant DNA technology: The role of the schools in developing public understanding. Paper prepared for the Office of Technology Assessment, unpublished, 1987b).

3. DNA Learning Center, Cold Spring Harbor Laboratory. D.A. Micklos, Director. Cold Spring Harbor, N.Y.

4. Biological Sciences Curriculum Study. Joseph D. McInerney, Director. Colorado Springs, Colo.

5. Project Genethics. Jon R. Hendrix, Founder and Co-director. Ball State University, Muncie, Ind.

6. University of Kansas Medical Center—Medical Genetics. Debra Collins, Director. Kansas City, Kans.

7. A complaint was recently filed with the Federal Trade Commission about a radio talk show on Los Angeles' KFI in which a prominent broadcaster was criticized for her decision to give birth to a child with the same genetic disorder that affects the mother (ectrodactylism, the absence of digits in both hands and feet) (reported in the *Washington Post,* October 20, 1991, p. D1, and on a number of television talk shows and news programs).

8. Two National Institutes of Health (NIH) clinical trials on the use of growth hormone for short stature have raised broad concerns; both trials are now being reevaluated by outside advisory groups appointed by the NIH.

9. Controversy over racial and other ethical, legal, and social implications of a planned conference on genetic factors in crime raised questions about the appropriate goals and purposes of genetics, and the use and misuse of knowledge from behavioral genetics. The controversy resulted in the withdrawal of funding for the conference by the director of NIH, and the appointment by NIH of an outside advisory group to suggest program modifications (*Washington Post,* September 5, 1992, p. A1), even though the conference had been approved by a peer-review group appointed by NIH.

REFERENCES

ABC News Poll. 1990. Public Opinion Online Database. Roper Center for Public Research, Storrs, Conn., May.

American Association for the Advancement of Science (AAAS). 1989a. Pp. 89-90 in Project 2061: Science for All Americans. Washington, D.C.

American Association for the Advancement of Science (AAAS). 1989b. Science for All Americans. Washington, D.C.

Astin, A., et al. 1991. The American Freshman: National Norms for Fall 1991. Cooperative Institutional Research Program, University of California, Los Angeles.

Bandura, A. 1986. Social Foundations of Thought and Action. Englewood Cliffs, N.J.: Prentice Hall.

Biological Sciences Curriculum Study (BSCS). 1978. Guidelines for educational priorities and curricular innovations in human and molecular genetics. BSCS Journal 1(1):20-29.

Bybee, R. (ed.). 1986. NSTA Yearbook: Science Technology Society. National Science Teachers Association. Washington, D.C.

Cunningham, G. 1992 (published in 1994). Statewide governmentally administered prenatal blood screening: A case study in cost-effective prevention. In Fullarton, J. (ed.) Proceedings of the Committee on Assessing Genetic Risks. Washington, D.C.: National Academy Press.

Ebert, J. 1993. National Research Council News Report. National Committee on Science Education Standards and Assessment, Washington, D.C.

Farquhar, J. 1992. Presentation before the Committee on Prevention of Mental Disorders, Institute of Medicine, Washington, D.C.

Holtzman, N. 1989. Pp. 156-157 in Proceed with Caution. Baltimore, Md.: The Johns Hopkins University Press.

Hurd, P. 1985. Science education for a new age: The reform movement. National Association of Secondary School Principals Bulletin 69(482):83.

Kaback, M. 1992 (published in 1994). Genetic knowledge and attitudes: A multi-ethnic study. In Fullarton, J. (ed.) Proceedings of the Committee on Assessing Genetic Risks. Washington, D.C.: National Academy Press.

Keller, E. 1992. Nature, nurture, and the Human Genome Project. In Kevles, D., and Hood, L. (eds.) The Code of Codes. Cambridge, Mass.: Harvard University Press.

Kevles, D., and Hood, L. (eds). 1992. The Code of Codes. Cambridge, Mass.: Harvard University Press.

Levi-Pearl, S. 1992 (published in 1994). From a consumer's perspective. In Fullarton, J. (ed.) Proceedings of the Committee on Assessing Genetic Risks. Washington, D.C.: National Academy Press.

Lippman, A. 1992 (published in 1994). Presentation at the Workshop on Prenatal Diagnosis Proceedings, IOM Committee on Assessing Genetic Risks, Irvine, Calif. In Fullarton, J. (ed.) Proceedings of the Committee on Assessing Genetic Risks. Washington, D.C.: National Academy Press.

Lippman-Hand, A., and Fraser, F. 1979. Genetic counseling: Parents' responses to uncertainty. Birth Defects: Original Article Series 15:325-339.

March of Dimes Birth Defects Foundation News Release. 1992a. White Plains, N.Y., September 29.

March of Dimes Birth Defects Foundation. 1992b. Genetic Testing and Gene Therapy National Survey Findings. Louis Harris and Associates, White Plains, N.Y.

McInerney, J. 1987a. Curriculum development at the Biological Sciences Curriculum Study. Educational Leadership 44(4):24.

McInerney, J. 1987b. Testing for human genetic disorders using recombinant DNA technology: The role of the schools in developing public understanding. Unpublished paper prepared for the Office of Technology Assessment.

Micklos, D. 1992 (published in 1994). Public education in genetics. In Fullarton, J. (ed.) Proceedings of the Committee on Assessing Genetic Risks. Washington, D.C.: National Academy Press.

Micklos, D., and Kruper, J. 1991. Preparing for the gene age: A profile of innovative high school science teachers in 22 states. Unpublished manuscript.

Miller, J. 1992. The Public Understanding of Science and Technology in the United States, 1990. Report to the National Science Foundation, Washington, D.C.

Motulsky, A. 1992. Book Review of Backdoor to Eugenics by T. Duster. American Journal of Human Genetics.

Motulsky, A., and Murray J. 1983. Will prenatal diagnosis with selective abortion affect society's attitude toward the handicapped? Pp. 277-291 in Berg, K., and Tranoy, K. (eds.) Research Ethics. New York: Liss.

National Academy of Sciences (NAS). 1975. Genetic Screening: Programs, Principles, and Research. Committee for the Study of Inborn Errors of Metabolism. Washington, D.C.: NAS.

National Opinion Research Center (NORC). 1990. General social science survey 9/1990. Public Opinion Online Database. Roper Center for Public Research, Storrs, Conn.

National Opinion Research Center (NORC). 1991. General social science survey 9/1991. Public Opinion Online Database. Roper Center for Public Research, Storrs, Conn.

Office of Technology Assessment (OTA). 1987. Public Perceptions: New Developments in Biotechnology. Washington, D.C.: U.S. Government Printing Office.

President's Commission for the Study of Ethical Problems in Medicine and Biomedical and Behavioral Research. 1983. Screening and Counseling for Genetic Conditions: The Ethical, Social, and Legal Implications of Genetic Screening, Counseling, and Education Programs. Washington, D.C.

Press, N., and Browner, C. 1992 (published in 1994). Policy issues in maternal serum alpha-fetoprotein. In Fullarton, J. (ed.) Proceedings of the Committee on Assessing Genetic Risks. Washington, D.C.: National Academy Press.

Reilly, D. 1989. A knowledge base for education: Cognitive science. Journal of Teacher Education 40(3):9-13.

Rosenburg, M. 1992. Presentation before the Committee on Prevention of Mental Disorders, Institute of Medicine, Washington, D.C.: U.S. Government Printing Office.

Rosenstock, I., et al. 1988. Social learning theory and the health belief model. Health Education Quarterly 15(2):175-183.

Rothman, B. 1992 (published in 1994). The tentative pregnancy: Then and now. In Fullarton, J. (ed.) Proceedings of the Committee on Assessing Genetic Risks. Washington, D.C.: National Academy Press.

Rutherford, J., and Ahlgren, A. 1988. Rethinking the science curriculum. In Brandt, R. (ed.) Content of the Curriculum. Alexandria, Va.: Association for Supervision and Curriculum Development.

Saunders, W. 1992. The constructivist perspective: Implications and teaching strategies for science. School Science and Mathematics 92(3):136-141.

U.S. Department of Health and Human Services (USDHHS) and U.S. Department of Energy (US-DOE). 1990. Understanding Our Genetic Inheritance. The Human Genome Project: The First Five Years FY 1991-1995. NIH Publication No. 90-1580. National Center for Human Genome Research, Bethesda, Md.

U.S. Department of Health and Human Services (USDHHS) and U.S. Department of Energy (US-DOE). 1991. Request for Applications: Ethical, Legal, and Social Implications of the Human Genome Project. National Institutes of Health, Bethesda, Md.; Request for Proposals, Department of Energy, Oak Ridge, Tenn.

Walker, R., et al. 1980. Sequenced instruction in genetics and Piagetian cognitive development. American Biology Teacher 42(2):104-105.

Watson, J. 1992. Seminar presented at the Department of Energy-sponsored workshop on Human Genetics and Genome Analysis for Public Policy Makers and Opinion Leaders, Cold Spring Harbor Laboratory, February 26.

Yager, R. 1991. The constructivist learning model. The Science Teacher 58(6):53-57.

6

Personnel Issues in
Human Genetics

Historically, genetic tests have been administered and interpreted by highly trained health professionals working in academic health settings, usually with a strong genetics research and service record. In the future, however, genetic tests will become available for a growing variety of monogenic and complex diseases and for susceptibility to more common disorders such as breast, colon, and other cancers. Testing on such a broad scale will necessarily move us beyond the models of service delivery and professional roles that have characterized genetic testing and screening in the past. Increasingly, genetic tests will be offered and interpreted within the context of the mainstream of medicine in primary care practice—including pediatrics, obstetrics, internal medicine, and family practice in a variety of individual and group practice settings.

This exciting and challenging prospect for the future involves a large pool of potential personnel for genetic testing, screening, education, and counseling, but will they be prepared to play this role? How will primary care practitioners be trained to provide these services appropriately and to understand the complexities and limitations of genetic tests? How will they be trained to provide the nondirective counseling that is absolutely essential in reproductive decisions and in testing for disorders for which there is no effective treatment? Once trained, how will primary care practitioners keep up with the exponential growth in knowledge about the role of genetics in health and about genetic tests?

This chapter presents an overview of available data on specialized genetics personnel and primary care practitioners, as well as information on their training in and knowledge of genetics. The chapter also examines the personnel implications arising from the trends in genetic testing and screening discussed elsewhere in the report. The committee considered whether there will be enough adequately trained health professionals in the future to handle the potential volume, diversity, and complexity of genetic tests, and to perform specific functions in genetic services, such as laboratory testing, taking family history, diagnosis, education, counseling, technical support, and research.[1] This chapter addresses the separate issues of specialized genetics education for specialists and genetics education for generalists (primary care practitioners), recognizing that both will be needed as more genetic tests become available. The following section focuses on current and future supplies of genetic specialists and their certification. The latter half of the chapter addresses, more broadly, the issues surrounding genetics education in medical school and general practice, and the potential role of other health professionals in providing genetics services. The chapter concludes with recommendations intended to help prepare the nation for changes likely to be brought about by widespread genetic testing. These recommendations include suggestions for research to better inform policy makers as they prepare for that future.

GENETIC SPECIALISTS

Many types of professionals provide specialized genetic services: physicians, Ph.D. clinical geneticists, genetic counselors, nurses, and social workers. Other individuals trained as research scientists are involved in genetics research. A large medical center that provides genetic services and conducts research is likely to employ individuals at all levels—master's, Ph.D., and M.D. Smaller private or community-based hospitals are likely to employ master's-level genetic counselors or nurses and physicians trained in genetics. Until recently, Ph.D. geneticists and genetic counselors were not able to see patients without the oversight of an M.D., but changes in the certification status of these individuals may change their roles in the clinical setting (see below). Although available data indicate that the numbers of individuals graduating from human genetics training programs are increasing, it is not clear that this increase is occurring at the rate necessary to ensure adequate and appropriate levels of support for genetic services in the future.

Furthermore, the geographic distribution of genetic specialists will be critical in ensuring access to individuals needing genetic services. Currently, genetics professionals tend to be clustered in the Northeast and on the West Coast, as well as in the Chicago area. A survey of genetic counselors and nurses working in genetics showed a heavy concentration of counselors in five states, with 43 percent of respondents located in California, Illinois, New Jersey, New York, and Pennsylvania (OTA, 1992b). This uneven distribution of scarce genetic practitioners is even more limiting given the specialized expertise of many genetic centers in a relatively small number of genetic disorders. As a result, families must often travel long distances to receive specialized genetic services for a particular genetic disorder.

Reimbursement policies regarding genetic testing also have a significant effect on personnel issues. Currently, genetic counselors cannot be reimbursed directly; genetic counseling must be authorized and billed by a physician for insurance reimbursement. If these reimbursement practices continue, it is not clear whether full genetics services will be provided as needed, including essential education and counseling. Because primary care practitioners are able to obtain reimbursement for genetic consultation as a type of office visit, patients might be more inclined to seek care through this route than through a route that could involve out-of-pocket expenses (see Chapter 7).

Some of the controversy about personnel needs stems from uncertainty about who will be providing genetic services in the future. For example, one study estimated that a minimum of 651,000 counseling hours would be required annually if the maximum estimate of 6 to 8 million preconceptional couples are screened for cystic fibrosis (CF) carrier status (Wilfond and Fost, 1990). Given the current number of practicing genetic counselors in the United States today, this translates to 17 weeks per year from each genetic counselor just to serve CF-related clients. This study concluded that CF screening could not be offered solely through specialized genetics centers; it is likely that this and genetic tests of significance in making reproductive decisions, such as carrier screening, will be offered increasingly by obstetrician-gynecologists.

Background Data on Genetics Professionals

As early as 1985—prior to the initiation of the Human Genome Project—concerns were raised about the availability of clinical genetics personnel. In a survey of 476 programs providing genetic services in the United States, 195 programs supplied data on predoctoral and postdoctoral trainees (Finley et al., 1987). A total of 524 students were enrolled in medical genetics training in the 195 training programs; of these, 224 (43 percent) were postdoctoral candidates, 193 (37 percent) were doctoral candidates, and 107 (20 percent) were master's candidates. The study also asked about the number of job vacancies, both current and anticipated, for the next five years: in 1985, there were 150 vacancies, of which 36 percent were for cytogenetic technicians, 27 percent for M.D. clinical geneticists, and 19 percent for genetic counselors. Over the period 1986 through 1990, more than 600 vacancies were anticipated by these 195 programs (Finley et al., 1987).

The American Society of Human Genetics (ASHG)—a nonprofit professional society founded in 1948—serves as the primary scientific and professional society for all human geneticists in North America. It routinely surveys its membership as well as the graduate and postgraduate training programs from which its members come. Its 1989 survey gathered data on its approximately 4,000 members (Garver and Lent, 1990). Membership distribution according to highest degree obtained is 44 percent Ph.D.'s, 29 percent M.D.'s, 20 percent master's, and 7 percent M.D.-Ph.D.'s. Graduate degree distributions appear to be changing (Table 6-1).

In terms of current enrollment in human genetics training programs, 64 percent of the students are in Ph.D. programs (both predoctoral and postdoctoral), 22

TABLE 6-1 Graduates from Human Genetics Training Programs, 1984-1992

Degree	1984-1985	1986-1987	1988-1989	1991-1992
Masters, Genetic Counseling	147	156	168	155
Other Masters	97	62	81	118
Subtotal	234	218	249	273
Doctoral, Ph.D. in Human Genetics	155	129	132	185
Postdoctoral				
M.D.	108	134	159	157
Ph.D.	81	88	122	185
M.D./Ph.D.	3	1	6	7
Subtotal	192	223	287	349
Grand total	581	570	662	807

SOURCES: Riccardi and Smith, 1986; Friedman and Riccardi, 1988; Murray and Toriello, 1990; Blitzer, 1992.

percent are in master's-level programs, and 14 percent are in M.D. or M.D-Ph.D. programs (Blitzer, 1992). Although there has been steady growth in the number of graduates of human genetics training programs since 1985 (807 individuals completed training in 1992, compared with 581 in 1985), postdoctoral fellows account for approximately 74 percent of the growth (Riccardi and Smith, 1986; Murray and Toriello, 1990). Many of these programs are not oriented to delivering clinical genetics services, particularly preparation in the behavioral sciences essential for genetic counseling. Also, since most Ph.D.-level geneticists enter into research- or laboratory-oriented activities, the growing number of Ph.D. postdoctoral students appears to indicate a trend toward research or laboratory careers.

From limited available data, it appears that only a relatively small percentage of people attaining these doctorates enters medical genetics, although some of these Ph.D. geneticists are also likely to work in clinical laboratories. Since the majority of genetic testing is currently being done in research laboratories, some of this pool of Ph.D. geneticists is likely to be involved in human genetics and genetic testing and screening as part of research programs; however, most Ph.D.'s will not be providing traditional genetics services or practicing in traditional medical genetics settings. Since they do not have the clinical training required for some aspects of medical genetics, Ph.D.'s have often been discouraged from entering medical genetics.

Individuals with M.S. degrees from established programs in genetic counseling are more likely to pursue traditional clinical genetics service careers. However, the number of graduates with an M.D. or M.S. has remained relatively stable, with only slight increases in the numbers of physicians specializing in genetics.

Of those M.D.'s who do complete their training in genetics, most are in pediatrics (59 percent), followed by internal medicine (12 percent), obstetrics (10 percent), and "other" (16 percent). As genetic tests for presymptomatic and predispositional assessment become more widely available, therefore, there may not be enough physicians trained to provide the necessary specialized genetics services, including the education and genetic counseling that will be essential if and when more widespread genetic testing and screening develop in the future. This will require close attention over the next three to five years.

Another growing area of concern involves the effects of market forces on the training and career paths of genetics professionals. Anecdotal evidence suggests that commercial laboratories are drawing personnel away from academic laboratories. This poses problems for the future training of genetics professionals, since commercial facilities are less likely to provide advanced clinical training than academic centers. For example, the committee heard reports that commercial laboratories recently have begun to buy genetic testing laboratories in academic institutions and to discontinue fellowships and other advanced genetics training in those laboratories.

Although there is a need for trained genetics personnel for research and laboratory testing, the readily available funding for research training appears to be leading more genetics students to enter career paths leading to potential research careers rather than to clinical genetics careers.

Training Programs

The total number of human genetics training programs increased slightly between 1984 and 1992, from 99 to 111 (see Table 6-2) (Riccardi and Smith, 1986; Friedman and Riccardi, 1988; Murray and Toriello, 1990; Blitzer, 1992). Approximately 40 percent of human genetics graduates have come from 10 percent of the human genetics training programs. The American Board of Medical Genetics (ABMG) accredits most U.S. human genetics training programs, although it accredits only the clinical training *sites* of the master's-level genetic counseling programs. ABMG certification by subspecialty is shown in Figures 6-1 and 6-2 and Table 6-3.

TABLE 6-2   Number of North American Human Genetics Training Programs

Programs	1984-1985	1986-1987	1988-1989	1990-1991	1992-1993
Total listings	99	106	120	120	111
Degree-granting	68	66	83	83	69
Nondegree-granting	31	40	37	37	42

SOURCES: Riccardi and Smith, 1986; Friedman and Riccardi, 1988; Murray and Toriello, 1990; Blitzer, 1992.

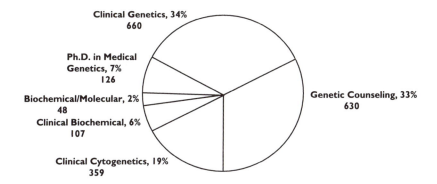

FIGURE 6-1 Number of certificates awarded by the American Board of Medical Genetics by subspecialty area, 1981-1990.

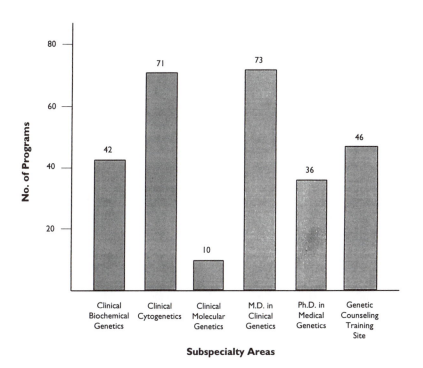

FIGURE 6-2 Number of training programs and genetic counseling training sites accredited by the American Board of Medical Genetics (AMBG). Based on AMBG data as of May 1991.

TABLE 6-3 ABMG Certification by Year and Subspecialty Area

Subspecialty	No. of Diplomates per Exam Year				Total No. of Certificates	% of Diplomates[a]
	1981	1984	1987	1990		
Clinical biochemical	57	24	26	48[b]	155	9
Clinical cytogenetics	125	71	100	63	359	22
Genetic counseling	169	143	177	141	630	38
Clinical genetics	286	127	111	136	660	40
Ph.D. medical genetics	56	31	26	13	126	8
Total	693	396	440	401	1,930	

[a]Percentage of total number of diplomates (N = 1,639); certification in more than one subspecialty possible.

[b]Certified as biochemical-molecular geneticists (1990 only); since 1993 a separate subspecialty exam in molecular genetics has been available.

SOURCE: Records of the American Board of Medical Genetics (1991).

The curriculum of doctoral or postdoctoral training in human genetics has not been extensively reviewed. However, as part of the process of accreditation for their clinical training through ABMG, human genetics training programs must submit extensive data on their programs (see Box 6-1).

Master's-Level Genetic Counselors

The master's-level genetic counselor is a relatively new addition to the human genetics community. There are approximately 1,000 master's-level genetic counselors practicing in the United States, 100 times more than the 10 first graduated in 1971. To date, genetic counselors have been certified by the ABMG (currently 68 percent are certified), and their training has both reflected and shaped the requirements of that board.

Genetic counselors formed their own professional organization in 1979, the National Society of Genetic Counselors (NSGC). Current membership includes more than 1,000 individuals working in the United States and several foreign countries. More than 80 percent of the members are in clinical practice, with most working in a university medical center or a private hospital (OTA, 1992b; Uhlmann, 1992).

The curriculum of master's-level genetic counseling training programs has evolved over time and is a balance of medical genetics, practical and theoretical counseling, and behavioral sciences. During the 1970s, a series of meetings were held to discuss the role and educational needs of the genetic associate or genetic counselor (Genetics Associates, 1979). Then, in 1989, a conference held in Asilomar reevaluated recommendations for the minimum program curriculum of master's-level training in genetic counseling (Walker et al., 1990). The recommenda-

---

BOX 6-1   ABMG Accreditation Requirements

The American Board of Medical Genetics (ABMG) conducts an extensive review of doctoral and postdoctoral training in programs applying for its accreditation. Its application process includes:

- a brief history of the training program and program objectives;
- a list of faculty (where trained, degree, year of degree, and area of research);
- a description of each required and optional course offered, the number of contact hours, and to whom it is offered;
- a list of seminars offered in the last two years;
- an outline of weekly schedules and annual plans of activities for each subspecialty;
- a list of trainees over the last five years, including information on past history, number of years in training, present position, source of funding, and research area during training;
- a list of current trainees;
- data concerning clinical caseload such as number of cases by etiology and number of cases for inpatient consult, prenatal diagnosis, initial visits, or return visits;
- data concerning laboratory caseload (cytogenetic, biochemical, or molecular); and
- laboratory participation in and results of quality control audits.

---

tions were based in part on requirements for certification through the ABMG. The need for and desirability of training beyond the master's level in genetic counseling (i.e., doctoral study) was also discussed along with alternatives to master's-level training to overcome a projected shortage of genetic counseling personnel. A 1989 survey of NSGC members indicated that just over half of those responding saw a need for a doctoral (Ph.D.) degree in the field of genetic counseling, while 30 percent were undecided (Gaupman et al., 1991). To date, there is one program (University of Pittsburgh) offering a doctoral degree in genetic counseling.

The Asilomar conference recommended a minimum curriculum at the master's level that includes seven specific didactic course work content areas, as well as a broad scope of clinical experience; these include

1. principles and application of human genetics and related sciences;
2. principles and practice of clinical and medical genetics;
3. genetic laboratory methods;
4. theory and application of interviewing and counseling;
5. social, ethical, legal, and cultural issues;
6. health care delivery systems and principles of public health; and
7. teaching.

The scope of clinical experience includes participation as primary genetic counselor in at least 50 cases, in three or more clinic settings (e.g., general genetics, prenatal diagnosis, specialty diseases); supervision by a geneticist or ABMG-certified genetic counselor; and demonstration of competence in the skills of genetic counseling.

Experience in several additional areas was deemed desirable, but not mandatory, for minimum clinical experience, including service delivery, screening programs, cross-cultural issues, community and professional education, and clinic administration. Master's-level genetic counselors receive specialized multidisciplinary training and experience to prepare them for counseling related to a wide variety of genetic disorders, including late-onset adult disorders, as well as birth defects. The committee strongly recommends the incorporation of these essential areas into all genetic counseling curricula, particularly as new programs develop.

Over the past 20 years, master's-level graduate programs in genetic counseling have increased to 14 in the United States, and one in Canada (see Table 6-4). Combined, they produce approximately 81 graduates each year (77 in the United States and 4 in Canada), but 30 percent of all graduates in a given year come from one training program, Sarah Lawrence College (New York), the oldest program in the United States.

TABLE 6-4   Master's-Level Programs in Genetic Counseling in the United States and Canada

School	Average No. of Graduates per Year
Howard University	3
Medical College of Virginia	1
Northwestern University	4
Sarah Lawrence College	23
University of California, Berkeley	8
University of California, Irvine	3
University of Cincinnati	2
University of Colorado	5
University of Michigan	4
University of Minnesota	3
University of Pittsburgh	12
University of South Carolina	3
University of Texas, Houston	1
University of Wisconsin, Madison	5
McGill University, Canada	4
Total	81

SOURCE: Riccardi and Smith, 1986; Friedman and Riccardi, 1988; Murray and Toriello, 1990; Blitzer, 1992.

BOX 6-2   Genetic Counseling Personnel in New York State

A recent, limited pilot survey was conducted by Zinberg and Greendale (1991) to assess whether a shortage of genetic counselors existed in New York State in 1990. In their study, 57 comprehensive and specific genetic disease centers were asked about their level of genetic counselor staffing. A total of 103 ABMG-certified or board-eligible genetic counselors were employed at the 57 centers. Ninety-four percent of these were graduates from an NSGC-recognized genetic counseling training program.

This study also examined the overall attrition rate and found it to be very high. In the previous two years, 56 genetic counselors had been hired, the majority of whom were to fill 34 positions left vacant in New York by staff departures.

Recognizing the need for additional genetic counselors, the state of New York developed two new initiatives to meet personnel demands. First, a new certificate program is offered by the Division of Medical and Molecular Genetics at Mt. Sinai Medical Center to prepare individuals with master's degrees in related fields for ABMG certification in genetic counseling. Second, as part of their request for funding for genetic services, New York genetics providers may now obtain partial support, in the form of salary, stipend, or scholarship, for a graduate student enrolled in a master's-level program in genetic counseling. Once graduated, the student would be committed to work at the sponsoring institution for a period of three years.

Training support for master's-level genetic counselors has been minimal. The U.S. Department of Health and Human Services (DHHS) provides no financial support for the training of genetic counselors or for improving genetics education in medical schools (Holtzman, 1989). However, the Maternal and Child Health Program of DHHS's Health Resources and Services Administration provides support to the Council of Regional Networks for Genetic Services (CORN) for some continuing professional education programs for physicians and postdoctoral students, but not for master's-level counselors. The same explosion of new genetic information affects genetic counseling, and continuing education is just as essential for genetic counselors (NSGC, 1991; Gettig, 1992).

Although an average of 77 graduates entered the nation's work force annually from 1984 to 1992, the demand for genetic counselors continues to exceed the available supply. According to the NSGC executive office, from 1988 to 1991 there were at least 35 unfilled genetic counseling positions listed with its Jobs Hotline at any given time. The total number of unfilled positions nationwide is unknown. However, an attempt to answer this question for the state of New York suggests that the number is high (see Box 6-2). Finally, there appears to be some attrition of existing master's-level genetic counselors into full-time administration or away from the profession altogether. Not nearly enough is known at this time about how many master's-level genetic counselors are now or will be needed, since so many uncertainties exist about the nature and scope of their role in the future.

Non-Master's-Level Counselors

Research to examine a "train-the-trainer" model for increasing the availability of genetic counseling in the United States is being supported by the Ethical, Legal, and Social Implications (ELSI) Program of the National Center for Human Genome Research at the National Institutes of Health (NIH). As the profession has developed, master's-level counselors have begun taking on the role of trainers of other health professionals. In some clinical settings, master's-level genetic counselors are training non-master's-level individuals to meet the demand for patient education related to a single diagnostic category of disease. In other settings, non-master's-level individuals assist genetic counselors in overcoming cultural, linguistic, geographic, or economic barriers.

Individuals who assist genetic counselors, often called "single-gene counselors," "single-disorder counselors," or "non-master's-level counselors," do not have the same training as master's-level genetic counselors and have not been eligible for ABMG certification. With the growth of genetic services and increasing demands on the time and resources of traditionally trained counselors, the use of these individuals has stimulated debate. A number of programs have been developed to train non-master's-level educators or counselors (see Box 6-3).

Advocates for the use of single-disorder counselors cite the limited number of practicing genetic counselors and the increasing development of genetic testing as reasons to support this type of training. Single-disorder counselors could also improve the quality of service in underserved, culturally diverse populations that are disproportionately affected by a particular genetic disease (OTA, 1992a).

Those opposed to single-disorder counselors express concern about what they view as a lack of genetics and genetic counseling training. There is also concern about whether single-disorder counselors have a broad enough view of clinical genetics to identify complex and obscure risks of other genetic disorders in their patients. Since taking a family history often exposes previously unknown or undiagnosed genetic disorders or predispositions, individuals who focus on one category of disease might not recognize the need to further investigate peripheral information.

An NSGC task force made the following recommendations to the society:

• acknowledge the current and predicted personnel needs for genetic counselors, as well as the shortage of master's-level genetic counselors;

• recognize the existing use of non-master's-level counselors and the benefits they offer;

• educate NSGC membership regarding the potential use of these individuals;

BOX 6-3 Single-Disorder Educator-Counselor Programs

Genetic counselors have been involved in developing and conducting training programs in several states. In California and Massachusetts, established programs lasting four days to one month, respectively, provide training to become a sickle cell educator-counselor or a hemoglobin trait counselor. Students are trained and supervised by master's-level genetic counselors. In addition to training, the California program also provides certification for sickle cell educators-counselors. The sickle cell educators must attend a four-day training course and pass a final certification examination. The sickle cell counselor must meet these same requirements plus attend an additional two-day counseling course and counseling practicum.

San Francisco General Hospital utilizes genetic aides to provide patient advocacy and education, and to act as liaisons between non-English-speaking patients and the genetic counselor. These bilingual or multilingual individuals are trained and supervised by genetic counselors, who continue to serve as case managers. A similar genetic aide program also exists at the University of California at San Diego. To date, the numbers of trained genetic aides remain relatively small. However, with the increasing Southeast Asian population in California, the need for multilingual individuals to provide state-supported genetic services is increasing. Actual job titles of such individuals vary according to their role or function and include, but are not limited to, single-gene counselor, single-disorder counselor, hemoglobin trait counselor, sickle cell educator, sickle cell counselor, genetic counseling aide, genetics educator, and genetic interpreter.

- support the use of non-master's-level counselors in specific settings where genetic counselors can be involved in training, evaluating, and supervising these individuals; and
- establish a committee to collaborate with other organizations.

Certification and Accreditation of Genetics Specialists

Genetics professionals who are physicians are licensed by the states as physicians. Certification procedures for specialties are voluntary but might be a requirement for employment or reimbursement in some settings. Genetic counselors and Ph.D. geneticists are not licensed by states, but until 1992 were certified by the ABMG (see Box 6-4). Ph.D. geneticists continue to be certified by the ABMG.

As of the 1990 exam cycle, 1,639 total diplomates had been certified. A breakdown of the number of diplomates by year and subspecialty is shown in Table 6-3. The percentage of certificates awarded according to subspecialty area is depicted in Figure 6-1.

**BOX 6-4   Certification by the American
Board of Medical Genetics**

The ABMG was incorporated in 1980 at the request of the American Society of Human Genetics to provide accreditation of training programs and certification of individuals in the United States who provide medical genetics service. Until 1992, certification was available for the following subspecialties: clinical geneticist, Ph.D. medical geneticist, genetic counselor, clinical biochemical geneticist, and clinical cytogeneticist. Four exam cycles have occurred: 1981, 1984, 1987, and 1990. During the 1990 cycle, dual certification as a clinical biochemical/molecular geneticist was available; independent certification as a clinical molecular geneticist has been available since 1993.

Eligibility to sit for ABMG examinations requires application and credential review. Eligibility criteria include, but are not limited to, training in a required set of clinical experiences and verification of training in an ABMG-accredited clinical genetics training program. For the subspecialties of M.D. clinical geneticist, Ph.D. medical geneticist, clinical biochemical geneticist, clinical cytogeneticist, and clinical molecular geneticist, a minimum of two years of postdoctoral training experience through appropriate ABMG-accredited training programs is required. The genetic counselor subspecialty requires at least one year of clinical experience in one or more ABMG-accredited genetic counseling training sites, although the master's-level genetic counseling programs per se are not accredited by ABMG as they are for other subspecialties.

In Canada, an equivalent certifying body to the U.S. ABMG, the Canadian College of Medical Geneticists, also provides certification in clinical genetics, Ph.D. medical genetics, cytogenetics, biochemical genetics, and molecular genetics, but not for genetic counselors.

The status of certification changed in 1992 when the American Board of Medical Specialties (ABMS) agreed to admit the American Board of Medical Genetics to its ranks, the first such admission since 1979. ABMS has never admitted a board that certifies non-doctoral-level individuals and had, to this date, only admitted one other board that certified doctoral-level specialists who were not physicians. In order to gain admission, the ABMG had to agree not to certify master's-level genetic counselors in the 1993 examination.

Acceptance of both M.D.'s and Ph.D.'s in the ABMS was considered a victory by some, as was the admission to ABMS, which had previously not recognized medical genetics as a bona fide medical specialty. This precedent also paves the way for the newly formed American College of Medical Genetics (ACMG) to seek recognition by the American Medical Association (AMA) and to be granted a seat in the AMA House of Delegates, which is essential for the development of additional current procedural terminology (CPT) codes for genetic procedures (used in billing and insurance reimbursement policy)(see Chapter 7). Others are concerned that this medical subspecialization may further isolate medical genetics from general medicine at a time when it most needs to be integrated into routine medical education and practice, and that it is motivated to improve revenues for genetic services. For the first time, Ph.D. clinical geneticists will be able to set fees, be reimbursed by insurance companies, and not be under the supervision of an M.D. Genetic counselors who were not already certified by the ABMG have established an American Board of Genetic Counseling.

Beginning in 1993, the ABMG will provide accreditation of U.S. clinical genetics training programs for all six subspecialties; prior to 1990, molecular genetics accreditation was not available. Accreditation of Canadian training programs is available through the Canadian College of Medical Genetics (CCMG) in the same areas, except genetic counseling. As of May 1991, 81 programs had received accreditation through the ABMG in at least one of the six subspecialty areas (Table 6-4). The CCMG has accredited eight training programs. A breakdown of the training programs accredited by ABMG and CCMG is shown in Table 6-5.

At present, there is no national certification or standard for training, supervision, or job responsibilities for genetics service providers without graduate training. The state of California provides both training and certification for sickle cell educators and sickle cell counselors. Certification is based on completion of the California training program requirements and passing the certification examination. Other states are looking at this program as a model. In addition, a proposal to initiate a national effort to provide training accreditation and certification of sickle cell counselors-educators was endorsed by CORN at its fall 1990 meeting, but this proposal has not yet been implemented.

Related Genetics Certification and Training: Cytogenetics

In 1981, the Association of Cytogenetic Technologists (ACT), in conjunction with the National Certification Agency of Medical Laboratory Personnel (NCAM-LP), developed and administered a technologist certification examination in cyto-

TABLE 6-5 Accredited Clinical Genetics Training Programs by Subspecialty Area

Subspecialty	ABMG	CCMG	Total
Clinical biochemical genetics	42	44	6
Clinical cytogenetics	71	6	77
Clinical molecular genetics	10	3	13
M.D. clinical genetics	73	8	81
Ph.D. medical genetics	36	3	39
Genetic counseling training site	46	NA	46

SOURCES: ABMG Executive Office, personal communication, May 1991; Murray and Toriello, 1990.

genetics. More than 1,500 individuals have been certified. Recertification is also available, either by accumulation of continuing education units or by retaking and passing the certification examination.

The majority of cytogenetic technologists have university degrees in scientific fields. Historically, however, cytogenetic training has been acquired on the job. With rapid developments in the field of cytogenetics in recent years, there has been an increasing demand for trained cytogenetic technologists. Training programs in cytogenetic technology were established in 1980 to meet this demand.

The annual number of graduates has been approximately 60 to 80 (1987 data). Job surveys conducted by ACT in cooperation with other groups document a demand that exceeds the supply of qualified people in clinical cytogenetics. Since 1987, more than 400 jobs have been available each year, with only 60 to 80 graduates. The current number of graduates is anticipated to meet only 10 to 15 percent of the human resource needs of clinical cytogenetic laboratories in the future (Fatemi and Gasparini, 1990).

GENETICS INSTRUCTION IN MEDICAL SCHOOLS

Increasingly, primary care physicians will be called on to interpret tests results, relay this information to the patient in an accurate and sensitive manner, and deal with the sometimes profound impact such information can have on the patient's psychological well-being. Attention to genetics education in the nation's medical schools has not increased to meet this growing demand (see Box 6-5). The emergence of a variety of genetic indicators of the more common multifactorial conditions, such as diabetes and heart disease, means that genetics will increasingly touch nearly every discipline in medicine. Yet perhaps the persistent notion that genetic diseases are inevitable and untreatable has delayed more rapid integration of genetics into medical school curricula (Motulsky, 1983; Davidson and Childs, 1987).

Few studies have examined physicians' knowledge of genetics or their awareness of the availability of tests for genetic disorders (Naylor, 1975; Lemkus et al., 1978; Kapur et al., 1983; Firth and Lindenbaum, 1992; Hofman et al., 1993). Recent data show that there is a significant upward trend in total genetics knowledge as a function of year of graduation from medical school. In fact, year of graduation is the most powerful predictor of knowledge (Hofman et al., 1993). Having a required genetics course in medical school was also a significant predictor of genetics knowledge.

The level of instruction in genetics in medical schools has been a source of concern and recommendation for nearly 20 years (NAS, 1975; Childs et al., 1981; Riccardi and Schmickel, 1988; Graham et al., 1989). The 1975 National Academy of Sciences report reported on a survey that included questions on past medical education and identification of potential barriers to genetic screening by physicians (pediatricians, internists, and obstetrician-gynecologists). Nearly 75

**BOX 6-5   Reflections on the Inclusion of
Genetics in Medical Education**

By Barton Childs

One way of discussing the assimilation of genetics into medical education is to ask how genetic risks should be presented in the curriculum. Should it be in practical ways: for example how to calculate risks and impart them to actual patients and their relatives? Or should genetic risks be presented first as inherent in the way nature deals with the perpetuation of the species? Posing the two approaches in this manner highlights the tension in medical education between training and education; tension that exists because the exigency of medicine tends to give primacy to training. Education embodies the principles and ideas of disease and health, whereas training represents exercises in problem solving and dealing with disease whether or not its mysteries can be solved.

There is a widespread and profound uneasiness in the minds of medical educators, a sense that something has gone wrong even when so much about medical practice seems to have gone right. Two aspects of this concern stand out; a) technology seems to have gotten itself interposed between the doctor and the patient so that students are perhaps less likely to be brought up in an atmosphere of deep humane concern for the feelings and fears of sick people than once they were; and b) the volume of knowledge to be absorbed is enormous and sometimes results in a lack of coherence for the student. The challenge for medical education is how to proceed from the facts of reductionism, with its arcane language of acronyms, letters and numbers, through the many levels of integration by which these fundamental units coalesce into the systems that inform the unity of the organism.

Genetics courses given to first and second year students should serve two missions; to teach the rudiments of genetics to students with variable background, and at the same time to make clear that there *is* such a thing as medical genetics as a separate entity. There is always the risk that the latter will be over emphasized, or that the students will draw the conclusion for themselves that the main application of genetics is to a medical specialty called medical genetics. Since most entering students today have been exposed to the basics of mendelism, a shift could be effected from emphasis on the facts of genetics to the ideas of genetics, to the preparation of the mind to receive at a later time the quite different ideas of practice. This would necessarily move emphasis from mendelizing disorders to multifactorial conditions which comprise most of medicine. SOURCE: Childs, 1992.

---

percent of responding physicians reported that no courses in genetics had been available during their medical training; even among those in practice less than six years, only half reported that such courses had been available to them. This survey also identified substantial differences among specialties in the perceived frequency of genetic defects; pediatricians and obstetricians believed genetic diseases to be more common than did family practitioners. The conclusion of the 1975 report was that "the medical profession as represented by the three subspecialties studied is not as a whole ready to accept the importance of genetic disease and of screening for it at the present time." However, the readiness of physicians could be increased "if physicians had greater knowledge of genetics, deeper appreciation of the impact of untreated genetic disease on families, and more direct experience with genetic disease" (NAS, 1975, p. 164).

Another survey in 1977 examined the level and nature of genetics instruction in U.S. medical schools (Childs et al., 1981) (see Box 6-6). Nearly two-thirds of the schools reported required courses in genetics, but most courses were entirely lectures, with discussion groups in only one-third and laboratory hours in less than one-quarter. Most teaching of genetics was offered in schools with a department or division of genetics, and most teaching faculty members were pediatricians. Very little teaching of genetics occurred in departments of preventive, community, or family medicine.

In 1985, Riccardi and Schmickel (1988) conducted a less elaborate survey of all medical schools in the United States, Canada, and Puerto Rico. Even seven years later, there had been little improvement in the number of course hours devoted to genetics. They found that nearly half (47 percent) of medical schools had nonexistent or inadequate human genetics teaching, with only 21 percent having good or excellent teaching in this area.

In response to the results of this 1985 survey and the 1984 report *Physicians for the Twenty-First Century* (AAMC, 1984), a multidisciplinary task force of members of the American Society of Human Genetics (Graham et al., 1989) was convened to examine the challenges of teaching human genetics in medical schools. The group agreed on a set of core content areas that should be understood by medical students by the time of graduation (see Box 6-6).

Finally, the Association of American Medical Colleges (AAMC) maintains a data base on courses offered at all U.S. medical schools. A review of curricula for 1992 showed that more medical schools are including some human and medical genetics in their curriculum in required courses (AAMC, 1991).

Some progress has been made in increasing physicians' knowledge of genetics and genetic testing and their ability to take good family histories, particularly in specialties that involve more genetic tests (e.g., pediatrics and obstetrics) and among more recent medical graduates. Nevertheless, not enough progress has been made—certainly not enough to prepare physicians-in-training for the increasing requirements for genetic testing, education, and counseling projected for the future. More research is needed on ways for medical education to begin to incorporate a genetic point of view throughout its curriculum, but especially in the critical clinical years, and on the knowledge of genetics and skills needed for genetics education and genetic counseling among all of these professional groups so that proper reforms can be implemented.

The Council on Resident Education in Obstetrics and Gynecology (CREOG) has also published standards for minimal skills that an obstetrics-gynecology res-

BOX 6-6 Genetics Instruction in Medical Schools

1977: A survey was conducted in 1977 (Childs et al., 1981) to determine the level and nature of genetics instruction in U.S. medical schools (100 responders). It found that

- 72 percent of schools listed required courses in genetics, ranging from 6 to 54 hours, with an average of 24 hours;
- most courses were entirely in lecture format, although one-third included discussion groups and 22 percent included from one to five laboratory hours (only 12 schools offered no courses in genetics);
- courses were more likely to be offered in schools with a department or division of genetics, and most faculty were pediatricians;
- very little teaching of genetics occurred in departments of preventive, community, or family medicine.

1985: Riccardi and Schmickel (1988) conducted a less elaborate survey of all medical schools in the United States, Canada, and Puerto Rico (119 out of 140 schools responding). A review of 79 course schedules, 41 syllabuses, and 40 sets of examination questions revealed the following:

- The mean number of hours of genetics teaching was 21.3 (18 hours if schools with no hours were included in the calculation).
- Responsibility for teaching genetics was assumed more often by departments of pediatrics than by all other departments combined.
- "The lack of basic science information about genes [in the syllabuses] is striking" (Riccardi and Schmickel, 1988, p. 641).
- Of the schools surveyed, 47 percent had what the authors judged to be nonexistent or poor human genetics teaching, with only 21 percent appearing to provide good or excellent teaching in this area.
- Little progress had been made since the previous survey reported in 1981 in improving the position of genetics in the medical school curriculum.

1989: In response to the results of the 1985 survey, a multidisciplinary task force of members of the American Society of Human Genetics was convened to examine the challenges of teaching human genetics in medical schools (Graham et al., 1989). The group agreed that the following content areas should be understood by medical students before graduation:

- the gene and chromosomes;
- Mendelian and multifactorial inheritance
- congenital malformations;
- adult-onset disorders;
- teratology;
- linkage analysis;
- DNA polymorphisms;
- gene mapping;
- evaluation and calculation of genetic risk;
- sexual differentiation and its disorders;

- biochemical genetics;
- cancer genetics;
- genetic screening;
- prenatal diagnosis;
- pharmacogenetics;
- neurogenetics;
- behavior genetics;
- genetic heterogeneity; and
- ethics.

continued

BOX 6-6—Continued

1991: The Association of American Medical Colleges maintains a data base on courses offered at all U.S. medical schools. A review of curricula for 1992 shows that in terms of courses required, more medical schools are including human and medical genetics in their curriculum (AAMC, 1991).

During 1991-1992, 79 of 126 medical schools (63 percent) required a human or medical genetics course. Of these, 70 percent required the course in the first year and 30 percent required it in the second year. The number of hours spent in the course ranged from 4 to 74, with the average course entailing 30 hours.

---

ident should possess in dealing with prenatal genetic counseling. The resident was expected to be able to discuss the principles of and give examples for Mendelian inheritance, define multifactorial inheritance, understand and be able to discuss chromosomal anomalies, obtain a genetic history and construct a family history chart, know the indications for amniocentesis, discuss the principles of cell biochemical analysis for the detection of inborn errors of metabolism, discuss maternal serum alpha-fetoprotein (MSAFP) screening, and discuss the value of population screening for genetic disorders as well as the prerequisites for such a screening program (CREOG, 1984). In June 1992, CREOG issued its revised core curriculum, including requirements for genetic counseling, which includes much more detailed and extensive knowledge and skills in genetics required for obstetrics-gynecology residents (CREOG, 1992) (see Box 6-7).

The Association of Professors of Gynecology and Obstetrics (APGO) proposed similar standards in its 1992 *Guide to Basic Science Prerequisites to a Clerkship in Obstetrics and Gynecology* to assist basic science departments of medical schools with developing essential curricular materials (APGO, 1992). The recommended proficiencies essential to genetics are listed in Table 6-6.

Continuing Medical Education

Continuing education credits for physicians wanting to learn more about medical genetics have been in existence for some time. Many medical centers offer courses, as do specialized centers such as the Jackson Memorial Laboratories in Bar Harbor, Maine, and the annual March of Dimes birth defects meetings. Such courses could also help to attract human and molecular geneticists into clinical genetics. The effects of such training on changes in clinical genetics practice are not known.

Physicians can also voluntarily engage in self-assessment activities in specific disciplines. For example, the American College of Physicians (ACP) offers a Medical Knowledge Self-Assessment Program in Genetic and Molecular Medi-

BOX 6-7   CREOG Standards for Training of Ob-Gyn Residents

EDUCATIONAL OBJECTIVES:
CORE CURRICULUM FOR RESIDENTS IN
OBSTETRICS AND GYNECOLOGY

GENETIC COUNSELING

1. **History and assessment of risk factors**
   a. Pedigree analysis
   b. Risks related to individual and family history and ethnic background for delivery of infants with inherited disorders
      i. Advanced maternal/paternal age
      ii. Maternal disease or exposure to known teratogens
      iii. Ethnic or racial background
      iv. Recessive disorders (X linked and autosomal)
      v. Dominant disorders (X linked and autosomal)
      vi. Family history of multiple spontaneous abortion and anomalous, live-born children (balanced translocation)
      vii. Multifactorial disorders
      viii. Disorders of metabolism
   c. Manifestations of common genetic disorders
      i. Trisomy 21 (Down syndrome)
      ii. 5p syndrome (cri du chat syndrome)
      iii. Trisomy 18 (Edwards syndrome)
      iv. Trisomy 13 (Patau syndrome)
      v. 47,XXY (Klinefelter syndrome)
      vi. 45,X (Turner syndrome)
      vii. Congenital adrenal hyperplasia
      viii. Neurofibromatosis
      ix. Tuberous sclerosis
      x. Duchenne muscular dystrophy
      xi. Fragile X syndrome
      xii. Cystic fibrosis
2. **Physical examination:** Physical characteristics that may indicate associated genetic disorders
   a. Fetal growth retardation
   b. Oligohydramnios
   c. Polyhydramnios
3. **Diagnostic studies**
   a. Screening tests
      i. Routine: Maternal serum alpha-fetoprotein testing
      ii. Targeted
         (a) Hexosaminidase A for Tay-Sachs disease (Jews of Eastern European descent)
         (b) Sickle cell preparation for sickle cell disease (blacks)
         (c) Hemoglobin electrophoresis for hemoglobinopathy (patients of Mediterranean or Asian descent with anemia)
         (d) Creatinine phosphokinase, DNA analysis, etc., for Duchenne muscular dystrophy (potential carriers)
         (e) Cystic fibrosis

continued

BOX 6-7—*Continued*

b. Prenatal diagnosis
   i.   Ultrasound
   ii. Amniocentesis: DNA and chromosomal analysis, acetylcholinesterase
   iii. Chorionic villus sampling
   iv. Percutaneous umbilical cord blood sampling
c. Institution of fetal death protocol

4. **Diagnosis**: Analysis of data gathered to identify potential genetic syndromes or inherited disorders

5. **Management**
   a. Possible interventions
      i.   Medical/nonoperative (e.g., intrauterine treatment of congenital adrenal hyperplasia to prevent masculinization of female fetus
      ii. Surgical (e.g., induced abortion)
      iii. Preconceptional counseling
   b. Factors influencing decisions regarding intervention
      i.   Age of patient
      ii. Maternal health
      iii. Severity of fetal disease or anomaly
      iv. Long-term implications
      v.   Patient's preferences
      vi. Cost factors related to proposed intervention or nonintervention
   c. Potential complications of intervention
      i.   Medical/nonoperative: Maternal or fetal drug side effects (systemic or local)
      ii. Operative
           (a) Complications of induced abortion
           (b) Outcome of neonatal surgery for neural tube defect (e.g., paralysis)
   d. Potential complications of nonintervention
      i.   Birth of a child affected with genetic disorder
      ii. Maternal complications of undelivered fetal death
      iii. Genital ambiguity in female affected with congenital adrenal hyperplasia not treated during pregnancy

6. **Follow-up**
   a. Inclusive management plan for specific diagnoses
      i.   Drug/hormone therapy and dosage
      ii. Operative procedure
   b. Counseling the couple and family
      i.   Mode of inheritance, risk of occurrence or recurrence
      ii. Associated anomalies or medical problems
      iii. Course and prognosis of genetic disorder
      iv. Family studies and examinations
      v.   Preconceptional and prenatal diagnosis
      vi. Grief counseling

PRENATAL CARE
1. **History**
   a. Menstrual history
   b. Past pregnancies
   c. Medical history
   d. Genetic screening
   e. Infection history

SOURCE: Council on Resident Education in Obstetrics and Gynecology, 1992, pp. 52-54.

TABLE 6-6   Basic Science Prerequisites in Genetics for a Clerkship in Obstetrics and Gynecology

---

I. Define the following basic genetic terms and mechanisms
  A. The structure of the nucleic acids
  B. Cell division
  C. Chromosomal abnormalities
  D. Molecular genetics
  E. Linkage, crossing over, and chromosome mapping
  F. Diagnostic techniques

II. Describe the manifestations and mechanisms for detection of abnormal inheritance
  A. Single-gene inheritance
  B. Sex chromosomal anomalies (risk, characteristics)
  C. Autosomal anomalies

III. Describe laboratory and special studies
  A. Tissue culture techniques
  B. Karyotype construction and interpretation
  C. DNA testing

SOURCE: Association of Professors of Gynecology and Obstetrics, 1992.

cine, among other subjects. This home-study program can also provide continuing medical education credits for participating physicians.

In addition to continuing medical education, informal learning occurs in contacts between genetics specialists and referring physicians. This is particularly true for physicians frequently exposed to genetic conditions, such as obstetricians and pediatricians, who tend to score higher on tests of genetic knowledge than do physicians with little clinical exposure (Hofman et al., 1993). The clinical "need to know" may be the best motivator for genetics education. As more genetic tests are available, the need to know will inevitably grow.

Professional Statements, Guidance, and Proficiencies

Many medical and scientific organizations issue standards and guidelines for practice regarding drugs and procedures, including genetic tests and procedures that might serve an educational purpose. For some physicians, these guidelines and directives might be influential in their decision making regarding incorporation of new tests and procedures. Concerns about protection from professional liability may play an important role in the development of professional standards and guidelines, and may influence the speed with which genetic tests are adopted into clinical practice.

The American Society of Human Genetics and the American College of Obstetricians and Gynecologists (ACOG) have issued several statements in the past decade recommending particular courses of action (or inaction) regarding genetic tests and procedures. For example, the ASHG (1992) has issued statements regarding cystic fibrosis carrier screening, and MSAFP screening (see also Garver, 1989; Caskey et al., 1990).

In 1986, ACOG suggested that obstetricians discuss the availability of the MSAFP test with their pregnant patients, but recommended against routine use of MSAFP screening in all pregnancies; ACOG issued a medical liability "alert" recommending that obstetricians offer every pregnant woman screening for elevated MSAFP to detect increased risk of certain genetic disorders (ACOG, 1985, 1986, 1991).

In 1987, ACOG issued guidelines for the use of antenatal diagnosis of genetic disorders. This technical bulletin (ACOG, 1987) serves as an educational aid to obstetrician-gynecologists and contains information on taking a genetic history, indications for prenatal genetic studies, technical considerations for amniocentesis, chorionic villus sampling, fetal visualization, fetoscopic tissue sampling, and molecular genetics in prenatal genetics. The standards require that physicians obtain the following information in evaluating genetic risk: (1) advanced parental age; (2) previous offspring with a chromosomal aberration; (3) chromosomal abnormality in either parent, particularly a translocation; (4) family history of a sex-linked condition; (5) family history of an inborn errors of metabolism; (6) family history of a neural tube defect; (7) family history of hemoglobinopathies; and/or (8) ancestry, indicating risk for Tay-Sachs disease, beta-thalassemia, or alpha-thalassemia.

OTHER HEALTH PROFESSIONALS

Other professional groups could (and sometimes do) provide essential genetic counseling and support services. Other health professionals now playing or likely to play a critical role in providing genetic services include nurses, social workers, and public health workers. Key issues concern the training of other professionals to provide essential genetic services and how their services will be overseen.

Nurses in Genetics

There are nearly 2 million registered professional nurses in the United States, many involved in maternal and child health nursing, providing a unique potential to contribute to the effective delivery of genetic services. In some settings—such as community, occupational, or school health—nurses may be the only link with the health care system (Forsman, 1988; Jones, 1988). Thus, nurses can assist in the identification, education, counseling, and follow-up of patients (Fibison, 1983; Jones, 1988; Thomson, 1992). Yet although nurses can be a valuable part of genetics services, to date they are a largely untapped resource (Forsman, 1988).

For nearly 30 years, it has been suggested that human genetics be included in the nursing curriculum (Brantl and Esslinger, 1962). A 1980 workshop on education in genetics for nurses and social workers developed academic criteria; didactic course work and clinical experience requirements for training as a master's-level clinical nurse specialist in genetics were developed in graduate programs in schools of nursing, were developed (Forsman and Bishop, 1981) (see Box 6-8). Candidates must meet the same academic admission requirements defined by the National League for Nursing accredited maternal child nursing program with a clinical nurse specialist option.

Despite this attention to the importance of genetics in nursing education, a 1984 survey of nursing instructors revealed that most schools dedicated less than 10 hours to genetics instruction, with little clinical experience (Forsman, 1988). Only four of the 200 universities in the United States that offer graduate degrees in nursing have established programs providing a master's-level genetics major (Forsman, 1988). A small number of nurses, particularly those in maternal and child health nursing, have been certified in genetic counseling by the ABMG (Forsman, 1988; OTA, 1992b). More than 100 nurses are employed in genetics, according to the International Society of Nurses in Genetics (ISONG).

Social Workers in Genetics

Social workers can play an important role in genetics services delivery, particularly in underserved communities. Social workers also have contact with many clients with genetic conditions in medical settings, such as facilities for high-risk infants, or pediatric, neurological, endocrine, and other specialty clinics. Other social work settings that might require some genetics expertise include family planning services, adoption and child welfare agencies, child guidance clinics, public health programs, agencies serving the mentally retarded and their families, and departments that serve developmentally and physically disabled clients (Schild and Black, 1984).

A 1980 conference (see Box 6-8) recommended that *all* social workers be provided a working knowledge of genetic diseases, their etiology, and consequences. In 1986, the Council on Social Work Education published a guide to genetic content for graduate social work education (Rauch, 1986). Nevertheless, only 9 of almost 100 accredited social work graduate programs in the United States offer special courses on genetic topics (Friedman and Blitzer, 1991). A course in genetics is offered to nurses and social workers in Washington, D.C. (see Box 6-8).

Public Health

Similarly, public education in genetics requires increased commitment at the public health level (also see discussion in Chapter 5). This requires educating

BOX 6-8   Education in Genetics for
Nurses and Social Workers

NURSING

In 1980, a workshop "Education in Genetics for Nurses and Social Workers" was sponsored by the Office of Maternal and Child Health to explore training and recommend service needs for nurses and social workers in genetics. The conference recommended that *all* nurses be provided a working knowledge of genetic diseases, their etiology, and consequences, and developed academic criteria, a list of didactic course work in human and medical genetics, and clinical experience required for training as an MSN clinical nurse specialist in genetics (Forsman and Bishop, 1981). Training occurs in graduate programs in schools of nursing. Candidates must meet the same academic admission requirements defined by the National League for Nursing accredited maternal child nursing program with a clinical nurse specialist option.

Didactic course work in both human and clinical medical genetics is required, including:

- patterns of inheritance
- cytogenetics
- immunogenetics
- biochemical genetics
- developmental genetics

- population genetics
- pharmacogenetics
- chromosomal disorders
- Mendelian disorders
- congenital malformation

- prenatal diagnosis
- genetic counseling
- ethical, legal, and social issues in genetics

Although genetics is generally a part of the nursing school curriculum, but again, programs vary (Forsman, 1988). Of the 200 universities in the United States that offer graduate degrees in nursing, only four have established programs providing a master's-level major in genetics (Forsman, 1988).

A course in genetics is offered to nurses and social workers in Washington, D.C., and is funded by the Genetics Services Branch, Division of Maternal and Child Health, Office of Research and Training, Health Resources and Services Administration, in the Department of Health and Human Services. The course introduces the fundamental concepts of human genetics and provides for learning the skills of screening and identification, referral, case management, and health education.

A small number of nurses, particularly those in maternal and child health nursing, have specialized in genetics in order to sit for the genetic counseling examination given by the ABMG (Forsman, 1988; OTA, 1992b; Thomson, 1992). According to ISONG, more than 100 nurses are employed in genetics; 48 percent of its members have a master's degree and 11 percent doctoral degrees; 43 percent have achieved certification in genetics or a nursing specialty; 37 percent have had 10 or more years of experience in genetics; and 85 percent have had 10 or more years of experience in nursing.

SOCIAL WORK

This conference also recommended a working knowledge of genetics for *all* social workers, including an understanding of the etiology and implications of genetic disorders. The Council on Social Work Education published a guide to genetics education for social workers (Rauch, 1986) public health professionals about pertinent issues related to medical genetics and changing the attitudes and staffing patterns of key state agencies (Cunningham and Kizer, 1990; Davis, 1990). Yet a survey of curricula at member schools of the Association of Schools of Public Health indicated a decrease in the number of schools offering human genetics as a major area of study (Friedman and Blitzer, 1991). Few schools of public health offer genetics as part of their curriculum, and in none is it required (Schull and Hanis, 1990). The limited attention given to genetics in schools of public health is troubling. Genetic testing will become an increasingly important aspect of health and social policy as more tests are developed. Some genetic testing programs—especially newborn screening—directly involve public health agencies.

FINDINGS AND RECOMMENDATIONS

As the availability of genetic tests increases and testing becomes more commonplace, it is likely that genetic testing will follow the path of other technological innovations in health care, and will be ordered and interpreted by primary care physicians, including pediatricians, obstetrician-gynecologists, internists, and general practitioners. There seems to be no prospect, in the foreseeable future, of having enough highly specialized genetics personnel to handle all genetic testing, including essential genetics education and genetic counseling. Although the number of individuals being certified in clinical genetics has been increasing, it is not clear that this is occurring quickly enough to ensure adequate and appropriate levels of support for greatly expanded genetic testing, education, and counseling in the future. Indeed, much of the manpower increase has gone to research, rather than to clinical genetics.

As a result, the role of the genetic specialist as the primary provider of genetic services is likely to change in the future. Genetic specialists will be called upon to play an important and expanded role in three areas: (1) continuing to provide genetic testing and counseling for disorders with the most complex interpretations and implications; (2) training and continuing education for other professionals in genetics and genetic counseling (Waples et al., 1988); and (3) seeing people in need of specialized genetic services referred by many more professionals (see discussions in Chapters 2 and 4). As genetic tests penetrate increasingly into the repertoire of primary care providers, it is likely that genetic specialists—be they master's-level genetic counselors, Ph.D.'s, or physicians—will continue to receive referrals from primary care providers of individuals with positive test results or psychosocial concerns that require more intensive follow-up. With training from genetic specialists, other health professionals, such as nurses, nurse practitioners, social workers, psychologists, and physicians, could be integrated into the existing genetics network.

Two issues should be addressed in terms of professional education in order for new genetic tests to be assimilated into medical practice in an appropriate manner. First, the committee recommends efforts to train more genetics professionals with the skills needed for adequate and accurate education, diagnosis, and counseling to (1) expand the pool of teachers in human genetics; and (2) meet the expected increase in referrals from primary care practitioners. This means increasing support (and funding, as appropriate) for the following:

• *Training of master's-level genetic counselors.* The committee recommends that, at least, the current number of genetic counseling graduates be maintained annually. This area will require close consideration over the next few years as genetic testing, education, and counseling services expand. In addition, the committee recommends funds for the training of master's-level genetic counselors, including stipends to attract minority students to this field. Because of the rapid development of new knowledge in genetic testing, the committee also recommends the development of formal continuing education programs for genetic counselors.

• *Development and evaluation of programs for single-disorder educators-counselors.* Programs should use innovative methods and personnel including the use of single-disorder educator-counselors drawn from the populations they are intended to serve. Evaluation should focus particularly on the types of methods or personnel necessary to provide specific kinds of genetic education and counseling, settings in which these services should be provided, and the training and support required if these innovative approaches are to be successful.

The committee recommends that genetic counseling and education be considered essential components of the standard of care, not only for specialized genetics personnel, but also for physicians, particularly primary care practitioners, who offer and interpret genetic tests. The committee endorses the core content areas identified by the ASHG task force, particularly the inclusion of ethics. However, the committee strongly recommends the addition of attention to patient education and counseling in genetics to this list of core subjects that should be understood by medical students by the time of graduation, and that national board examinations and specialty examinations for primary care specialists include more questions on genetics. The committee also commends CREOG and APGO for establishing standards and basic proficiencies for genetic counseling, and it recommends that other specialties follow their example.

The committee strongly recommends the expansion of continuing medical education programs in clinical genetics, including those geared to the primary care practitioner, and the development of additional continuing medical education programs to improve the knowledge and skills of currently practicing physicians in genetic testing, education, and counseling. This should include physician fellowships and postdoctoral support for training in clinical genetics, not only support for research training and research careers; postdoctoral education in human genetics in the form of intensive two-week courses or summer courses; and predoctoral graduate students in genetics and molecular biology to take appropriate human genetics classes intended to increase the understanding of medical genetics (such as those offered by medical school faculties).

To ensure that genetic tests are administered in an appropriate manner, the committee recommends

- **reform of the education of physicians and other health professionals who are not trained as geneticists to include increased attention to basic genetics;**
- **in particular, training of medical students to deal with the sensitivities of genetics education and the need for nondirectiveness, especially in counseling about reproductive options and about disorders for which no treatment exists;**
- **reform of medical education should begin to incorporate a genetic point of view throughout its curriculum to enable physicians to recognize that human variability exists in the pathogenesis of human disease;**
- **training for genetics professionals and others** *offering or referring* **for genetic testing in the ethical, legal, and social issues surrounding genetic diagnosis, testing, and screening;**
- **training for laboratory personnel in order to understand the complexities of genetic testing so as to adequately interpret tests with a knowledge of test limitations and a sensitivity to the social issues surrounding genetic testing;**
- **more research on knowledge of genetics and skills needed for genetics education and genetic counseling among all of the professional groups discussed in this report so that proper reforms can be implemented, and**
- **establishment of basic proficiencies in genetics for physicians, nurses, and social workers.**

The committee also recommends the development of formal continuing education and training for genetic counselors and other professionals. Geneticists should also take a leadership role in genetics education for the public. Other health care professionals should also participate in programs intended to increase public awareness and education about genetics.

The committee believes that with proper training, the integration of other health professionals such as nurses, nurse practitioners, social workers, psychologists, and primary care physicians, into the existing genetics services network will supplement the time and skills of the traditional genetic counselor. **Consequently, the committee strongly recommends expanded undergraduate and graduate training of nurses and social workers in the special requirements of genetics, genetics education, and genetic counseling. The committee recommends that public health professionals have training to ensure that they understand the underlying science of genetics and genetic testing, as well as the ethical, legal, and social issues outlined in this report.**

The committee recommends the recruitment of more minorities for training programs in all aspects of clinical genetics. This will be especially important in providing culturally sensitive and appropriate genetic testing, education, and counseling services in the future when so-called minority groups will comprise a majority of the population of the United States (see Chapter 4).

The committee also recommends the development and evaluation of innovative on-line computer and interactive computer systems to disseminate the latest information on genetic disorders and on recommendations and guidelines for genetic testing. This is one way to improve the quality of genetic testing, education, and counseling services in the future (e.g., through the program of the National Library of Medicine (NLM) and the American College of Physicians for ACP members to have on-line access to the resources of the NLM). The committee believes that the NLM is an excellent mechanism for providing access to critical information on genetics and recommended criteria for genetic testing, genetic counseling, and follow-up care to members of ACP and other interested professional groups. The ELSI program should coordinate with professional genetics organizations and the NLM to develop such a genetics education and dissemination program for interested health professionals.

NOTE

1. In its deliberations, the committee had the benefit of a 1991 background paper on professional personnel issues in human genetics developed by Ann C.M. Smith, M.S. (a consultant to the committee), and committee staff members, Jane Fullarton (Study Director) and C. Elaine Lawson (Research Assistant). Additional data (for 1992) were provided by Kathi Hanna, D.P.A., who provided technical consulting to the committee on parts of this chapter. The committee particularly benefited from access to new data on physician knowledge of basic genetics (Hofman et al., 1993).

REFERENCES

Acton, R., et al. 1989. Use of self-administered family history of disease instruments to predict individuals at risk for cardiovascular diseases, hypertension and diabetes. American Journal of Human Genetics 45(S):A275.

American College of Obstetricians and Gynecologists (ACOG). 1985. Professional Liability Implications of AFP Testing (Liability Alert). May. Washington, D.C.

American College of Obstetricians and Gynecologists (ACOG). 1986. Prenatal Detection of Neural Tube Defects. ACOG Technical Bulletin No. 99. December 1986 (replaced Technical Bulletin No. 67. October 1982). Washington, D.C.

American College of Obstetricians and Gynecologists (ACOG). 1987. Antenatal Diagnosis of Genetic Disorders. ACOG Technical Bulletin No. 108. September 1987 (replaced No. 34, January 1976). Washington, D.C.

American College of Obstetricians and Gynecologists (ACOG). 1991. Alpha-Fetoprotein. ACOG Technical Bulletin No. 154. April. Washington, D.C.

American Society of Human Genetics (ASHG). 1992. Statement of the American Society of Human Genetics on cystic fibrosis carrier screening. American Journal of Human Genetics S1:1443-1444.

Association of American Medical Colleges (AAMC). 1984. General professional education of the physician: Physicians for the twenty-first century. Journal of Medical Education 59:1-208.

Association of American Medical Colleges (AAMC). 1991. 1991-92 AAMC Curriculum Directory. Washington, D.C.

Association of Professors of Gynecology and Obstetrics (APGO). 1992. Guide to Basic Science Prerequisites for a Clerkship in Obstetrics and Gynecology. Washington, D.C.

Blitzer, M. 1992. Guide to North American Graduate and Postgraduate Training Programs in Human Genetics, 1992-93 (2nd Ed.). Bethesda, Md.: American Society of Human Genetics.

Brantl, V., and Esslinger, P. 1962. Genetic implications for the nursing curriculum. Nursing Forum (Spring 1):90-100.

Caskey, T., et al. 1990. The American Society of Human Genetics statement on cystic fibrosis screening. American Journal of Human Genetics 46:393.

Childs, B. 1992 (published in 1994). Genetics and medical education. In Fullarton, J. (ed.) Proceedings of the Committee on Assessing Genetic Risks. Washington, D.C.: National Academy Press.

Childs, B., et al. 1981. Human genetics teaching in U.S. medical schools. American Journal of Human Genetics 33:1-10.

Cole, J., et al. 1978. Genetic family history questionnaire. Journal of Medical Genetics 15:10-18.

Council on Resident Education in Obstetrics and Gynecology (CREOG). 1984. American College of Obstetrics and Gynecology. Washington, D.C.

Council on Resident Education in Obstetrics and Gynecology (CREOG). 1992. American College of Obstetrics and Gynecology. Washington, D.C.

Cunningham, G., and Kizer, K. 1990. Maternal serum alpha-fetoprotein screening activities of state health agencies: A survey. American Journal of Human Genetics 47:899-903.

Davidson, R., and Childs, B. 1987. Perspectives in the teaching of human genetics. In Harris, H., and Hirschhorn, K. (eds.) Advances in Human Genetics 16. New York: Plenum Press.

Davis, J. 1990. Invited editorial: State-sponsored maternal serum alpha-fetoprotein activities: Current issues in genetics and public health. American Journal of Human Genetics 47:896-898.

Fatemi, C., and Gasparini, R. 1990. 1990 salary statistics for cytogenetic technologists and supervisors throughout the United States. Applied Cytotechnology 16(4):85-90.

Fibison, W. 1983. The nursing role in the delivery of genetic services. Issues in Health Care of Women 4:1-15.

Finley, W., et al. 1987. Letter to the editor: Survey of medical genetics personnel. American Journal of Human Genetics 40(4): 374-377.

Firth, H., and Lindenbaum, R. 1992. U.K. clinicians' knowledge of and attitudes to the prenatal diagnosis of single gene disorders. Journal of Medical Genetics 29:20-23.

Forsman, I. 1988. Education of nurses in genetics. American Journal of Human Genetics 43:552-558.

Forsman, I., and Bishop, K. 1981. Education in Genetics: Nurses and Social Workers: Proceedings of a Workshop. HHS Pub. No. 81-51120A. U.S. Department of Health and Human Services. Rockville, Md.

Friedman, J., and Blitzer, M. 1991. ASHG/NSGC activities related to education: Workshop on human genetics education. American Journal of Human Genetics 49:1127-1128.

Friedman, J., and Riccardi, V. (eds.). 1988. Guide to North American Graduate and Postgraduate Training Programs in Human Genetics (2nd Ed.). Rockville, Md.: American Society of Human Genetics.

Garver, K. 1989. Update on MSAFP policy statement from the American Society of Human Genetics. American Journal of Human Genetics 45:332-334.

Garver, K., and Lent, K. 1990. American Society of Human Genetics membership survey results, 1989. American Journal of Human Genetics 47:345-348.

Gasparini, R., et al. 1988. Undergraduate and postgraduate training programs for cytogenetic technologists. American Journal of Human Genetics 42: 200-203.

Gaupman, K., et al. 1991. ASHG/NSGC activities related to education: The doctoral degree in genetic counseling: Attitudes of genetic counselors. American Journal of Human Genetics 49:488-493.

Genetics Associates: Their, Training, Role and Function (Conference Proceedings). 1979. Williamsburg, Va.: U.S. Department of Health, Education, and Welfare.

Gettig, E. 1992 (published in 1994). Recommendations on minimum criteria for genetic counseling. In Fullarton, J. (ed.) Proceedings of the Committee on Assessing Genetic Risks. Washington, D.C.: National Academy Press.

Graham, J., et al. 1989. Report of the task force on teaching human genetics in North American medical schools. American Journal of Human Genetics 44:161-165.

Hofman, K., et al. 1993. Physicians' knowledge of genetics and genetic tests. Academic Medicine 68(8):625-631.

Holtzman, N. 1989. Proceed with Caution: Predicting Genetic Risks in the Recombinant DNA Era. Baltimore, Md.: The Johns Hopkins University Press.

Holtzman, N. 1991. The interpretation of laboratory results: The paradoxical effect of medical training. Journal of Clinical Ethics 2(4):1-2.

Hunt, S., et al. 1986. A comparison of positive family history definitions for defining risk of future disease. Journal of Chronic Disease 39:809-821.

Jones, S. 1988. Decision making in clinical genetics: Ethical implications for perinatal practice. Journal of Perinatal and Neonatal Nursing 1(3):11-23.

Kapur, S., et al. 1983. Medical practice and genetics in the mid-Michigan area. Journal of Medical Education 58:186-193.

Lemkus, S., et al. 1978. Genetic and congenital disorders: Knowledge and attitudes of the public, nurses, and medical practitioners in South Africa. South African Medical Journal 53:491-494.

Motulsky, A. 1983. Role of medical genetics in United States academic medicine. In Bowers, J., and King, E. (eds.) Academic Medicine: Present and Future. North Tarrytown, N.Y.: Rockefeller Archive Center.

Murray, J., and Toriello, H. (eds.). 1990. Guide to North American Graduate and Postgraduate Training Programs in Human Genetics (3rd Ed.). American Society of Human Genetics. Bethesda, Md.

Napier, J., et al. 1972. Limitations of morbidity and mortality data from family histories: A report from the Tecumseh community health study. American Journal of Public Health 62:30-35.

National Academy of Sciences. 1975. Genetic Screening: Programs, Principles, and Research. Washington, D.C.: National Academy of Sciences.

National Society of Genetic Counselors (NSGC). 1991. Code of Ethics. Chicago, Ill.

Naylor, E. 1975. Genetic screening and genetic counseling: Knowledge, attitudes, and practices in two groups of family planning professionals. Social Biology 22:304-314.

Office of Technology Assessment (OTA). 1992a. U.S. Congress. Cystic Fibrosis and DNA Tests: Implications of Carrier Screening. OTA-BA-532. Washington, D.C.: U.S. Government Printing Office.

Office of Technology Assessment (OTA). 1992b. U.S. Congress. Genetic Counseling and Cystic Fibrosis Carrier Screening: Results of a Survey. OTA-BP-BA-97. Washington, D.C.: U.S. Government Printing Office.

Pew Health Professions Commission. 1991. Healthy America: Practitioners for 2005: An Agenda for Action for U.S. Health Professional Schools. Durham, N.C.

Rauch, F. 1986. Guide to Graduate Social Work Education in Genetics. New York: Council on Social Work Education.

Riccardi, V., and Schmickel, R. 1988. Human genetics as a component of medical school curricula: A report of the American Society of Human Genetics. American Journal of Human Genetics 42:639-643.

Riccardi, V., and Smith, A.C.M. (eds.). 1986. Guide to Human Genetics Training Programs in North America (1st Edition). Bethesda, Md.: American Society of Human Genetics.

Robert Wood Johnson Foundation. 1991. Environment for Learning: An Interim Report of the Robert Wood Johnson Foundation Commission on Medical Education: The Sciences of Medical Practice. Philadelphia, Pa.

Schild, S., and Black, R. 1984. Social Work and Genetics: A Guide for Practice. New York: Hawthorne Press.

Schull, W., and Hanis, C. 1990. Genetics and public health in the 1990s. Annual Review of Public Health 11:105-125.

Singer, E. 1991. Public attitudes toward genetic testing. In Population Research and Policy Review 10:235-255.

Thomson, E. 1992 (published in 1994). Issues in genetic counseling: The nursing perspective. In Fullarton, J. (ed.) Proceedings of the Committee on Assessing Genetic Risks. Washington, D.C.: National Academy Press.

Uhlmann, W.R. 1992. Professional status survey results. Perspectives in Genetic Counseling, Suppl. 14(2):7-10, Summer.

Walker, A., et al. 1990. Report of the 1989 Asilomar Meeting on education in genetic counseling. American Journal of Human Genetics 46:1223-1230.

Waples, C., et al. 1988. Resources for Genetic Disorders. Genetics Applications: A Health Perspective. Lawrence, Kans.: Learner Managed Designs.

Wilfond, B., and Fost, N. 1990. The cystic fibrosis gene: Medical and social implications for heterozygote detection. Journal of the American Medical Association 263:2777-2783.

Williams, R., et al. 1988. Health family trees: A tool for finding and helping young family members of coronary and cancer prone pedigrees in Texas and Utah. American Journal of Public Health 1878:1283-1286.

Zinberg, R., and Greendale, K. 1991. Do we have a shortage of genetic counselors in New York State? The Newsletter of the Genetics Network of the Empire State 3(3):1.

7

Financing of Genetic Testing and Screening Services

The cost and financing of genetic testing and counseling have had a profound impact on access to these services in the United States (OTA, 1992b). No matter what aspect of genetics is discussed, it is almost impossible to keep the discussion from turning to issues related to financing of genetic testing services, in particular the role of health insurance in genetic testing and counseling.

The United States is the only developed country in the world without a social insurance or statutory system to cover basic expenses for medical services for most or all of its population (Fields and Shapiro, 1993).[1] This creates problems of access and equity, especially for low-income or high-risk individuals who are self-employed, work part-time, or are employed by small businesses and who may not be able to afford or obtain health insurance. More than 36 million people are without health insurance coverage in the United States (EBRI, 1993, p. 1).

Current activities in health insurance reform may obviate some concerns about health insurance discrimination related to genetic testing and the use of genetic information. The Ethical, Legal, and Social Implications Program (ELSI) Task Force on Insurance and Genetic Testing (ELSI Insurance Task Force, 1993)[2] has already submitted its concerns to President Clinton's health insurance reform committee. Health insurance reform proposals will need to be evaluated to determine whether they adequately protect genetic information and persons with genetic disorders from discrimination and other potential social, legal, and ethical harms related to health insurance and the use of genetic information (see Chapter 8).

Even for those who have health insurance, coverage for most preventive, screening, and counseling services may be excluded. These limitations of U.S. health care coverage particularly affect genetics services, which have an important counseling component. As discussed below, insurance reimbursement or other financing for genetic diagnosis, testing, and screening, and essential genetic counseling, is not generally available now in the United States.

Moreover, the committee heard testimony at its public forum that individuals whose insurance does cover some or all genetic services may be reluctant or unwilling to file claims for such services. They may fear that the information they seek might be used to evaluate and deny their future applications for health or life insurance coverage, or might lead to higher premiums or limited coverage. Because much coverage in the United States is employment based, people may also worry that their employer will have access to the information and use it (overtly or covertly) to discriminate against them (Fields and Shapiro, 1993).

Even the casual conversation of medical personnel, human resources staff, and others about genetic information may affect insurance coverage if such information is reflected in medical records or in the personnel system of self-insured companies. To avoid such impact on insurability, some genetic counselors report that they routinely advise their counselees not to seek insurance reimbursement because of the potential risk to future health and life insurance coverage for them and their families (OTA, 1992c). However, if the information is subsequently sent to primary care practitioners for follow-up care and entered in the patient's medical record, insurers may then have access to that information even if they did not reimburse for the test itself. Many people seeking genetic testing and/or genetic counseling now pay "out-of-pocket" for such services, either because they do not have insurance coverage for such services, or because they fear the consequences of having such information known to their insurance companies or to others. To keep information about genetic testing from reaching insurers, physicians are sometimes being requested to set up separate patient records (as is now sometimes done for records of treatment for AIDS or mental disorders).

When people do pay out-of-pocket for genetic diagnosis and testing, they often pay a substantial sum, especially if the testing requires complex linkage analysis. The cost of complex family studies involving linkage analysis ranges from $500 to $4,000, depending in part on the number of tests and the size of the family. The person seeking the testing must be able to pay the full costs of the testing for *all* relatives, or the testing may not be performed.

Direct DNA testing of individuals can be considerably less expensive; such tests now cost from $50 to more than $900 per test. Future costs for DNA tests could be even lower with automation and more widespread testing, and costs of $50 to $150 for a panel of six or more DNA tests are now being discussed; however, patents and royalties resulting from the patenting and licensing of genes and gene products have the potential greatly to increase the cost of such testing, as has already occurred in DNA tests for cystic fibrosis (Beaudet, 1992). These cost estimates for direct DNA analysis do not include any of the costs of interpretation, education, and genetic counseling prior to and/or following direct DNA testing (see Chapter 4).

Genetic counseling is generally not reimbursed directly by health insurers unless the counseling is provided or billed by a physician, although the counseling may be done by a counselor or nurse under the supervision of the physician. However, genetic education and counseling are time-consuming activities, and some physicians may not take the time or have the training required to provide these critical genetic testing services, and they also may not have appropriately trained staff. Genetic counseling is, in some instances, reimbursed indirectly as a hidden cost of the genetic testing process. Under the current reimbursement approach, genetic counseling is not recognized by third-party payers as a necessary component of any genetic diagnosis, testing, or screening procedure. Because of these reimbursement limitations, genetic testing and counseling are often accessible only to the middle class and wealthy—those with enough discretionary income to pay for genetics services out-of-pocket.

WHO PAYS FOR GENETIC
TESTING AND COUNSELING?

Although only limited data have been available on who now pays for genetic testing and genetic counseling, third-party reimbursement for genetics services has been relatively rare. Problems of underinsured and uninsured families, and financial support for genetics services, were ranked as among the top priority issues in their respective states by state genetics services coordinators who were asked about the most important issues in genetics services facing patients and families in a 1991 Council of Regional Networks for Genetic Services survey (CORN, 1991).

Many genetics services have difficulty meeting traditional standards for reimbursement by third-party payers. Until their value has been established scientifically, new genetics services are excluded as "investigational" (see below). Yet even when a service is no longer investigational, insurers may refuse reimbursement on the grounds that it is not "medically necessary" for the diagnosis or treatment of an illness. Genetic testing and screening services generally differ from diagnostic medical testing that occurs after a patient develops symptoms. Because genetic testing is often performed on *asymptomatic* people with a family history of the disorder, many patients report that their claims for insurance reimbursement are denied (OTA, 1992b).

Geneticists, in contrast, may feel that such tests are necessary based not only on the patient's family history, but also on (1) membership in a population subgroup (by race or ethnicity) that is at a higher risk than the general population for developing a particular disorder themselves or in their offspring; (2) increased risk associated with pregnancies in women of advanced age (usually age 35 and over); and (3) screening of pregnancies for increased risk of neural tube defects, regardless of the mother's age, in order to determine whether increased risk warrants offering further prenatal genetic testing. In the future, population-wide genetic screening may be warranted, and that will require the development of appropriate reimbursement policy as well. Genetic screening may thus follow the path of certain other screening and preventive services such as mammography or immunization, which are increasingly becoming part of health insurance plans; however, counseling raises another dimension for reimbursement of genetic testing services that differs from these other screening and preventive health services.

Newborn screening is another type of genetic testing for which insurance reimbursement has been limited. In the past, most states paid directly for newborn screening tests, but now more than half the states bill the birth hospital (or more rarely the birth physician or even the parents) for the cost of newborn screening (CORN, 1992). They leave the hospital (or doctor) to collect from whatever third-party coverage the parents may have. Insurance companies, however, have resisted paying for such screening in many states, so the hospitals must somehow absorb the expense (S. Panney, Maryland Department of Health and Mental Hygiene, personal communication, 1993).

There are a few sources of noninsurance funding for genetics services that will reimburse out-of-pocket costs for persons without health insurance or whose insurer will not reimburse for genetic testing and counseling. Some academic laboratories have special research funding, some programs have state grants-in-aid (including funding from the Maternal and Child Health block grant funds to the states), some programs have limited private foundation funding, and some programs receive financial assistance available from genetic support groups. Such alternative sources of funding are not consistently available.

However, much of the complex genetic linkage analysis today is performed in academic research laboratories, and some of these laboratories bill patients for such services. Even if the proband has insurance that would cover individual genetic testing and linkage analysis, his or her insurance company may not pay for genetic testing and linkage analysis for the whole family. Extended family members are likely to have different insurance coverage that may or may not cover such procedures, and if family members are unable or unwilling to pay the costs of their own genetic testing and linkage analysis, the procedures will not produce complete and useful results. Thus, the structure of the insurance system in the United States imposes an additional impediment to genetic testing that requires linkage analysis; patients must often pay out-of-pocket or not have access to such testing.

Another barrier to coverage is the fact that most testing now performed by academic laboratories has not been approved and is therefore "investigational" under the definitions of the Food and Drug Administration. "Investigational" or "experimental" services are almost never reimbursed by third-party payers. However, most of these laboratories have not applied for or received certification under the requirements of the Clinical Laboratory Improvements Amendments of 1988. Requiring these laboratories to comply with existing federal laws (see Chapter 3) will remove some of the genetic testing and counseling these laboratories currently provide as patient care from the investigational category. Thus, one additional barrier to insurance reimbursement would be reduced.

Recently, some laboratories began receiving insurance reimbursement, particularly those doing genetic testing for cancer. In addition, some patients have successfully challenged their insurer's initial refusal of payment. In a survey reported by the congressional Office of Technology Assessment (OTA, 1992b), about 40 percent of the patients were able to get their genetic test reimbursed after sending a letter from the testing laboratory to their insurer. Some patients report successfully obtaining third-party reimbursement for cystic fibrosis (CF) carrier screening, particularly during pregnancy (Bernhardt and Eierman, 1992). However, as discussed in Chapters 2 and 8, this may not be the ideal time for CF carrier testing.

PRIVATE SOURCES OF PAYMENT FOR GENETICS SERVICES

The majority of health insurance for the under-65 population in the United States is private health insurance, generally provided through employers (Fields and Shapiro, 1993).[3] In the United States, private commercial health insurance is usually a private business enterprise, run on basic business principles of responsibility to shareholders to maintain profitability (Pokorsky, 1989). Ensuring profitability for private health insurance means providing insurance to as many people as possible, while containing outlays through a variety of methods, including limits on coverage, copayments, and deductibles. Such insurance is generally provided through indemnity plans that do not cover all services.

Many health maintenance organizations (HMOs) are not for profit, but they cannot continue to operate if their coverage decisions, "open-enrollment" policies, and other practices combine to produce a continuing deficit. In this sense, even the not-for-profit insurers and managed care providers are concerned with controlling losses to their plans through coverage determinations and policies. If state insurance regulation permits, HMOs and other managed care practices may impose limits on open-enrollment periods (e.g., just a few weeks a year when they accept anyone who applies for membership) and limits on outside referrals for specialty care. The latter may impact on genetics services, which—for the most part—are outside the usual specialty services found in managed care plans. Although genetic education and counseling are essential components of any genetic testing *services* (see Chapters 1, 4, and 6), genetic counseling and education are not likely to be explicitly reimbursed without changes in reimbursement policies.

Self-Insurance by Employers

An increasing number of U.S. employers have moved to self-insurance in recent years, because it gives them more control over benefit systems and health care costs, as well as tax advantages. Federal legislation (the Employee Retirement Income Security Act, or ERISA) exempts employers from state benefits regulations. Consequently, employers may impose disease-specific dollar limits on particular diseases or conditions (see discussion of *H & H Music Company* case in Chapter 8), and are not required to meet specified state minimum benefit packages or to participate in high-risk insurance pools (for persons unable to get insurance otherwise). This complex subject is covered in a recent Institute of Medicine study, *Employment and Health Benefits* (Fields and Shapiro, 1993). It is estimated that from 50 to 60 percent of persons covered by employer-based health insurance plans participate in plans for which the company is self-insured (EBRI, 1993).

Above a certain dollar limit, the increased risk assumed by the employer for employee health expenses is then often "reinsured" against major losses through traditional insurance companies (so-called stop-loss insurance). Many businesses also contract with traditional health insurance companies to administer their health insurance plans.

Key Health Insurance Policy Barriers to Reimbursement for Genetics Services

Group health insurance coverage of genetic testing and counseling is highly variable. Most group health insurance plans—and for that matter, Medicare—limit coverage to services determined to be "medically necessary" for the treatment of a diagnosed illness or injury; they do not cover screening tests in the absence of symptoms, and thus exclude most preventive services and immunizations, in addition to much of genetic testing, education, and counseling. Where reimbursed, genetic tests may be subject to insurance company requirements for prior approval of procedures. Prenatal genetics services are more widely covered by third parties than other genetics services; many group health insurance plans and health maintenance organizations include coverage for prenatal diagnosis if recommended by the attending physician. Where coverage exists for prenatal diagnosis, however, it rarely includes full reimbursement for the time required for education and genetic counseling before and after genetic testing, and in some instances genetic education and counseling are not covered at all. Some select group plans include more liberal coverage of genetic testing.

Survey of Attitudes of Health Insurers About the Use of Genetic Information

The Office of Technology Assessment (OTA) surveyed commercial insurers, Blue Cross and Blue Shield (BC/BS) plans, and health maintenance organizations that offer individual or medically underwritten group policies (OTA, 1992b). A majority of insurers believe that the wide availability of genetic testing would have a negative financial impact on their companies unless they had access to the results for purposes of medical underwriting.[4] None of the responding companies reported that they had done any economic analysis of the costs and benefits of carrier testing or genetic tests as part of applicant screening, although one commercial company had done an analysis of prenatal coverage. Similarly, none of the companies reported any economic analysis of providing carrier screening or genetic counseling within their benefit package. However, the survey did confirm concerns about policies and practices of insurers regarding genetic testing for CF. "On balance, however, it appears that, for now, if no medical indication for the test exists, a third-party payor generally will not pay for the (CF screening) assay" (OTA, 1992a, p. 178) (see Table 7-1).

The Impact of CPT Codes on Reimbursement

CPT-4 (current procedural terminology) codes (standardized categories used for reimbursement of health services) do not exist for many genetic tests, since the technology is developing so rapidly. In the absence of CPT-4 codes, insurance reimbursement is not possible without special review by the insurer. Some genetic testing centers are using CPT-4 codes intended for biochemical precursors to seek reimbursement from insurers. As genetic testing becomes more widespread, the lack of CPT-4 codes for genetic testing and genetic counseling will be a major impediment to insurance reimbursement even for those people who have insurance coverage for genetic diagnosis (OTA, 1992c). A committee of the American Medical Association (AMA) establishes CPT codes, including the addition of new codes. Now that the new American College of Medical Genetics (ACMG) has been recognized by the American Board of Medical Specialties (ABMS) of the AMA, the ACMG may be able to influence the AMA committee responsible for CPT-4 codes to develop appropriate codes for genetic tests.

PUBLIC SOURCES OF PAYMENT FOR GENETICS SERVICES

In some instances, public financing for genetics services occurs through Medicaid, Medicare, or state genetics services programs.

Medicare

Medicare is primarily a program to reimburse medical expenses considered "medically necessary" for people over age 65 and certain categories of disabled persons. Medicare coverage decisions and reimbursement policies related to genetic testing now affect primarily the population of persons with disabilities, some of whom would find genetics services relevant and useful. In the future, Medicare may have a broader impact, as genetic tests are developed for more disorders common to older Americans, including complex common disorders such as heart disease, cancers, diabetes mellitus, and certain mental health disorders.

TABLE 7-1   Reimbursement for Cystic Fibrosis Carrier Tests and Genetic Counseling

Question: Do your standard individual policies and medically underwritten policies provide coverage for:

Respondent	At Patient Request	Medically Indicated Only	Not Covered	No Response[a]
Individual Policies				
Carrier tests for CF?				
Commercials	0 (0%)	12 (41%)	12 (41%)	5 (17%)
HMOs	2 (18%)	7 (64%)	0 (0%)	2 (18%)
BC/BS plans[b]	2 (8%)	16 (64%)	7 (28%)	0 (0%)
Prenatal tests for CF?				
Commercials	0 (0%)	12 (41%)	14 (48%)	3 (10%)
HMOs	1 (9%)	7 (64%)	1 (9%)	2 (18%)
BC/BS plans	3 (12%)	19 (76%)	3 (12%)	0 (0%)
Genetic counseling?				
Commercials	2 (7%)	6 (21%)	18 (62%)	3 (10%)
HMOs	1 (9%)	6 (55%)	1 (9%)	3 (27%)
BC/BS plans	1 (4%)	9 (36%)	13 (52%)	2 (8%)
Medically Underwritten Policies				
Carrier tests for CF?				
Commercials	0 (0%)	24 (65%)	10 (27%)	3 (8%)
HMOs	1 (5%)	13 (65%)	2 (10%)	4 (20%)
BC/BS plans	2 (10%)	11 (52%)	8 (38%)	0 (0%)
Prenatal tests for CF?				
Commercials	1 (3%)	23 (62%)	10 (27%)	3 (8%)
HMOs	2 (10%)	14 (70%)	0 (0%)	4 (20%)
BC/BS plans	3 (14%)	14 (67%)	4 (19%)	0 (0%)
Genetic counseling?				
Commercials	2 (5%)	16 (43%)	17 (46%)	2 (5%)
HMOs	2 (10%)	12 (60%)	1 (5%)	5 (25%)
BC/BS plans	1 (5%)	7 (33%)	12 (57%)	1 (5%)

[a]Percentages may not add to 100 due to rounding.
[b]OTA also inquired about reimbursement practices for BC/BS open enrollment nongroup policies and reports these data elsewhere.

SOURCE: Office of Technology Assessment, 1992a, p. 181.

One consequence of the Deficit Reduction Act of 1984 was a change in how Medicare pays for clinical laboratory tests and services furnished to outpatients and nonpatients by hospitals, and also to patients by independent laboratories and physician offices (e.g., for certain CPT-4 codes covering laboratory processes involved in conducting and reporting certain genetic tests). Medicare fee schedules were substantially reduced, and this reduction has subsequently been adopted by many state Medicaid programs. The low rates have reduced the number of providers who will perform these tests if Medicaid-Medicare reimbursement is the only available payment (Arkansas Medicare carrier, unpublished letter, October 1, 1991). The provisions of this 1984 legislation continues to affect reimbursement for all clinical laboratory services, including genetic tests.

Medicaid

Medicaid is a joint federal-state program to reimburse health care expenses for qualified low-income individuals and families. Preliminary data indicate variable coverage of genetic testing and counseling by state Medicaid programs (OTA, 1992a).

OTA surveyed state Medicaid directors about their coverage and reimbursement levels for selected genetics services: amniocentesis, ultrasound, chorionic villus sampling (CVS), maternal serum alpha-fetoprotein (MSAFP) screening tests, DNA analysis, chromosomal analysis, and genetic counseling. Of the 46 states whose data are included in the OTA (1992a, p. 183) report,

* 44 state Medicaid programs cover MSAFP, with average reimbursement of $21.76 (and 1 requires special review);
* 45 state Medicaid programs cover amniocentesis, with average reimbursement of $59.32;
* 44 state Medicaid programs cover fetal ultrasound, with average reimbursement of $83.13 (2 require special review of "individual considerations" to decide on coverage);
* 31 state Medicaid programs cover CVS; 10 do not cover CVS (4 require special review and 1 did not know if CVS was covered); average CVS reimbursement was $145.90;
* 41 state Medicaid programs cover chromosomal analysis from amniotic fluid or chorionic villus (1 does not cover it and 4 require special review); average reimbursement is $235.68; and
* 26 state Medicaid programs cover DNA analysis; 6 do not cover it (8 did not know if DNA analysis was covered; 6 require special review; and "family DNA testing" is covered in New York); average reported reimbursement is $33.39.

State Medicaid programs varied in whether they provided coverage of genetic counseling. As is common for many counseling services in a medical setting, genetic counseling might be covered if it were included in a general office visit code (either provided by the physician or provided by other professionals such as genetic counselors under the supervision of a physician). In 11 states, Medicaid coverage for genetic counseling is reported as part of an office visit or consultation; 19 states did not cover genetic counseling; 3 states did not know if genetic counseling was covered; and 2 states required special review. The average reimbursement of $68.87 reported for genetic counseling actually reflected the range of reimbursements for different levels of physician office visits, rather than for genetic counseling per se (OTA, 1992a, p. 182).

Medicaid reimbursement is available for some genetic laboratory testing services, but the Medicare reimbursement practice of setting "maximum allowable charges" for particular tests and then reimbursing a percentage (generally 80 percent of maximum allowable charges) has had a negative impact on Medicaid practices (Arkansas Medicare carrier, unpublished letter, October 1, 1991). Although good data are not available, estimates indicate that Medicaid pays less than half of the actual charges for some of the genetic tests for which it reimburses. It is frequently difficult to find providers of genetic testing services who will accept patients for whom Medicaid is the only reimbursement available. In addition, not all genetics centers accept state Medicaid reimbursement. "Those genetic service providers that accept Medicaid patients must subsidize the costs" (OTA, 1992a, p. 184).

CHAMPUS

The federal government also finances some genetic testing and screening services through the Civilian Health and Medical Program of the Uniformed Services (CHAMPUS), the primary health insurer for military dependents and retirees. CHAMPUS has adopted basic concepts similar to those of private insurers and state Medicaid programs for genetic testing and related services. It covers genetic testing for couples identified as "high risk," for example, due to prior births of affected children, but specifically excludes routine screening of low-risk pregnancies (Charo, 1992).

State Genetics Services Programs

State genetics services programs vary widely (CORN, 1991). Some states provide limited genetics services directly; most states coordinate at least some genetics services, particularly with Medicaid, Medicare (which sets reimbursement rates used by state Medicaid programs), and other possible funding sources (such as programs for persons with mental retardation or developmental disabilities, or for children with special needs) to help secure funding for people who cannot afford needed genetics services. All of the 41 states responding to a recent CORN survey reported some level of coordinated state genetics services, and 60 percent of these have a full-time state genetics services coordinator (CORN, 1991). Coordinators are located in a wide variety of state agencies, although nearly 80 percent are in the state health department, usually in the maternal and child health (MCH) program.

Of the 41 state programs that responded to the CORN survey, 84 percent were initially established with federal funding under the Genetic Diseases Act of 1976.[5] Most (77 percent) still receive some support for genetics services from the state through federal Maternal and Child Health block grant funds (Public Law 997-35), to which funding from the Genetic Diseases Act was transferred in 1981. However, MCH block grants generally represented less than 25 percent of total state funding. Nearly half the programs reported a decrease in block grant funding when inflation is taken into account (CORN, 1991). Many state genetics services programs historically paid for newborn screening, but the majority now charge birth hospitals, attending physicians, or parents for newborn screening.

A few state programs have more extensive authorization and funding that permits them to provide or pay for genetic testing or genetic counseling. State genetics services programs also vary in their policies toward the use of genetic testing information for abortion counseling (Clayton, 1993). Several states specifically attempt to limit use of available state genetics services when the goal is selective abortion of affected fetuses. Minnesota and Missouri provide extensive genetic testing services, but almost no funding for abortion services; Tennessee's extensive prenatal diagnosis program is limited to conditions leading to treatment in the mother or the baby, but its legislation states that "use of this program to abort unborn children is against the public policy of the State of Tennessee" (Tennessee Code Annotated, 1991, §§ 68-5-501-505).

Thus, the committee sees (1) wide variation in policy, practice, and funding within state programs; (2) differences in reimbursement policies and practices among third-party payers concerning reimbursement for genetic testing and counseling services; and (3) regulatory, administrative, and funding barriers to coverage and reimbursement of appropriate genetics services.

Federal Support for Genetics Services Programs

The federal government still maintains a small amount of direct project grant funding for Special Projects of Regional and National Significance (SPRANS) through the Genetic Services Branch, Maternal and Child Health Services Bureau, Health Resources and Services Administration, in the Department of Health and Human Services. These special project grants are available on a competitive basis for genetics projects of special regional or national significance, but are not intended to replace the ongoing state funding that was transferred to block grants in 1981. These grants have funded special projects around the nation as well as many activities of the Council of Regional Networks for Genetic Services (CORN), including its genetics services data collection, newborn screening, and laboratory quality assurance activities. Special project funds have also supported activities of the Alliance of Genetic Support Groups. Federal funding has reached slightly more than $9 million for fiscal year 1993 for SPRANS grants, essentially the same level of funding received for 1992.

RECOMMENDATIONS

The committee believes that education and counseling are essential components of any genetic testing (see Chapter 4). In order to develop appropriate reimbursement for genetic testing and counseling services, the committee recommends that greater efforts be made for joint undertakings among private and public health plans and geneticists to develop guidelines for the appropriate reimbursement of genetics services. Such guidelines should address the issue of how each new genetic test should be assessed for its sensitivity and specificity in light of the availability of effective treatment, the consequences of the test, the evaluation of pilot study results, and when new tests are appropriate for use in routine clinical practice.

The insurance concept of what is reimbursable (so-called medically necessary) should be defined to include appropriate genetic testing and related education and counseling, and these genetics services be reimbursed under health insurance plans. Medical necessity can often be established by a family history of the disorder. In pregnancy, medical necessity should be considered established for cytogenetic testing in pregnancies in women of advanced maternal age or those considered at high risk based on other methods of assessing risk. The committee also recommends that newborn screening and appropriate MSAFP screening in pregnant women of any age be considered within the insurance definition of what is medically appropriate, and be reimbursed under health insurance plans.

To facilitate such coverage and reimbursement for genetic testing, education, and counseling, the committee recommends the establishment and updating of appropriate and specific CPT-4 diagnostic codes for these genetic testing and counseling services. Now that the ACMG has become part of the ABMS of the AMA, the ACMG should take the lead in working with the AMA committee responsible for CPT-4 codes.

Finally, the committee recommends that health insurance reform proposals be evaluated to determine whether they adequately protect genetic information and persons with genetic disorders from discrimination and other potential social, legal, and ethical harms related to health insurance and the use of genetic information (see Chapters 7 and 8).

NOTES

1. The Committee on Assessing Genetic Risks had the benefit of the advice of Marilyn Field, Study Director of the Institute of Medicine (IOM) Committee on Employer Based Benefit Plans in preparing its analysis of issues of health insurance and its impact on access to genetic testing and counseling services.

2. The full report of the ELSI Task Force on Insurance and Genetic Testing covers many of these issues in more detail and was released in May 1993 (ELSI Insurance Task Force, 1993). Committee staff followed the work of the ELSI Task Force so that the IOM committee had the benefit of this work in its own deliberations.

3. For additional information, see the recent IOM report *Employment and Health Benefits: A Connection at Risk* (Fields and Shapiro, 1993).

4. Medical underwriting is the evaluation of a person's insurability, usually assessed through a combination of answers to a written questionnaire and physical examination to identify certain conditions determined by medical underwriters (and underwriting manuals) to reduce life expectancy or increase medical care costs beyond actuarial norms. Standards for medical underwriting vary substantially by insurance company, and underwriting decisions are considered crucial business decisions by insurers, and are thus considered "trade secrets" not subject to public disclosure.

5. The National Sickle Cell Anemia, Cooley Anemia, Tay-Sachs, and Genetic Diseases Act of 1976 (Public Law 94-278) consolidated separate 1972 legislation for sickle cell anemia (Public Law 92-294) and Cooley anemia (Public Law 92-414) and added other genetic conditions into the provisions of the law. It required the development of information and education materials "to persons providing health care, to teachers and students, and to the public in general in order to rapidly make available the latest advances in the testing, diagnosis, counseling and treatment of individuals respecting genetic disease." It also required that federally assisted programs for the disorders included were to be entirely voluntary. Although this legislation was repealed in 1981, with the passage of the Maternal and Child Health Services Block Grant Act (Public Law 97-35), the requirement that programs supported with block grant funds be entirely voluntary was never repealed.

REFERENCES

Beaudet, A. 1992 (published in 1994). General perspectives on DNA diagnosis drawn from the cystic fibrosis experience. In Fullarton, J. (ed.) Proceedings of the Committee on Assessing Genetic Risks. Washington, D.C.: National Academy Press.

Bernhardt, B., and Eierman, L. 1992. Reimbursement for cystic fibrosis (CF) DNA testing (Abstract). Meeting of the American Society of Human Genetics. San Francisco. November.

Charo, A. 1992 (published in 1994). Impact of abortion law on genetic screening. In Fullarton, J. (ed.) Proceedings of the Committee on Assessing Genetic Risks. Washington, D.C.: National Academy Press.

Clayton, E. 1993. Reproductive genetic testing: Regulatory and liability issues. Fetal Diagnosis and Therapy 8:(suppl. 1):39-59.

Council of Regional Networks for Genetic Services (CORN). 1991. Survey of state genetic services coordinators (unpublished data). New York, N.Y.

Council of Regional Networks for Genetic Services (CORN). 1992. Newborn Screening Report: 1990 (Final report, February 1992). New York, N.Y.

Employee Benefit Research Institute (EBRI). 1993. Sources of health insurance and characteristics of the uninsured, Analysis of the March 1992 Current Population Survey. Issue 133. Washington, D.C.

Field, M., and Shapiro, H. 1993. Employment and Health Benefits: A Connection at Risk. Washington, D.C.: National Academy Press.

Insurance Task Force. 1993. Genetic Information and Health Insurance. Report of the Task Force on Genetic Information and Insurance. HIH-DOE Working Group on Ethical, Legal, and Social Implications of Human Genome Research. Bethesda, Md.: National Institutes of Health (Pub. No. 93-3686). May.

Office of Technology Assessment (OTA). U.S. Congress. 1992a. Cystic Fibrosis and DNA Tests: Implications of Carrier Screening. OTA-BA-532. Washington, D.C.: U.S. Government Printing Office.

Office of Technology Assessment (OTA). U.S. Congress. 1992b. Genetic Tests and Health Insurance: Results of a Survey (background paper). OTA-BP-BA-98. Washington, D.C.: U.S. Government Printing Office.

Office of Technology Assessment (OTA). U.S. Congress. 1992c. Panel discussion; Panel on Population Screening for Cystic Fibrosis. Washington, D.C., March 11, 1992.

Pokorsky, R. 1989. Public and government relations issues. Pp. 10-11 in The Potential Role of Genetic Testing in Risk Classification. Report of the Genetic Testing Committee to the Medical Section of the American Council of Life Insurance, Hilton Head, S.C.

8

Social, Legal, and Ethical
Implications of Genetic Testing

Each new genetic test that is developed raises serious issues for medicine, public health, and social policy regarding the circumstances under which the test should be used, how the test is implemented, and what uses are made of its results. Should people be allowed to choose or refuse the test, or should it be mandatory, as newborn screening is in some states? Should people be able to control access to the results of their tests? If test results are released to third parties such as employers or insurers, what protections should be in place to ensure that people are not treated unfairly because of their genotype?

The answers to these questions depend in part on the significance given to four important ethical and legal principles: autonomy, confidentiality, privacy, and equity. A review of the meaning of those concepts and how they are currently protected by the law provides a starting point for the development of recommendations on the degree of control people should have in deciding whether to undergo genetic testing and what uses should be made of the results. The task is a pressing one. In a 1992 national probability survey of the public, sponsored by the March of Dimes, 38 percent of respondents said that new types of genetic testing should be stopped altogether until the privacy issues are settled.[1]

This chapter reviews some of the conflicts that will arise in the research and clinical settings, and suggests general principles that should be the starting point for policy analyses in this evolving field.

Since many of the references in this chapter are legal citations, its references appear in legal style as numbered end notes.

KEY DEFINITIONS

Autonomy

Ethical Analysis

Autonomy can be defined as self-determination, self-rule, or self-governance. Autonomous agents or actions presuppose some capacity of reasoning, deciding, and willing. Moral, social, and legal norms establish obligations to respect autonomous agents and their choices. Respect for personal autonomy implies that agents have the right or power to be self-governing and self-directing, without outside control. In the context of genetic testing and screening, respect for autonomy refers to the right of persons to make an informed, independent judgment about whether they wish to be tested and then whether they wish to know the details of the outcome of the testing. Autonomy is also the right of the individual to control his or her destiny, with or without reliance on genetic information, and to avoid interference by others with important life decisions, whether these are based on genetic information or other factors. Respect for autonomy also implies the right of persons to control the future use of genetic material submitted for analysis for a specific purpose (including when the genetic material itself and the information derived from that material may be stored for future analysis, such as in a DNA bank or registry file).

Even though respect for autonomy is centrally important in our society, it is not absolute. It can be overridden in some circumstances, for example, to prevent serious harm to others, as is the case in mandatory newborn screening for phenylketonuria (PKU) and hypothyroidism.

Legal Issues

The legal concept of autonomy serves as the basis for numerous decisions protecting a person's bodily integrity. In particular, cases have held that competent adults have the right to choose whether or not to undergo medical interventions.[2] Before people make such a choice, they have a right to be informed of facts that might be material to their decision,[3] such as the nature of their condition and its prognosis,[4] the potential risks and benefits of a proposed test or treatment,[5] and the alternatives to the proposed intervention.[6] In the genetics context, health care providers have been held liable for not providing the information that a genetic test is available.[7]

People also have a right to be informed about and to control the subsequent use of tissue that has been removed from their bodies.[8] There is some leeway under the federal regulations governing research involving human subjects for researchers to undertake subsequent research on blood samples provided for genetic tests (as in the newborn screening context) as long as the samples are anonymous and as long as the subsequent use was not anticipated at the time the sample was collected.[9] If the additional test *was* anticipated at the time the sample was collected, informed consent for that use should be obtained prior to the collection of the original sample.

Such an approach is thought appropriate to avert conflicts of interest, such as a physician/researcher suggesting that a patient undergo a particular test when the researcher actually wanted the tissue for the researcher's own additional use in a research or commercial project. In such a situation, the patient's autonomy is compromised even if the sample is used anonymously in the subsequent use. A report from the Office of Technology Assessment similarly stressed the importance of knowledge and consent:

> The consent of the patient is required to remove blood or tissue from his or her body, and also to perform tests, but it is important that the patient be informed of all the tests which are done and that a concern for the privacy of the patient extends to the control of tissues removed from his or her body.[10]

Privacy

Ethical Analysis

Among the various definitions of privacy, one broad definition captures its central element: privacy is "a state or condition of limited access to a person."[11] People have privacy if others lack or do not exercise access to them. They have privacy if they are left alone and do not suffer unauthorized intrusion by others. Once persons undergo genetic tests, privacy includes the right to make an informed, independent decision about whether—and which—others may know details of their genome (e.g., insurers, employers, educational institutions, spouses and other family members, researchers, and social agencies).

Various justifications have been offered for rules of privacy. First, some philosophers argue that privacy rights are merely shorthand expressions for a cluster of personal and property rights, each of which can be explicated without any reference to the concept of privacy. In making this argument, Judith Jarvis Thomson holds that privacy rights simply reflect personal and property rights, such as the rights not to be looked at, not to be overheard, and not to be caused distress.[12]

A second justification holds that rights to privacy are important instruments or means to other goods, including intimate relations such as trust and friendship. Being able to control access to themselves enables people to have various kinds of relationships with different people, rather than being equally accessible to all others.

A third approach finds the basis for rights to privacy in respect for personal autonomy. Decisional privacy is often very close to personal autonomy. The language of personal autonomy reflects the idea of a domain or territory of self-rule, and thus overlaps with zones of decisional privacy.

Whatever their rationale or justification, rights of privacy are the subject of ongoing debate about their scope and weight. However, their scope is not unlimited, and they do not always override all other competing interests, such as the interests of others.

Legal Issues

In the legal sphere, the principle of privacy is an umbrella concept encompassing issues of both autonomy and confidentiality. The right to make choices about one's health care is protected, in part, by the right to privacy guaranteed by the U.S. Constitution, as well as state constitutions. This includes a right to make certain reproductive choices,[13] such as whether to use genetic testing.[14] It also includes a right to refuse treatment.

An entirely different standard of privacy protects personal information. A few court decisions find protection for such information under the constitutional doctrine of privacy,[15] but more commonly, privacy protection against disclosure of personal information is found under common law tort principles.[16] In addition, there is a federal privacy act,[17] as well as state statutes protecting privacy.

Confidentiality

Ethical Analysis

Confidentiality as a principle implies that some body of information is sensitive, and hence, access to it must be controlled and limited to parties authorized to have such access. The information provided within the relationship is given in confidence, with the expectation that it will not be disclosed to others or will be disclosed to others only within limits. The state or condition of nondisclosure or limited disclosure may be protected by moral, social, or legal principles and rules, which can be expressed in terms of rights or obligations.

In health care and various other relationships, we grant others access to our bodies. They may touch, observe, listen, palpate, and even physically invade. They may examine our bodies as a whole or in parts; and parts, such as tissue, may be removed for further study, as in some forms of testing. Privacy is necessarily diminished when others have such access to us; rules of confidentiality authorize us to control and thus to limit further access to the information generated in that relationship. For example, rules of confidentiality may prohibit a physician from disclosing some information to an insurance company or an employer without the patient's authorization.

Rules of confidentiality appear in virtually every code or set of regulations for health care relationships. Their presence is not surprising, because such rules are often justified on the basis of their instrumental value: if prospective patients cannot count on health care professionals to maintain confidentiality, they will be reluctant to allow professionals the full and complete access necessary for diagnosis and treatment. Hence, rules of confidentiality are indispensable for patient and social welfare; without those rules, people who need medical, psychiatric, or other treatment will refrain from seeking or fully participating in it. Another justification for rules of confidentiality is based on the principles of respect for autonomy and privacy, above. Respecting persons involves respecting their zone of privacy and accepting their decisions to control access to information about them. When people grant health care professionals access to them, they should retain the right to determine who else has access to the information generated in that relationship. Hence, the arguments for respect for autonomy and privacy support rules of confidentiality. Finally, duties of confidentiality often derive from explicit or implicit promises in the relationship. For instance, if the professional's public oath or the profession's code of ethics promises confidentiality of information, and the particular professional does not specifically disavow it, then the patient has a right to expect that information generated in the relationship will be treated as confidential.[18]

There are at least two distinct types of infringements of rules of confidentiality. On the one hand, rules of confidentiality are sometimes infringed through deliberate breaches. On the other hand, rules of confidentiality are often infringed through carelessness, for example, when health care professionals do not take adequate precautions to protect the confidential information. Some commentators argue that both carelessness and modern practices of health care have rendered medical confidentiality a "decrepit concept," since it is compromised routinely in the provision of health care.[19]

It is widely recognized that the rules of confidentiality are limited in at least two senses: (1) some information may not be protected, and (2) the rules may sometimes be overridden to protect other values. First, not all information is deemed confidential, and patients do not have a right to expect that such information will be protected from disclosure to others. For example, laws frequently require that health care professionals report gunshot wounds, venereal diseases, and other communicable diseases such as tuberculosis. Second, health care professionals may also have a moral or legal right (and sometimes even an obligation) to infringe rules of confidentiality, for example, to prevent a serious harm from occurring. In such cases, rules of confidentiality protect the information, but they can be overridden in order to protect some other value. Judgments about such cases depend on the probability of serious harm occurring unless confidentiality is breached. Any justified infringements of rules of confidentiality should satisfy the conditions identified earlier in the discussion of justified infringements of the principle of respect for autonomy.

Legal Issues

The legal concept of confidentiality focuses on the information that people provide to their physicians. The protection of confidentiality is thought to serve an important public health goal in encouraging people to seek access to health care. It is thought that the patient's interest can be served only in an atmosphere of total frankness and candor.[20] Without the promise of confidentiality, people might avoid seeking medical treatment, thus potentially harming themselves as well as the community. In fact, the first doctor-patient confidentiality statute was passed in 1828 in New York during the smallpox epidemic to encourage people to seek health care. Various legal decisions have protected confidentiality of health care information,[21] as have certain state and federal statutes.

Confidentiality of health care information is also protected because disclosure of a person's medical condition can cause harm to him or her. An alternative set of legal principles—those penalizing discrimination (see below)—protects people against unfair uses of certain information.

Equity

Ethical Analysis

Issues of justice, fairness, and equity crop up in several actions, practices, and policies relating to genetic testing. It is now commonplace to distinguish formal justice from substantive justice. Formal justice requires treating similar cases in a similar way. Standards of substantive or material justice establish the identity of the relevant similarities and differences and the appropriate responses to those similarities and differences. For instance, a society has to determine whether to distribute a scarce resource such as health care according to persons' differences in need, social worth, or ability to pay.

One crucial question is whether genetic disorders or predispositions provide a basis for blocking access to certain social goods, such as employment or health insurance. Most conceptions of justice dictate that employment be based on the ability to perform particular tasks effectively and safely. For these conceptions, it is unjust to deny employment to someone who meets the relevant qualifications but also has a genetic disease. Frequently these questions of employment overlap with questions of health insurance. Practices of medical underwriting in health insurance reflect what is often called "actuarial fairness"—that is, grouping those with similar risks together so insurers can accurately predict costs, and set fair and sufficient premium rates. Although actuarial fairness may be intuitively appealing, critics argue that it does not express moral or social fairness. According to Norman Daniels, there is "a clear mismatch between standard underwriting practices and the social function of health insurance" in providing individuals with resources for access to health care[22] (see Chapter 7).

The fundamental argument for excluding genetic discrimination in health insurance amounts to an argument for establishing a right to health care. One of the central issues in debates about the distribution of health care is one's view of the "natural lottery," in particular, a "genetic lottery."[23] The metaphor of a lottery suggests that health needs result largely from an impersonal natural lottery and are thus undeserved. But even if health needs are largely undeserved because of the role of chance, society's response to those needs may vary, as H. Tristram Engelhardt notes, depending on whether it views those needs as *unfair* or as *unfortunate*.[24] If health needs are unfortunate, but not unfair, they may be the object of individual or social compassion. Other individuals, voluntary associations, and even society may be motivated by compassion to try to meet those needs. If, however, the needs are viewed as unfair as well as unfortunate, society may have a duty of justice to try to meet those needs.

One prominent argument for the societal provision of a decent minimum of health care is that, generally, health needs are randomly distributed and unpredictable, as well as overwhelming when health crises occur.[25] Because of these features of health needs, many argue that it is inappropriate to distribute health care according to merit, societal contribution, or even ability to pay. Another version of the argument from fairness holds that health needs represent departures from normal species functioning and deprive people of fair equality of opportunity. Thus, fairness requires the provision of health care to "maintain, restore, or compensate for the loss of normal functioning" in order to ensure fair equality of opportunity.[26]

Several committee members expressed concerns that these stated arguments are somewhat weakened by the fact that a number of diseases are not the result of random events, but are brought on or exacerbated by dispensable habits such as cigarette smoking and excessive alcohol ingestion. While our and other societies attempt to discourage such habits by education and taxation, there is general agreement that access to full health care must be ensured once illness develops. If a tendency to abuse alcohol, for example, were to have a genetic predisposition, an additional argument could be made for providing the same level of health care to everyone since a person does not choose his or her genetic propensities.

The argument that society should guarantee or provide a decent minimum of health care for all citizens and residents points toward a direction for health policy, but it does not determine exactly how much health care the society should provide relative to other goods it also seeks. And, within the health care budget, there will be difficult allocation questions, including how much should be used for particular illnesses and for particular treatments for those illnesses. Questions of allocation cannot be resolved in the abstract. In democratic societies, they should be resolved through political processes that express the public's will. In specifying and implementing a conception of a decent minimum, an adequate level, or a fair share of health care in the context of scarce resources, as the President's Commission noted in 1983, it is reasonable for a society to turn to fair, democratic political procedures to choose among alternative conceptions of adequate health care, and in view of "the great imprecision in the notion of adequate health care . . . it is especially important that the procedures used to define that level be—and be perceived to be—fair."[27]

Legal Issues

The concept of equity serves as the underpinning for a variety of legal doctrines and statutes. Certain needy people are provided health care, including some genetics services, under government programs such as Medicaid (see Chapter 7). In addition, some legislative efforts have been made to prohibit discrimination based on genotype. For example, some states have statutes prohibiting discrimination in employment based on one's genotype.[28] And nearly all people over age 65 are deemed to have a right to care (under Medicare).

CURRENT PRACTICE OF PROTECTION IN GENETICS

The development of genetic testing has raised numerous concerns about autonomy, confidentiality, privacy, and equity that are exacerbated by the range of contexts in which such tests are undertaken, the sheer volume of tests that could be offered, the many uses that can be made of test results, and the variety of institutions that store genetic information. To date, most genetic testing has been done in the reproductive context or with newborns, to identify serious disorders that currently or soon will affect the fetus or infant. However, the types of genetic conditions or predispositions that can potentially be tested for are much broader than those signaling serious, imminent diseases. These include characteristics (such as sex or height) that are not diseases, potential susceptibility to diseases if the person comes into contact with particular environmental stimuli, and indications that a currently asymptomatic person will suffer later in life from a debilitating disease such as Huntington disease. The genetic anomalies that can be tested for range widely in their manifestations, their severity, their treatability, and their social significance. People's ability to define themselves, to manage their destiny and self-concept, will depend in large measure on the control they have over whether they and others come to know their genetic characteristics.

Most medical testing is done within a physician-patient relationship. With genetic testing, however, the potential range of contexts in which it can be undertaken is large. Already, in the public health context, more than 4 million newborns are tested annually for metabolic disorders so that effective treatment can be started in a few hundred. Researchers are inviting people to participate in family studies and undergo genetic testing, including collection of DNA samples for present or future analyses. There are a growing number of nonmedical applications of genetic testing as well. In the law enforcement context, DNA testing is undertaken to attempt to identify criminal offenders. At least 17 states have DNA fingerprint programs for felons.[29] The armed services are collecting DNA samples from all members of the military, the primary purpose of which is to identify bodies of deceased soldiers. Employers and insurers may require people to undergo testing for genetic disorders for exclusionary purposes. One challenge for policy posed by this wide array of testing settings is that many of the existing legal precedents about autonomy, confidentiality, and privacy apply only to the traditional doctor-patient relationship. For example, some state statutes governing confidentiality deal only with information provided to physicians and might not cover information provided to Ph.D. researchers or employers.

There seems to be great variation among institutions and among providers in the amount of attention paid to autonomy, confidentiality, and privacy. For example, some obstetricians recognize the patient's autonomy by providing them the information about maternal serum alpha-fetoprotein (MSAFP) screening but acknowledging the patient's right to decide whether or not to undergo the test. Other obstetricians run the test on blood gathered from the woman for other purposes, so the woman does not even know she has been the subject of the test unless the obstetrician delivers the bad news that she has had an abnormal result.

Geneticists differ with respect to the emphasis they place on the confidentiality of the results of genetic testing. In a survey by Dorothy Wertz and John Fletcher,[30] numerous geneticists suggested that there were at least four situations in which they would breach confidentiality and disclose genetic information without the patient's permission, even over the patient's refusal: (1) 54 percent said they would disclose to a relative the risk of Huntington disease; (2) 53 percent said they would disclose the risk of hemophilia A; (3) 24 percent said they would disclose genetic information to a patient's employer; and (4) 12 percent said they would disclose such information to the patient's insurer. Primary care physicians may be even more likely to disclose such information.[31] Health care providers should explain their policies for disclosure in advance, including for disclosure to relatives.

Institutions that store DNA samples[32] or store the results of genetic tests also differ in the amount of respect they give to autonomy, confidentiality, and privacy.[33] Some institutions do additional tests on DNA samples without the permission of the person who provided the sample. Some share samples with other institutions. Some store samples or information with identifiers attached, rather than anonymously. Indeed, storage conditions themselves differ widely. Some newborn screening programs store filter papers in a temperature-controlled, secure setting; others merely pile them in a file cabinet or storage closet. Programs also differ in the length of time the sample or the test results are maintained.

Once DNA material has been submitted, there are few safeguards concerning other present or future uses that may be made of the material. DNA from the blood spots collected for newborn screening can now be extracted for further testing.[34] No standards or safeguards currently exist to govern the appropriate use of DNA analysis and storage from newborn screening tests. These possibilities raise questions about the need to obtain consent for additional and subsequent uses (particularly since consent is almost never obtained initially in newborn screening), as well as questions about the duty to warn if disorders are detected in the blood by using the new DNA extraction testing techniques.

The issue of confidentiality of genetic information will be underscored with the introduction of "optical memory cards," a credit card-sized device that stores medical information.[35] These cards have already been introduced for use in Houston city health clinics. There is sufficient computer memory on the cards to include genetic information about the person and, in the future, to include a person's entire genome.

Congressional legislation has been introduced that would require all patients to use optical memory cards. This bill, the Medical and Health Insurance Information Reform Act of 1992, would mandate a totally electronic system of communication between health care providers and insurers. Such a system would be based either on the optical memory card (with a microchip capable of storing data) or on a card similar to an Automated Teller Card (which simply provides access to data stored elsewhere).

APPLYING THE PRINCIPLES
TO GENETIC TESTING

The principles of autonomy, privacy, confidentiality, and equity place great weight on individuals' rights to make personal decisions without interference. This is due, in part, to the importance placed on individuals in our culture and our legal system. However, individual rights are not without bound, and the area of genetics raises important questions of where individual rights end and where responsibilities to a group—such as one's family or the larger society—begin.

Medicine is generally practiced within this culture of individual rights (with provisions for patients' right to refuse treatment and right to control the dissemination of medical information about themselves), but there have been circumstances in which the medical model has been supplanted by the public health model, which encourages the *prevention* of disease—for example, by requiring that certain medical intervention (such as vaccinations) be undertaken and by warning individuals of health risks (e.g., through educational campaigns against smoking or through contact tracing with respect to venereal diseases). Some commentators have suggested that the public health model be applied to genetics,[36] with mandatory genetic screening and even mandatory abortion of seriously affected fetuses. A related measure might be warning people of their risk of genetic disorders.

There are several difficulties with applying the public health model to genetics, however. Certain infectious diseases potentially put society as a whole at immediate risk since the diseases can be transmitted to a large number of people in a short time. The potential victims are existing human beings who may be total strangers to the affected individual. In contrast to infectious disease, the transmission of genetic diseases does not present an immediate threat to society. Whereas infectious disease can cause rapid devastation to a community, the transmission of genetic disorders to offspring does not necessarily have an immediate detrimental effect, but rather creates a potential risk for a future generation in society.[37] U.S.

Supreme Court cases dealing with fundamental rights have held that harm in the future is not as compelling a state interest as immediate harm.[38]

Moreover, the very concept of "prevention" does not readily fit most genetic diseases. In the case of newborn screening for PKU, treatment can prevent mental retardation. However, with many genetic diseases today, the genetic disease itself is not being prevented, but rather the birth of a particular individual with the disease is prevented (e.g., when a couple, each of whom is heterozygous for a serious recessive disorder, chooses not to conceive or chooses to terminate the pregnancy of a fetus who is homozygous for the disorder). This sort of prevention cannot be viewed in the same way as preventing measles or syphilis, for example. There is a great variation among people in their view of disability and what constitutes a disorder to be "prevented." Many people will welcome a child with Down syndrome or cystic fibrosis into their family. In addition, some individuals have religious or other personal moral objections to abortion; even mandatory carrier status screening or prenatal screening without mandatory abortion may be objected to because people who object to abortion are concerned that the abortion rate will rise among those in the general population who learn of genetic risks to their fetus. Furthermore, some people with a particular disability or genetic risk may view mandatory genetic testing for that risk or disability as an attempt to eradicate their kind, as a disavowal of their worth.

Mandatory genetic testing might also have devastating effects on the individuals who are tested. Unlike infectious disease (which can be viewed as external to the person), genetic disease may be viewed by people as an intractable part of their nature. Persons who learn, against their will, that they carry a defective gene may view themselves as defective. This harm is compounded if they did not choose to learn the information voluntarily. This assault on personal identity is less likely with infectious diseases, although AIDS and genital herpes (for example) can also have a negative impact on self-image. Moreover, most genetic defects, unlike most infectious diseases, generally cannot now be corrected.[39] Thus, the unasked-for revelation that occurs through mandatory genetic testing can haunt the person throughout his or her life and can have widespread reverberations in the family, including others who may be at risk or related as partners. The information can serve as the basis for discrimination against the individual.

Additionally, policy concerns raised by attempts to stop the transmission of genetic diseases differ from those addressed to infectious diseases because genetic diseases may differentially affect people of different races or ethnic backgrounds. For that reason, some commentators contest the applicability of the infectious disease model to government actions regarding genetic disorders. Catherine Damme notes that "unlike infectious disease which [generally] knows no ethnic, racial, or gender boundaries, genetic disease is the result of heredity"— leaving open the possibility for discriminatory governmental actions.[40]

The government has discretion with respect to which infectious diseases it tackles. For example, it can decide to require screening for syphilis but not chlamydia, or to require vaccinations for smallpox but not for diphtheria. Government action with respect to genetic diseases is likely to be regarded much differently, especially with respect to disorders for which an effective treatment does not exist and, consequently, the only medical procedure available is the abortion of an affected fetus. Minority groups who have been discriminated against in the past may view a screening program that targets only disorders that occur within their racial or ethnic group as an additional attack, and may view abstention from reproduction or the abortion of offspring based on genetic information as a form of genocide.[41]

Those commentators who argue that the infectious disease precedents justify mandatory genetic screening fail to recognize that even in the case of infectious disease, very few medical procedures are mandated for adults. Adults are not forced to seek medical diagnosis and treatment even if they have a treatable infectious disease. Laws that required compulsory infectious disease screening prior to marriage (e.g., for venereal disease) are being repealed. For example, New York abolished its requirements for premarital gonorrhea and syphilis testing. One of the reasons for the abolition of the requirements was that they were not the most appropriate way to reach the population at risk.[42]

Mandating diagnosis and treatment for genetic disorders is particularly problematic when the concept of disease is so flexible. Arno Motulsky has noted that "[t]he precise definition of 'disease' regardless of etiology, is difficult."[43] He notes that maladies such as high blood pressure and mental retardation are based on arbitrary cutoff levels. David Brock similarly noted that most disorders lie between the extremes of Tay-Sachs disease and alkaptonuria; what a physician advises "depends as much on the physician's ethical preconceptions as his medical experience."[44]

Despite the fact that the public health model does not fit the situation of genetics, the individual rights model should not be seen as absolute. There are certain situations in which the values of autonomy, privacy, confidentiality, and equity should give way to prevent serious harm to others. Determining the exceptions to these general principles is no easy matter, however. There may be instances in which harm can be prevented by violating one of these principles, but in which the value of upholding the principles will nonetheless outweigh the chance of averting harm. In each instance, it will be necessary to assess several factors: How serious is the harm to be averted? Is violating one of the principles the best way to avert the harm? What will be the medical, psychological, and other risks of violating the principle? What will be the financial costs of violating the principle?

The following section addresses the issues raised by the application of these principles—autonomy, privacy, confidentiality, and equity—in the contexts of clinical genetics, other medical practices, genetics research, and so forth. It also provides guidance for determining the appropriate circumstances for exceptions to these principles. The chapter concludes with the committee's recommendations on these issues.

ISSUES IN GENETIC TESTING

Autonomy

One important way to ensure autonomy with respect to genetic testing is to provide adequate information upon which a person can make a decision whether or not to undergo testing. A proper informed consent in medicine generally involves the presentation of information about the risks, benefits, efficacy, and alternatives to the procedure being undertaken. In addition, recent cases and statutes have recognized the importance of disclosures of any potential conflicts of interest that the health care professional recommending the test may have, such as a financial interest in the facility to which the patient is being referred. In the genetics context, this would include disclosure about equity holdings or ownership of the laboratory, dependence on test reimbursement to cover the costs of counseling, patents, and so forth. It would also include disclosure of any planned subsequent uses of the tissue samples, even if such uses are to be anonymous.

Various kinds of information are relevant to people who are attempting to exercise their autonomy by deciding whether or not to undergo genetic testing. This includes information about the severity, potential variability, and treatability of the disorder being tested for. If, for example, carrier status testing is being proposed for a pregnant woman or prenatal testing is being proposed for her fetus, she should be told whether the disorder at issue can be prevented or treated, or whether she will be faced with a decision about whether or not to abort (see Chapters 2, 4, and 5). The proposed informed consent guidelines for research involving genetic testing suggested by the Alliance of Genetic Support Groups provide an excellent starting point for the development of informed consent policies in the genetics area (see Chapter 4).

The potential development of multiplex testing adds another wrinkle to the issue of informed consent for genetic testing. If 100 disorders are tested from the same blood sample, it may be difficult to apply the current model of informed consent in which a health care provider gives information about each disorder and the efficacy of each test to the patient in advance of the testing. The difficulty in applying the traditional mechanisms for achieving informed consent does not provide an excuse for failing to respect a patient's autonomy and need for information, however. New mechanisms may have to be developed to protect these rights. It will be possible to have results reported back to the physician and patient only about those tests (or types of tests) the patient chooses. The choices can be made by the patient, based, for example, on the patient learning through a computer program about the various disorders and the various tests. Or the choices can be made according to general categories—for example, the patient might choose to have multiplex testing but choose *not* be informed of the results of testing for untreatable or unpreventable disorders[45] (see Chapters 1, 3, and 4).

In addition to the recognition that people are entitled to information before they make decisions, a second application of the autonomy principle comes with the recognition that the decision to participate in genetic testing and other genetics services must be voluntary. Voluntariness has been a recognized principle in past recommendations and practices involving genetics. This is in keeping with the recognized right of competent adults to refuse medical intervention, as well as the right to refuse even the presentation of medical information in the informed consent context.[46] If, for example, it becomes possible to accurately screen fetal cells isolated from a pregnant woman's blood in order to determine the genetic status of the fetus, state public health departments might be interested in requiring the test on the grounds that it is a minimally invasive procedure that can provide information to the woman (perhaps leading her to abort an affected fetus and saving the state money for care of that infant). Mandating such a test, however, would show insufficient respect for the woman's autonomy and would violate her right to make reproductive decisions.

Special Issues in the Screening and Testing of Children

The expansion of available tests fostered by the Human Genome Project will present complicated issues with respect to the testing of newborns and other children. Although there are clear legal precedents stating that adults are free to refuse even potentially beneficial testing and treatment, legal precedents provide that children can be treated without their consent (and over their parents' refusal) to prevent serious imminent harm. The U.S. Supreme Court has said that, while parents are free to make martyrs of themselves, they are not free to make martyrs of their children.[47] Medical intervention over parents' objection has been allowed in situations in which a child's life was in imminent danger and the treatment posed little risk of danger in itself.[48] Blood transfusions have been ordered for the children of Jehovah's Witnesses when the child's life was imminently endangered.[49]

All states have programs to screen newborns for certain inborn errors of metabolism for which early intervention with treatment provides a clear medical benefit to the child, such as phenylketonuria. Currently, the statutes of at least two jurisdictions (the District of Columbia and Maryland) clearly provide that newborn screening is voluntary.[50] In at least two states (Montana and West Virginia), screening is mandatory and there is no legal provision for parental objection or refusal based on religious grounds.[51] In the rest of the states, there are grounds for parental refusal for religious or other reasons. However, although the majority of states allow objection to screening on some grounds, very few statutes require that the parents or guardians of an infant either be sufficiently informed that they can choose whether or not their infant should submit to the screening or be told they have the right to object. Two states (Missouri and South Carolina) have criminal penalties for parents who refuse newborn screening of their children.[52]

The idea behind mandatory newborn screening is a benevolent one—to try to ensure that all children get the benefits of screening for PKU and hypothyroidism, for which early treatment can make a dramatic difference in the child's well-being by preventing mental retardation. Yet there is little evidence that it is necessary to make a newborn screening program mandatory to ensure that children are screened under the program. Recent studies show that the few states with voluntary newborn screening programs screen a higher percentage of newborns than some states with mandatory newborn screening programs; for 1990, voluntary programs reported reaching 100 percent of newborns in their states, while some states with mandatory programs report reaching 98 percent, and some even less than 96 percent.[53] Relevant research has suggested that even when a newborn screening program is completely voluntary and parents may refuse for any reason, the actual refusal rate is quite low, about 0.05 percent (27 of 50,000 mothers). In that study, most nurses reported that it required only one to five minutes to inform a mother about newborn screening.[54]

Newborn screening for PKU—like a necessary blood transfusion for a child over the parents' refusal—has been justified on the basis of the legal doctrine of *parens patriae*, where the state steps in to order an intervention to protect a child from substantial, imminent harm. In the era of the Human Genome Project, when additional tests are being developed, some people are promoting newborn screening in part for less immediate and less clear benefits. Proposed guidelines have suggested that another benefit of newborn screening "might take the form of inscription in registries for later reproductive counseling (material PKU) or of surveillance of phenotypes (congenital adrenal hyperplasia)."[55] To achieve such an outcome, the resulting children would need to be followed until the age when reproductive counseling was appropriate—or when symptoms manifest—a daunting task in this age of mobility.

The first newborn screening programs were for disorders in which early treatment of the newborn was effective. Increasingly, however, testing is suggested for untreatable disorders. In such instances, the justification is not the benefit to the newborn but the benefit to the parents for future reproductive plans. For such reasons, several countries—and some states in the United States (e.g., Pennsylvania)—screen newborns for Duchenne muscular dystrophy. This medical intervention has no immediate medical benefit for the newborn, and carrier screening of the parents could be obtained through other methods, even when (as in the case of Duchenne muscular dystrophy and some other conditions) they may not realize they are at risk.

Moreover, screening newborns for genes for untreatable disorders or carrier status may have disadvantages. The children may be provided with information that, at the age of consent, they would rather not have. Parents might treat them differently if the results are positive. Parents may stigmatize or reject children with the abnormal genes, or may be less willing to devote financial resources to education or other benefits for such children. In addition, release of the test results might cause them to be uninsurable, unemployable, and unmarriageable.

There are additional benefits from voluntariness in newborn screening. Informing parents about newborn screening in advance of testing allows quality assurance: parents can check to see if the sample was actually drawn. As children are being released from the hospital increasingly early, due to insurance pressures, they might receive a false negative result because blood levels of phenylalanine have not yet risen sufficiently to be detected if elevated. Informed motivated parents may need to bring their babies to be screened after release from the hospital in order to ensure an accurate test result. The recommended informed consent process can provide the necessary education and motivation that will be required to make the return trip far better than mandatory programs.

In the postgenome era, people will be facing the possibility of undergoing many more genetic tests in their lifetimes, and will need to master a wealth of genetic information that is relevant to their health, their reproductive plans, and the choices they make about what to eat, where to live, and what jobs to take. The more settings in which they can be informed about genetics, the more able they will be to make these decisions. In addition, when newborn screening programs are voluntary, there is a greater chance that parents will be provided with material in advance about the disorder and have their questions answered, thus presenting the possibility that they will view it more seriously and will make a greater effort to ensure that the child receives proper treatment if a condition is detected. The disclosure of information to parents about newborn screening prior to newborn screening can be an important tool for public education about genetics.

Mandatory newborn screening should only be undertaken if there is strong evidence of benefit to the newborn from effective treatment at the earliest possible age (e.g., PKU and congenital hypothyroidism). Under this principle, screening for Duchenne muscular dystrophy would not be justified. In addition, mandatory newborn screening for cystic fibrosis would currently not be justified.[56] A prospective double-blind study in Wisconsin (the only controlled study on the subject) has not found benefits of early detection in newborn screening for CF; the treatment of children could be initiated with just as successful results based on the occurrence of symptoms. In addition to its lack of clear benefit, newborn screening for CF has a clear downside. Screening by its nature is overly broad; in newborn screening for cystic fibrosis, for example, "only 6.1 percent of infants with positive first tests [in the Colorado and Wyoming program] were ultimately found to have cystic fibrosis on sweat chloride testing."[57] Yet one-fifth of parents with false positives on newborn screening for cystic fibrosis "had lingering anxiety about their children's health."[58] Of the parents whose infants had initial, later disproven positive reports of CF in the Wisconsin study, 5 percent still believed a year later that their child might have CF.[59] Such a reaction may influence how parents relate to their child. A report on the Wisconsin newborn screening for CF stated that of the 104 families with false positives, 8 percent planned to change their reproductive plans and an additional 22 percent were not sure whether they would change their reproductive plans.[60] In fact, in France, the newborn screening program for cystic fibrosis was terminated at the request of parents who objected to the high number of false positives.[61] Denmark stopped screening for alpha-1-antitrypsin deficiency because of negative long-term effects on the mother-child interactions associated with identifying the infant's alpha-1-antitrypsin deficiency.[62]

Even in cases where a treatment is available for a disorder detectable through newborn screening, it may not be of unequivocal benefit if started after symptoms appear. Treatment of children identified through screening for maple syrup urine disease may have only limited effectiveness at best, and parents may face a quandary about whether or not to treat. Even if hypothetical benefits exist, newborn screening programs need close scrutiny to determine if the necessary treatments are actually provided to the children. In states that support screening but not treatment, families may be unable to afford treatment and thus children may not benefit from screening. Many children with sickle cell anemia, for example, do not get their necessary penicillin prophylaxis.[63] Although most states provide education about diet and nutrition to parents of infants with PKU, not all states provide the expensive essential diet or other food assistance.

Beyond the issue of the testing of newborns in state-sponsored programs, there are more general issues regarding the genetic testing of children in clinical settings. Some technologies designed to identify affected individuals will also provide information about carrier status. If an infant is tested for sickle cell anemia, for example, the test will reveal whether the infant is a carrier. In that case, the carrier status information is a by-product of the test for sickle cell anemia since obtaining information on carrier status is not the primary purpose of the testing. Questions arise as to whether that information should be reported to the infant's parents.

One advantage to reporting the information is that it is relevant to the parents' future reproductive plans. If the infant is a carrier, at least one of the parents is a carrier. If both are carriers, then they are at 25 percent risk of having an affected child. On the other hand, there are disadvantages to the reporting of such information to parents. Unless education and counseling are available, they may erroneously worry that the child will be affected with a disease related to the carrier status. They may stigmatize the child or otherwise treat the child as different. In addition, the disclosure of the child's carrier status may result in disruption to the family if neither of the social parents is a carrier (which most often indicates that another man fathered the child).

Since numerous tests can be added in a newborn screening program using the initial filter paper spot, the pressure to add new tests may be difficult to resist. Under the American Society of Human Genetics (ASHG) guidelines, however, before tests are added, a rigorous analysis should be made about who will benefit, who will be harmed, and who consents. In state programs for newborn screening, subsequent anonymous uses of samples for research may be undertaken.

Voluntariness of Subsequent Uses

Many state newborn screening programs, as well as research and clinical facilities, store the filter paper spots or other DNA samples for long periods after their initial use in genetic testing. Some states use newborn screening spots to experiment with new tests, and this would seem permissible as long as the samples are not identified and the uses were not anticipated prior to the initial test.[64] If the samples are identified, the person's permission would be required. However, researchers constitute just one group that might want access to the newborn screening spots. Such spots are of interest to law enforcement officials; in one case, police contacted a newborn screening laboratory when they were trying to identify a young murder victim.

The American Society of Human Genetics issued a statement on DNA banking and DNA data banking in 1990.[65] ASHG recommended the purposes for which samples are acquired for DNA analysis be defined in advance:

> Later access to DNA samples or to the profiles for *other* purposes should be permitted only when (a) a court orders the information to be released, (b) the data are to be anonymously studied, or (c) the individual from whom the sample was obtained provides written permission. In general, regardless of the purpose for which it was compiled, this information should be accorded at least the confidentiality that is accorded to medical records.[66]

Confidentiality

Confidentiality is meant to encourage the free flow of information between patient and physician so that the patient's sickness may be adequately treated. The protection of confidentiality is also justified as a public health matter, since ill people may not seek medical services in the first place if confidentiality is not protected. As a legal matter, confidentiality is generally protected in the doctor-patient relationship. However, genetic testing may not always occur within a doctor-patient relationship: a non-M.D. scientist may undertake the testing, or screening may occur in the employment setting. Moreover, it is not just the result of the test that raises concern about confidentiality. The sample itself may be stored (as in DNA banking or family linkage studies) for future use.

Genetic information is unlike other medical information. It reveals not only potential disease or other risks to the patient, but also information about potential risks to the person's children and blood relatives. The fact that geneticists may wish to protect third parties from harm by breaching confidentiality and disclosing risks to relatives is evidenced in the study by Wertz and Fletcher, cited earlier, in which half of the geneticists surveyed would disclose information to relatives over a patient's refusal. The geneticist's desire to disclose is based on the idea that the information will help the relative avoid harm. Yet this study indicated that about the same number of geneticists would disclose to the relative when the disorder was untreatable as when the disorder was treatable (53 percent would contact a relative about the risk of Huntington disease; 54 percent about the risk of hemophilia A). Since most people at risk for Huntington disease have not chosen testing to see if they have the genetic marker for the disorder,[67] geneticists may be overestimating the relative's desire for genetic information and infringing upon the relative's right not to know. They may be causing psychological harm if they provide surprising or unwanted information for which there is no beneficial action the relative can take.

In the legal realm, there is an exception to confidentiality: A physician may in certain instances breach confidentiality in order to protect third parties from harm, for example, when the patient might transmit a contagious disease[68] or commit violence against an identifiable individual.[69] In a landmark California case, for example, a psychiatrist was found to have a duty to warn the potential victim that his patient planned to kill her.[70]

The principle of protecting third parties from serious harm might also be used to allow disclosure to an employer when an employee's medical condition could create a risk to the public. In one case, the results of an employee's blood test for alcohol were given to his employer.[71] The court held the disclosure was not actionable because the state did not have a statute protecting confidentiality, but the court also noted that public policy would favor disclosure in this instance since the plaintiff was an engineer who controlled a railroad passenger train.

An argument could be made that health care professionals working in the medical genetics field have disclosure obligations similar to those of the physician whose patient suffers from an infectious disease or a psychotherapist with a potentially violent patient. Because of the heritable nature of genetic diseases, a health professional who—through research, counseling, examination, testing, or treatment—gains knowledge about an individual's genetic status often has information that would be of value not only to the patient, but to his or her spouse or relatives, as well as to insurers, employers, and others. A counterargument could be made, however, that since the health professional is not in a professional relationship with the relative and the patient will not be harming the relative (unlike in the case of violence or infectious diseases), there should be no duty to warn.

The claims of the third parties to information, in breach of the fundamental principle of confidentiality, need to be analyzed, as indicated earlier, by assessing how serious the potential harm is, whether disclosure is the best way to avert the harm, and what the risk of disclosure might be.

Disclosing Genetic Information to Spouses

The genetic testing of a spouse can give rise to information that is of interest to the other spouse. In the vast majority of situations, the tested individual will share that information with the other spouse. In rare instances, the information will not be disclosed and the health care provider will be faced with the issue of whether to breach confidentiality. When a married individual is diagnosed as having the allele for a serious recessive disorder, the spouse might claim that the health care provider has a duty to share that information with him or her to facilitate reproductive decision making.[72] A few court cases have allowed physicians to disclose medical information about an individual in order to protect a spouse or potential spouse.[73] The foundation for this approach is laid by cases allowing disclosure of communicable diseases.[74] In situations such as disclosure of information about venereal disease or AIDS, the argument is made that sacrificing confidentiality, by notifying spouses and lovers, is necessary for public health and welfare, and is essential as a warning to seriously endangered third parties where the risk of transmission is high.

Since genetic disorders are not communicable to the spouse, a counter argument could be made that there is no legitimate reason for disclosing them. However, the spouse might have a great interest in the genetic information because he or she would like to protect any potential children from risk. Consider the case of a doctor who learns that a young man will later suffer from Huntington disease. The wife would appear to have at least some claim to that information since, if she and her husband have children, there will be a 50 percent chance that each child would inherit the disease. Similarly, each spouse would seem to have a claim to the information that the other was a carrier of a single gene for a recessive defect. Because of the importance of reproductive decisions, such information is crucial to the spouse.

Another instance in which genetic risk information arises in the marriage context is through prenatal screening. A fetus may be found to have an autosomal recessive disorder, which occurs only if both parents transmit the particular gene. If, in the course of prenatal diagnosis, it is learned that the mother is a carrier of the gene but her husband is not, the health care professional has knowledge that the husband is almost certainly not the father of the child. A claim could be made that the health care professional has a duty, or at least a right, to advise the husband of his misattributed paternity, so that he will know that any future children he has will not be at risk for that particular disorder.

On the other hand, an argument could be made that spouses should not be entitled to genetic risk information about a patient, even if it is arguably relevant to their future reproductive plans.[75] The right of reproductive decision making is viewed as the right of the individual.[76] The U.S. Supreme Court has held that a woman can abort without her husband's consent even if this will interfere with her husband's reproductive plans.[77] More recently, the U.S. Supreme Court held that a husband was not even entitled to notice that his wife intends to abort.[78] The court expressed concerns that the husband might react to the disclosure with violence, with threats to withhold economic support, or with psychological coercion.[79] Similar reactions could occur with information about misattributed paternity, particularly because the primary purpose of the testing was not to get paternity information.

Disclosing Genetic Information to Relatives

Blood relatives of the patient may have a more convincing claim than spouses for requiring that health care providers breach confidentiality. They could argue that the information about genetic risks or the availability of genetic testing may be relevant to their own future health care.[80] The strongest case for a warning would exist when there is a high likelihood that the relative has the genetic defect, the defect presents a serious risk to the relative, and there is reason to believe that the disclosure is necessary to prevent serious harm (e.g., by allowing for treatment or by warning the person to avoid harmful environmental stimuli). Malignant hyperthermia is an autosomal dominant genetic condition causing a fatal reaction to common anesthesia. Prompt warning of families can literally save lives, especially from death due to minor surgeries such as setting broken bones in children.

If the patient does not want to inform relatives, however, questions arise as to whether the health care provider or counselor should contact the relative over the patient's refusal. The President's Commission for the Study of Ethical Problems in Medicine and Biomedical and Behavioral Research (1983) recommended that disclosure be made only if (1) reasonable attempts to elicit voluntary disclosure are unsuccessful; (2) there is a high probability of serious (e.g., irreversible or fatal) harm to an identifiable relative; (3) there is reason to believe that disclosure of the information will prevent harm to the relative; and (4) the disclosure is limited to the information necessary for diagnosis or treatment of the relative.[81]

Even in the more compelling situation of disclosure to relatives, the health care provider is not in a professional relationship with the relative, and previous legal cases regarding a duty to provide genetic information have all involved a health care provider in a professional relationship with the person to be informed. Although infectious disease cases provide a precedent for warning strangers about potential risks,[82] genetic diseases are simply different from infectious diseases. The only potential argument that the health care professional could make for contacting the relative is that through diagnosis of the patient, the health care professional has reason to believe that the relative is at higher risk than the general population of being affected by a genetic disorder. If disorders are highly likely and are treatable or preventable, many medical geneticists would overrule a patient's refusal to disclose, and would inform a relative. Although there may be no legal obligation to single out relatives as creating a special duty for physicians, the knowledge that a defined, unknowing relative is at high risk for a serious or life-threatening, treatable disease may allow rare exceptions to the principle of confidentiality.

Confidentiality and Discrimination When Third Parties Seek Genetic Information

Many entities may have an interest in learning about people's genetic information. Insurers, employers, bankers, mortgage companies, educational loan officers, providers of medical services, and others have an interest in knowing about a person's future health status. Already, people have been denied insurance, employment, and loans based on their genotype. Such discrimination has occurred both when the information has been obtained through genetic testing and when the information has been obtained in other ways (e.g., inadvertent release of a relative's medical record or disclosure from payment for medical service for a child).[83]

In the future, third parties may want access to genetic information or may wish to mandate genetic testing. In child custody cases, one spouse may claim that the other spouse should not get custody because of his or her genetic profile, for example, when the latter person has the gene for a serious, untreatable late-onset disorder. Professional schools (such as medical schools or law schools) may wish to deny admission to someone with such a disorder on the theory that such a person will have a shortened practice span.

Insurers underwriting individual health insurance currently use medical information to determine whether coverage should be granted and to determine how to price a particular policy. According to the Office of Technology Assessment, each year about 164,000 applicants are denied individual health insurance.[84] Far more Americans are covered by group plans—85 to 90 percent—with about 68 percent[85] covered by employment-based group plans rather than by individual plans. Although medical underwriting is not generally done as part of large employers' group policies, medical information is sometimes used against people in other ways in that context. People with medical problems or whose family members have medical problems have been refused jobs because employers do not want their insurance premiums increased due to payments for the care of the employee or the employee's family members.

In addition, employers that self-insure may choose to restrict coverage under their insurance plans so as not to pay for care for existing employees. One major airline already permanently excludes coverage for preexisting conditions for new employees.[86] Other employers have curtailed plan benefits once an employee has been diagnosed as having a particular disorder. In *McGann v. H. & H. Music Co.*, for example, a man was covered by employer-provided commercial insurance that had a million dollar medical benefit maximum.[87] Once the employee was diagnosed as having AIDS, however, the employer switched to self-insurance and established a $5,000 limitation for AIDS, while keeping the million dollar cap for other disorders. The court held that an employer who is self-insured could modify its plan in this way—an ominous decision when one considers that at least 65 percent of all companies and 82 percent of companies with more than 5,000 employees are self-insured.[88] The U.S. Supreme Court decided not to hear the case and let stand the lower court's decision. Employees who are covered by their employers' self-insurance are thus in a precarious position, akin to having no insurance at all:

When one considers that many employees contribute substantial amounts of money to purchase this "coverage," that many of them forego purchasing other insurance products in reliance on this coverage, and that few of them understand the precise nature of the self-insurance system, the entire system verges on fraud.[89]

This is particularly true, given that many people choose jobs because of the health benefits.[90] The Equal Employment Opportunity Commission is reportedly endeavoring to use the Americans with Disabilities Act to challenge companies' practices of setting caps on health insurance payouts for employees with AIDS.[91]

The advent of genetic testing, as well as the increasing identification of genetic diseases, makes genetic information, like other medical information, available for use as a basis for medical underwriting in health insurance. The danger, according to one study, is that "genetic testing made possible as we continue to map the human genome may result in many more individuals being denied private insurance coverage than ever before."[92] Genetic tests are not necessary to find out genetic information on applicants. Insurers already obtain genetic information from medically underwritten applicants through family histories and laboratory tests (e.g., cholesterol levels). This was of as much concern to the committee as the use of genetic information from other sources. Although insurers generally do not perform or require genetic tests when doing medical underwriting, they may seek to learn the results of any genetic tests from which an applicant may have information. This could deter people from seeking these tests.

The existence of medical underwriting can lead people to avoid needed medical services:

> If people worry that their use of health services may disqualify them from future insurance coverage, they may limit their use of needed services, fail to submit claims for covered expenses, or pressure physicians to record diagnoses that are less likely to attract an underwriter's attention. The last two actions add error to data bases used for health care research and monitoring.[93]

A survey of insurers undertaken by the Office of Technology Assessment (OTA) of the U.S. Congress found that insurers see a role for genetic information in medical underwriting. OTA surveyed commercial insurers, Blue Cross and Blue Shield companies, and large health maintenance organizations, which offered individual and medically underwritten small-group' health insurance coverage. Data were gathered on underwriting practices, including requirements for diagnostic tests or physical examinations before an insurance policy can be issued. Data on reimbursement practices, as well as general attitudes toward genetic testing, were also obtained.

Insurers generally believed that it was fair for them to use genetic tests to identify those at increased risk of disease; slightly more than one-fourth of medical directors indicated that they disagreed somewhat that such use was fair.

Three-quarters of the responding companies said they thought "an insurer should have the option of determining how to use genetic information in determining risk."[94]

OTA's survey of insurers found that genetic information is not viewed as a special type of information.[95] What seems important to insurers when making insurability and rating decisions is the particular condition, not that the condition is genetically based. OTA found that the majority of insurers did not anticipate using specific genetic tests in the future. However, a majority of medical directors from commercial insurers agreed with the statement that "it's fair for insurers to use genetic tests to identify individuals with increased risk of disease." In a comparison survey, OTA found that 14 percent of responding genetic counselors reported that they had clients who had experienced difficulties obtaining or retaining health care coverage as a result of genetic testing.

Surveys by Paul Billings and colleagues,[96] as well as by the Office of Technology Assessment,[97] uncovered specific examples of people being denied health insurance coverage based on their genotype. These incidents include cases in which a person with a positive test for a genetic disorder had his or her insurance canceled or "rated up" as a result;[98] where genetic disorders such as $alpha_1$-antitrypsin were defined as preexisting conditions, thus excluding payment for therapy; where a particular genetic condition resulted in exclusion from maternity coverage;[99] and where the birth of a child affected with a serious recessive disorder led to the inability of the parents and unaffected siblings to obtain insurance.[100]

Genetic information provides serious challenges to the traditional operation of insurance. Health insurance in this country is premised on the notion that risks can be predicted on a population-wide basis, but not well on an individual basis; thus insurance becomes a mechanism for spreading risks. If, through genetic testing or the use of genetic information acquired by other means, insurers can learn of people's actual future health risks (e.g., the risk of a serious late-onset disorder), the benefit of risk spreading will be lost; the individual will be charged an amount equal to future medical costs, which may in some cases make insurance prohibitively expensive.

Currently it is permissible in most states to do medical underwriting based on genetic information. However, the expansion of genetic testing presents a serious challenge to medical underwriting and could lead to an alternative policy approach in which medical underwriting is eliminated altogether. Originally, health insurance was based on health risks for entire communities, known as community rating, rather than on individual rating of health risks or conditions. Insurers gradually began to offer lower rates to employers based on the generally better health and lower risks of employed persons, and competition ensued among insurers to insure the "best" (i.e., lowest) risks. This has led to many of the problems in our current health insurance system in which some people have become permanently uninsurable.[101] In a system of community rating,

> . . . there would be no place for [the use of the results of] genetic testing, since applicants would not be rated according to their individual health risks and conditions.[102]

Rochester, New York has had a successful system of community rating; a key factor in its success has been the belief of large employers who would normally self-insure that their participation in a system that emphasizes risk sharing and collective strategies to contain costs, results in a system that will keep costs lower over the long term than they would be in a segmented, risk-rated competitive health insurance market.[103] The states of Maine and New York have recently passed legislation requiring health insurers offering policies in their states to return to community rating by 1993.[104] Several other states have introduced legislation to protect people from discrimination based on their genotype. In addition, more general antidiscrimination laws may provide some remedy for people who are discriminated against because of their genotype.

Much of this legislation has been a direct response to the debacle in the early 1970s with respect to sickle cell screening. When mandatory sickle cell screening laws were adopted, some insurers and employers began making decisions about insurance coverage and employment opportunities based on the results of the testing. In particular, carriers of sickle cell trait were denied jobs and charged higher insurance rates without evidence that possession of the *trait* placed a person at a higher risk of illness or death.[105] As a result, some states have adopted laws protecting people with sickle cell trait. At least two states prohibit denying an individual life insurance[106] or disability insurance,[107] or charging a higher premium,[108] solely because the individual has sickle cell trait. A few states have similarly adopted statutes to prohibit mandatory sickle cell screening as a condition of employment,[109] to prohibit discrimination in employment against people with sickle cell trait,[110] and to prohibit discrimination by unions against people with sickle trait.[111]

More recently, some states have adopted laws with a broader scope. A California statute prohibits discrimination by insurance companies against people who carry a gene that has no adverse effects on the carrier, but may affect his or her offspring.[112] Under a Wisconsin law,[113] insurers are prohibited from requiring that applicants undergo DNA testing to determine the presence of a genetic disease or disorder, or the individual's predisposition for a particular disease or disorder. Nor may insurers ask whether the individual has had a DNA test or what the results of the test were. Insurers are also prohibited from using DNA test results to determine rates or other aspects of coverage. However, insurance discrimination based on genetic information not obtained through DNA testing is not forbidden by the law.

There is also much concern about the use of genetic information in the employment context. The Council of Ethical and Judicial Affairs of the American Medical Association has taken the position that it is inappropriate for employers to perform genetic tests to exclude workers from jobs.[114] The opinion acknowledges that the protection of public safety is an important rationale for medical tests of employees. However, the opinion states:

> Genetic tests are not only generally inaccurate when used for public safety purposes, but also unnecessary. A more effective approach to protecting the public's safety would be routine testing of a worker's actual capacity to function in a job that is safety-sensitive.[115]

The opinion points out that capacity testing is more appropriate because it would not cause discrimination against someone who has the gene for a disorder but who is totally asymptomatic, yet it would "detect those whose incapacity would not be detected by genetic tests, either because of a false-negative test result or because the incapacity is caused by something other than the disease being tested for."[116]

In the employment context, a New Jersey law prohibits employment discrimination based on an "atypical hereditary cellular or blood trait."[117] In New York, a statute prohibits genetic discrimination based on sickle cell trait, Tay-Sachs trait, or Cooley anemia (beta-thalassemia) trait.[118] In Oregon, Wisconsin, and Iowa, even more comprehensive laws prohibit genetic screening as a condition of employment.[119]

At the federal level, it is still an open question whether the Americans with Disabilities Act (ADA)[120] will provide adequate protection against genetic discrimination. There are three definitions of persons considered to have a disability and, therefore, protected under the statute. Individuals currently with a disability comprise the first group, persons with a history of a disability comprise the second group, and persons who have the appearance of being disabled constitute the third. This lat_r category should protect carriers of genetic disease who are themselves healthy but could be refused employment because they have a high risk of giving birth to a child with a genetic disorder that might be expensive in insurance or health care costs to the employer. This third category for those with the appearance of disability should also protect persons with an increased risk of disease due to genetic susceptibility to breast cancer, or who have a gene for a late-onset disorder such as Huntington disease.

The NIH-DOE Joint Working Group on Ethical, Legal, and Social Implications (ELSI) of the Human Genome Project petitioned the Equal Employment Opportunity Commission (EEOC), which is responsible for implementing the law. ELSI requested that the EEOC broaden its proposed rulemaking to include these protections related to genetic testing and genetic disorders, or susceptibility to a genetic disorder.

However, according to an interpretation by the EEOC, the act does not protect carriers of genetic diseases who are themselves healthy but could be refused employment because they have a 25 percent risk of giving birth to a child with a genetic disorder. Also, the EEOC does not view a person with an increased risk of disease due to genetic factors, or who has the gene for a late-onset disorder such as Huntington disease, as having a disability and thus being protected by the law.

Legislation has been introduced to extend the definition of disability to a "genetic or medically identified potential of, or predisposition toward, a physical or mental impairment that substantially limits a major life activity."[121]

Another limitation of the ADA is that it allows employers to request any type of medical testing on an employee after a conditional offer of employment is made. In contrast, statutes in 11 states limit such testing to that which is job related.[122]

There may in fact be a narrow set of circumstances in which genetic testing may be appropriate to determine a person's ability to undertake a particular job. For example, a person with an active seizure disorder might be excluded from a job in which he or she could cause serious harm. Such a possibility would seem to be appropriate only if the potential harm were serious and screening were the most appropriate way to avert the harm. The committee was concerned, however, that employers might confuse having the gene for, or a genetic predisposition to, a particular disorder with currently being symptomatic. The possibility that someone, later in life, might become incapable of doing a job does not provide a sufficient rationale for not letting him or her undertake the job at the current time. Consequently, in most situations, periodic medical screening for symptoms rather than genetic screening will be a more appropriate means of determining whether an employee presents a serious risk of harm to third parties.[123]

FINDINGS AND RECOMMENDATIONS

Overall Principles

The committee recommends that vigorous protection be given to autonomy, privacy, confidentiality, and equity. These principles should be breached only in rare instances and only when the following conditions are met: (1) the action must be aimed at an important goal—such as the protection of others from serious harm—that outweighs the value of autonomy, privacy, confidentiality, or equity in the particular instance; (2) it must have a high probability of realizing that goal; (3) there must be no acceptable alternatives that can also realize the goal without breach of these principles; and (4) the degree of infringement of the principle must be the minimum necessary to realize the goal.

The committee recommends that regardless of the institutional structure of the entity offering genetic testing or other genetics services, there be a mechanism for advance review of the new genetic testing or other genetics services not only to assess scientific merit and efficacy, but also to ensure that adequate protections are in place for autonomy, privacy, confidentiality, and equity. The usual standards for review of research should be applied no matter what the setting. In particular, an institutional review board (IRB) should review the scientific and ethical issues related to new tests and services in academic research centers, state public health departments, and commercial enterprises.

These reviews should include any proposed investigational use of genetic tests, as well as more extensive pilot studies. In all instances the review body should include people from inside and outside the institution, including community representatives, preferably consumers of genetic services. In the clinical practice setting, professional societies should be encouraged to review studies and issue guidelines, thereby supplementing the guidance provided by IRBs (see Chapter 3).

The committee also recommends that the National Institutes of Health (NIH) Office of Protection from Research Risks provide guidance and training on how review bodies should scrutinize the risks to human subjects of genetic testing. IRBs may also need technical advice from a local advisory group on genetics (see Chapter 1). To the extent that a National Advisory Committee on Genetic Testing and its Working Group on Genetic Testing are established (see Chapter 9), these bodies should be consulted by IRBs and the NIH Office of Protection from Research Risks.

All laboratories offering genetic testing are included under the Clinical Laboratory Improvement Amendments of 1988 (CLIA88), and the committee recommends that the Health Care Financing Administration expand its existing lists of covered laboratory tests to include the full range of genetic tests now in use (see Chapter 3).

New tests, not validated elsewhere, that are added to the battery of tests should be considered investigational if they are used to make a clinical decision. The committee recommends that IRB approval be obtained in universities, commercial concerns, and other settings where new tests for additional disorders are being undertaken, even if the tests rely on existing technologies. IRB approval should be obtained before new tests are added to newborn screening.

Autonomy

Informed Consent

The committee recommends that for a proper informed consent to be obtained from a person who is considering whether to undergo genetic testing, the person should be given information about the risks, benefits, efficacy, and alternatives to the testing; information about the severity, potential variability, and treatability of the disorder being tested for; and information about the subsequent decisions that will be likely if the test is positive (e.g., whether the person will have to make a decision about abortion). Information should also be disclosed about any potential conflicts of interest of the person or institution offering the test (e.g., equity holdings or ownership of the laboratory performing the test, dependence on test reimbursement to cover the costs of counseling, patents). The difficulty in applying the traditional mechanisms for achieving informed consent should not be considered

an excuse for failing to respect a patient's autonomy and need for information.

The committee recommends that research be undertaken to determine what patients want to know in order to make a decision about whether or not to undergo a genetic test. People may have less interest in information about the label for the disorder and its mechanisms of action than they have in information about how certainly the test predicts the disorder, what effects the disorder has on physical and mental functioning, and how intrusive, difficult, or effective any existing treatment protocol would be. Research is also necessary to determine the advantages and disadvantages of various means of conveying that information (e.g., through specialized genetic counselors, primary care providers, single-disorder counselors, brochures, videos, audiotapes, and computer programs). People also need to know about potential losses of insurability or employability or social consequences that may result from knowledge about the disorder for which testing is being discussed.

Multiplex Testing

Performing multiple genetic tests on a single sample of genetic material—often using techniques of automation—has been called *multiplex testing*. **The committee recommends that informed consent be gained in advance of such multiplex testing.** New means (such as interactive or other types of computer programs, videotapes, and brochures) should be developed to provide people—in advance of testing—with the information described in the previous recommendations, such as descriptions of the nature of tests that are included in multiplex testing and the nature of the disorders being tested for (discussed in Chapter 4). A health care provider or counselor should also provide information about each of the tests, or if that is not possible because of the number of tests being grouped together, the provider or counselor should supply information about the categories of disorders so that the person will be able to make an informed decision about whether to undergo the testing.

The committee identified the area of multiplex testing as one in which more research is needed to develop ways to ensure that patient autonomy is recognized. The more general research the committee has advocated on determining what information should be conveyed and how it should be conveyed should be supplemented with additional research dealing with the unique case of multiplex testing where many disorders could be tested for at once, and those disorders may have differing characteristics. **In multiplexing, tests should be grouped so that tests requiring similar demands for informed consent and education and counseling may be offered together.** Only certain types of tests should be multiplexed; some tests should only be offered individually, especially tests for untreatable fatal disorders (e.g., Huntington disease). **The committee also recommends that research be undertaken to make**

decisions about which tests to group together in multiplex testing, based on the type of information the tests provide. The committee believes strongly that tests for untreatable disorders should not be multiplexed with tests for disorders that can be cured or prevented by treatment or by avoidance of particular environmental stimuli.

Voluntariness

The committee reaffirms that voluntariness should be the cornerstone of any genetic testing program. The committee found no justification for a state-sponsored mandatory public health program involving genetic testing of adults, or for unconsented-to genetic testing of patients in the clinical setting.

Screening and Testing of Children

The committee recommends that newborn screening programs be voluntary. The decision to make screening mandatory should require evidence that—without mandatory screening—newborns will not be screened for treatable illnesses in time to institute effective treatment (e.g., in PKU or congenital hypothyroidism). The committee bases its recommendation and preference for voluntariness on evidence from studies of existing mandated and voluntary programs that demonstrate that the best interests of the child can be served without abrogating the principle of voluntariness. Voluntary programs have delivered services as well or better than mandated programs. There is no evidence that a serious harm will result if autonomy is recognized, just as there is no evidence that mandating newborn screening is necessary to ensure that the vast majority of newborns are screened.

The committee recommends that newborn screening should not be undertaken in state programs unless there is a clear, immediate benefit to the particular infant being screened. In particular, screening should not be undertaken if presymptomatic identification of the infant and early intervention make no difference, if necessary and effective treatment is not available, or if the disorder is untreatable and screening is being done to provide information merely to aid the parents' (or the infant's) future reproductive plans. **The committee recommends that states that screen newborns have an obligation to ensure treatment of those detected with the disorder under state programs, without regard to ability to pay for treatment.**

The committee recommends that in the clinical setting, children generally be tested only for disorders for which a curative or preventive treatment exists and should be instituted at that early stage. Childhood screening is not appropriate for carrier status, untreatable childhood diseases, and late-onset diseases that cannot be prevented or forestalled by early treatment. Because only certain types of genetic testing are appropriate for children, tests specifically directed to obtaining information about carrier status, untreatable childhood diseases, or late-onset diseases, should not be included in the multiplex tests offered to children. Research should be undertaken to determine the appropriate age for testing and screening for genetic disorders in order to maximize the benefits of therapeutic intervention and to avoid the possibility that genetic information will be generated about a child when there is no likely benefit to the child in the immediate future.

The majority of the committee recommends that carrier status of newborns and other children be reported to parents only after the parents have been informed of the potential benefits and harms of knowing the carrier status of their children. Because of the risk of stigma for the newborn, such pretest information should be provided to parents when they are informed about newborn screening. Provision should be made for answering any questions the parents may have; these questions are best answered in the context of genetic counseling. The decisions of the parents about whether to receive such information should always be respected (see Chapter 4). **Where such information is not disclosed after parents are given the option to get such information and then knowingly refuse the information, the courts should take this policy analysis and the recommendation of this committee into consideration and not find liability if parents sue because the carrier status of their child was not disclosed and they subsequently give birth to an affected child.** Research is needed on the consequences of revealing carrier status in newborns to identify both harms and benefits from disclosing such information in the future.

Subsequent Uses

The committee recommends that before genetic information is obtained from individuals (or before a sample is obtained for genetic testing), they (or, in the case of minors, their parents) be told what specific uses will be made of the information or sample; how—and for how long—the information or sample will be stored; whether personal identifiers will be stored; and who will have access to the information or sample, and under what conditions. They should also be informed of future anticipated uses for the sample, asked permission for those uses, and told what procedures will be followed if the possibility for currently unanticipated uses develops. The individuals should have a right to consent or to object to particular uses of the sample or information.

Subsequent anonymous use of samples for research is permissible, including in state newborn screening programs. Except for such anonymous use, the newborn specimen should not be used for additional tests without informed consent of the parents or guardian.

If genetic test samples are collected for family linkage studies or clinical purposes, they should not be used for law enforcement purposes (except for body identification). If samples are collected for law enforcement purposes, they should not be accessible for other nonclinical uses such as testing for health insurance purposes.

Confidentiality

Disclosure to Spouses and Relatives

As a matter of general principle, the committee believes that patients should be encouraged and aided in sharing appropriate genetic information with spouses. Mechanisms should be developed to aid a tested individual in informing his or her spouse and relatives about the individual's genetic status and informing relatives about genetic risks. These mechanisms would include the use of written materials, referrals for counseling, and so forth.

On balance, the committee recommends that health care providers not reveal genetic information about a patient's carrier status to the patient's spouse without the patient's permission. Furthermore, information about misattributed paternity should be revealed to the mother but should not be volunteered to the woman's partner.

Although confidentiality may be breached to prevent harm to third parties, the harm envisioned by the cases generally has been substantial and imminent.[124] The spouse's claim of future harm due to the possibility of later conceiving a child with a genetic disorder would not be a sufficient reason to breach confidentiality. The committee found no evidence of a trend on the part of people to mislead their spouses about their carrier status. Moreover, since most people *do* tell their spouses about genetic risks, breaching of confidentiality would be needed only rarely.

The committee believes that patients should share genetic information with their relatives so that the relatives may avert risks or seek treatment. Health care providers should discuss with patients the benefits of sharing information with relatives about genetic conditions that are treatable or preventable or that involve important reproductive decision making. **The committee believes that the disadvantages of informing relatives over the patient's refusal generally outweigh the advantages, except in the rare instances described above.**

The committee recommends that confidentiality be breached and relatives informed about genetic risks only when attempts to elicit voluntary disclosure fail, there is a high probability of irreversible or fatal harm to the relative, the disclosure of the information will prevent harm, the disclosure is limited to the information necessary for diagnosis or treatment of the relative, and there is no other reasonable way to avert the harm. When disclosure is to be attempted over the patient's refusal, the burden should be on the person who wishes to disclose to justify to the patient, to an ethics committee, and perhaps in court that the disclosure was necessary and met the committee's test.

If there are any circumstances in which the geneticist or other health care professional could breach confidentiality and disclose information to a spouse, relative, or other third party—for example, to an employer—those circumstances should be explained in advance of testing; and, if the patient wishes, the patient should be given the opportunity to be referred to a health care provider who will protect confidentiality.

On a broader scale, the committee recommends that:

* **all forms of genetic information be considered confidential and not be disclosed without the individual's consent** (except as required by law), including genetic information that is obtained through specific genetic testing of a person as well as genetic information about a person that is obtained in other ways (e.g., physical examination, knowledge of past treatment, or knowledge of a relative's genetic status);
* **confidentiality of genetic information should be protected no matter who obtains or maintains that information,** including genetic information collected or maintained by health care professionals, health care institutions, researchers, employers, insurance companies, laboratory personnel, and law enforcement officials; and
* **to the extent that current statutes do not ensure such confidentiality, they should be amended so that disclosure of genetic information is not required.**

The committee recommends that codes of ethics of those professionals providing genetics services (such as those of the National Society of Genetic Counselors (NSGC), or of geneticists, physicians, and nurses) contain specific provisions to protect autonomy, privacy, and confidentiality. The committee endorses the NSGC statement of a guiding principle on confidentiality of test results:

> The NSGC support individual confidentiality regarding results of genetic testing. It is the right and responsibility of the individual to determine who shall have access to medical information, particularly results of testing for genetic conditions.[125]

The committee also endorses the principles on DNA banking and DNA data banking contained in the 1990 ASHG statement.

To further protect confidentiality, the committee recommends that

* **patients' consent be obtained before the patient's name is provided to a genetic disease registry and that consent be obtained before information is redisclosed;**
* **each entity that receives or maintains genetic information or samples have procedures in place to protect confidentiality,** including procedures limiting access on a need-to-know basis, identifying an individual who has responsibility for overseeing security procedures and safeguards, providing written information to each employee or agent regarding the need to maintain confidentiality,

and taking no punitive action against employees for bringing evidence of confidentiality breaches to light;

- **any entity that releases genetic information about an individual to someone other than that individual ensure that the recipient of the genetic information has procedures in place to protect the confidentiality of the information;**
- **any entity that collects or maintains genetic information or samples separate them from personal identifiers** and instead link the information or sample to the individual's name through some form of anonymous surrogate identifiers;
- **the person have control over what parts of his or her medical record are available to which people**; if an optical memory card is used, this could be accomplished through a partitioning-off of data on the card; and
- **any individual be allowed access to his or her genetic information in the context of appropriate education and counseling,** except in the early research phases during the development of genetic testing when an overall decision has been made that results based on the experimental procedure will not be released and the subjects of the research have been informed of that restriction prior to participation.

Discrimination in Insurance and Employment

In general, the committee recommends that principles of autonomy, privacy, confidentiality, and equity be maintained, and the disclosure of genetic information and the taking of genetic tests should not be mandated. Such a position, however, is in conflict with some current practices in insurance and employment.

Although more than half the U.S. population (approximately 156 million people) is covered by some kind of life insurance,[126] the use of genetic information in medical underwriting[127] decisions about life insurance appears to raise different and somewhat lesser concerns than the use of genetic information in health insurance underwriting. More of life insurance has historically been medically underwritten. Complaints of genetic discrimination in life insurance have been made.[128] Apparently, fewer Americans believe that life insurance is a basic right. In contrast, the Canadian Privacy Commission believes that life insurance is a basic right, and recommends that Canadians be permitted to purchase up to $100,000 in basic life insurance without genetic or other restrictions; underwriting for larger amounts of life insurance could be subject to a variety of life-style and health restrictions, including the use of genetic information.[129] **Most of the committee agrees with the spirit of the Canadian Commission's recommendation that a *limited* amount of life insurance be available to everyone without regard to health or genetic status. However, health insurance was considered a much more pressing ethical, legal, and social issue.**

The committee recommends that legislation be adopted so that medical risks, including genetic risks, not be taken into account in decisions on whether to issue or how to price health care insurance. Because health insurance differs significantly from other types of insurance in that it regulates access to health care, an important social good, risk-based health insurance should be eliminated. A means of access to health care should be available to every American without regard to the individual's present health status or condition, including genetic makeup. Any health insurance reform proposals need to be evaluated to determine their effect on genetic testing and the use of genetic information in health insurance (see Chapter 7).

The committee recommends that the unfair practices highlighted by the *McGann* case be prevented. Such situations could be eliminated by Congress in three ways. First, the antidiscrimination provision of the Employee Retirement Income Security Act (ERISA, see Chapter 7), section 510, could be amended to prohibit various types of employer conduct. For example, the legislation could prohibit: (1) the alteration of benefits or the alteration of benefits without a certain notice period; (2) the reduction of coverage for only a single medical condition; (3) the reduction of benefits after a claim for benefits already had been submitted, and so forth. At the very least, the committee recommends that an amendment be adopted making those practices illegal.

A second way of legislatively preventing *McGann*-type situations would be to amend the ERISA preemption provision, section 514. By amending this section to limit the preemptive effect of ERISA (e.g., that permits ERISA provisions to override state insurance regulations) or to eliminate ERISA preemption entirely, the result would be to allow the states to regulate self-insured employer benefits in the same way that state insurance commissions regulate commercial health insurance benefits. Although state regulation may be preferable to no regulation, it could lead to the burdensome multiplicity of state regulations that ERISA was intended to eliminate. For this reason, the committee believes that federal prohibition of the type of conduct in the *McGann* case would be preferable.

A third way to eliminate discrimination in employee health benefits by self-insured employers would be to amend section 501 of the ADA. The ADA is essentially neutral on the issue of health benefits; clauses on preexisting conditions, medical underwriting, and other actuarially based practices, to the extent permitted by state law, do not violate the ADA. Thus, the ADA could be amended to prohibit differences in health benefits that result in discrimination against individuals with disabilities. Amending the ADA in this manner would, in effect, mandate uniform coverage (although it is not clear what conditions would be covered) at community rates for employees. If Congress wanted to mandate that all employers offer a package of health benefits, a good argument could be made that it ought to do so separately and not via amendments to the ADA.

The committee recommends that legislation be adopted so that genetic information cannot be collected on prospective or current employees unless it

is clearly job related. Sometimes employers will have employees submit to medical exams to see if they are capable of performing particular job tasks. The committee recommends that if an individual consents to the release of genetic information to an employer or potential employer, the releasing entity should not release specific information, but instead answer only yes or no regarding whether the individual was fit to perform the job at issue.

The committee recommends that the EEOC recognize that the language of the Americans with Disabilities Act provides protection for presymptomatic people with a genetic profile for late-onset disorders, unaffected carriers of disorders that might affect their children, and people with genetic profiles indicating the possibility of increased risk of a multifactorial disorder. The committee also recommends that state legislatures adopt laws to protect people from genetic discrimination in employment. In addition, the committee recommends an amendment to the ADA (and adoption of similar state statutes) limiting the type of medical testing employers can request or the medical information they can collect to that which is job related.

Ultimately, new laws on a variety of other topics may also be necessary to protect autonomy, privacy, and confidentiality in the genetics field, and to protect people from inappropriate decisions based on their genotypes.[130] The ability of genetics to predict health risks for asymptomatic individuals and their potential offspring presents challenges in the ethical and social spheres. **The committee recommends that careful consideration be given to the development of policies for the implementation of genetic testing and the handling of genetic test results.**

NOTES

1. March of Dimes Birth Defects Foundation, *Genetic Testing and Gene Therapy: National Survey Findings* 18 (September 1992). New York.

2. See, e.g., *Satz v. Perlmutter*, 362 So.2d 160 (Fla. App. 1978) aff'd 379 So.2d 359 (Fla. 1980).

3. See, e.g., *Salgo v. Leland Stanford Jr. Univ. Bd. of Trustees*, 154 Cal. App. 2d 560, 317 P.2d 170 (1957); *Canterbury v. Spence*, 464 F.2d 772 (D.C. Cir.), cert. denied, 409 U.S. 1064 (1972).

4. *Gates v. Jensen*, 92 Wash. 2d 246, 595 P.2d 919 (1979).

5. *Salgo v. Leland Stanford Jr. Univ. Bd. of Trustees*, 154 Cal. App. 2d 560, 317 P. d 170 (1957).

6. *Kogan v. Holy Family Hospital*, 95 Wash.2d 306, 622 P.2d 1246 (1980).

7. See, e.g., *Becker v. Schwartz*, 46 N.Y.2d 401, 386 N.E.2d 807, 413 N.Y.S.2d 895 (1978). For a review of relevant cases, see Lori B. Andrews, "Torts and the Double Helix: Liability for Failure to Disclose Genetic Risks," 29 *U. Houston L. Rev.* 143 (1992).

8. L. Andrews, "My Body, My Property," 16(5) *Hastings Center Report* 28 (1986). See also *Moore v. Regents of the University of California.*

9. The federal regulations governing informed consent in the context of human experimentation provide that informed consent is not necessary for research on pathological or diagnostic specimens "if these sources are publicly available or if the information is recorded by the investigator in such a manner that subjects cannot be identified, directly or through identifiers linked to the subjects." 45 C.F.R. § 46.101(b)(5) (1991).

Similarly, some state human experimentation laws do not seem to extend their coverage to research on removed parts. In Virginia, for example, the law does not cover "the conduct of biological studies exclusively utilizing tissue or fluids after their removal or withdrawal from a human subject in the course of standard medical practice." Va. Code Ann. § 37.1-234(1) (1984). Under the New York law, human research is defined to exclude "studies exclusively utilizing tissue or fluids after their removal or withdrawal from a human subject in the course of standard medical practice." N.Y. Public Health Law § 2441(2) (McKinney 1977).

10. Office of Technology Assessment (OTA), U.S. Congress, *Human Gene Therapy* 72 (Washington, D.C.: U.S. Government Printing Office, 1984).

11. Ferdinand D. Schoeman, "Privacy: Philosophical Dimensions of the Literature," in *Philosophical Dimensions of Privacy: An Anthology*, ed., Ferdinand D. Schoeman (New York: Cambridge University Press, 1984).

12. See Judith Jarvis Thomson, "The Right to Privacy," *Philosophy and Public Affairs* 4(summer):315-333, (1975).

13. See, e.g., *Griswold v. Connecticut*, 381 U.S. 479 (1965); *Roe v. Wade*, 410 U.S. 113 (1973); *Planned Parenthood v. Casey*, ___ U.S. ___, 112 S.Ct. 2791 (1992).

14. *Lifchez v. Hartigan*, 735 F. Supp. 1361 (N.D. Ill. 1991), aff'd without opinion sub. nom.; *Scholber v. Lifchez*, 914 F.2d 260 (7th Cir. 1990), cert. denied, 111 S.Ct. 787 (1991).

15. *Carter v. Broadlawn Medical Center*, 667 F. Supp. 1269, 1282 (S.D. Iowa 1987). In that case, the court held that the privacy of patient records in a county hospital is protected by the Fourteenth Amendment's concept of personal liberty. See also *Whalen v. Roe*, 429 U.S. 589, 599 n. 23 (1977).

16. *Horne v. Patton*, 291 Ala. 701, 287 So.2d 824 (1973); *MacDonald v. Clinger*, 84 A.D.2d 482, 444 N.Y.S.2d 801 (1982).

17. Privacy Act of 1974, 5 U.S.C. § 552a (1991).

18. For further discussion of these arguments (and others in this section), see Tom L. Beauchamp and James F. Childress, *Principles of Biomedical Ethics*, 3rd ed. (New York: Oxford University Press, 1989, chap. 7).

19. Mark Siegler, "Confidentiality in Medicine—A Decrepit Concept," *N. Engl. J. Med.* 307: 1518-1521 (1982).

20. Research has found that people who are told that their answers would not be confidential provide less intimate information. Woods and McNamara, "Confidentiality: Its Effect on Interviewee Behavior," 11 *Prof. Psychology* 714, 719 (1980).

21. See, e.g., *Horne v. Patton*, 291 Ala. 701, 287 So.2d 824 (1973); *MacDonald v. Clinger*, 84 A.D.2d 482, 444 N.Y.S.2d 801 (1982). See W. Prosser and W.P. Keeton, *Prosser and Keeton on Torts* 856-863 (1984). See also S. Newman, "Privacy in Personal Medical Information: A Diagnosis," 33 *U. Fla. L. Rev.* 394-424 (1981). According to the latter article, the tort of invasion of privacy has been rejected only in Rhode Island, Nebraska and Wisconsin. *Id.* at 403. However, two of these states now recognize it by statute. R.I. Gen. Laws § 9-1-28 (1984); Wisc. Stat. § 895.50 (1985-86).

22. Norman Daniels, "Insurability and the HIV Epidemic: Ethical Issues in Underwriting," 68 *The Milbank Quarterly* 497-515 (1990). See also Mark A. Rothstein, "The Use of Genetic Information in Health and Life Insurance." In Friedman, T. (ed.) *Molecular Genetic Medicine* (New York: Academic Press, 1993).

23. On the natural lottery, see H. Tristram Engelhardt, Jr., *Foundations of Bioethics* (New York: Oxford University Press, 1986).

24. *Id.*

25. See Gene Outka, "Social Justice and Equal Access to Health Care," *Journal of Religious Ethics* 2 (1974). See also President's Commission for the Study of Ethical Problems in Biomedical and Behavioral Research, *Securing Access to Health Care*, Vol. 1: Report (Washington, D.C.: U.S. Government Printing Office, 1983).

26. Normal Daniels, "Equity of Access to Health Care: Some Conceptual and Ethical Issues," *Milbank Memorial Fund Quarterly/Health and Society* 60 (1982). See also Norman Daniels, *Just Health Care* (New York: Cambridge University Press, 1985).

27. President's Commission for the Study of Ethical Problems in Biomedical and Behavioral Research, *Securing Access to Health Care*, Vol. 1: Report (Washington, D.C.: U.S. Government Printing Office, 1983), p. 42.

28. Rothstein, "Genetic Discrimination in Employment and the American with Disabilities Act," 29 *Houston L. Rev.* 23, 31 (1992). See also the discussion *infra* in this chapter, "Discrimination."

29. Office of Technology Assessment (OTA), U.S. Congress, *Genetic Witness: Forensic Uses of DNA Tests* (Washington, D.C.: U.S. Government Printing Office, 1990).

30. D. C. Wertz and J.C. Fletcher, *Ethics and Human Genetics: A Cross-Cultural Perspective* (New York: Springer-Verlag, 1989); and D.C. Wertz and J.C. Fletcher, "An International Survey of Attitudes of Medical Geneticists Toward Mass Screening and Access to Results," 104 *Public Health Reports* 35-44 (1989).

31. G. Geller, E. Tambor, G. Chase, K. Hofman, R. Faden, N. Holtzman. "How Will Primary Care Physicians Incorporate Genetic Testing: Directiveness in Communication," 31 *Medical Care* 625-631 (1993).

32. There are several reasons why institutions store DNA samples, rather than just information from samples. The first is for future potential clinical benefit, such as when a new test may be developed that could provide a more accurate diagnosis. The second is for litigation purposes, so that the sample can be retested if the results are challenged. The third is for research purposes, to use the DNA for the development of additional tests.

33. Philip Reilly, Presentation to Ethical, Legal, and Social Implications Program Committee, January 1991.

34. Yoichi Matsubara, Kuniaki Narisawa, Keiya Tada, Hiroyuki Ikeda, Yao Ye-Qi, David M. Danks, Anne Green, Edward R.B. McCabe, "Prevalence of K329E Mutation in Medium-Chain Acyl-CoA Dehydrogenase Gene Determined from Guthrie Cards," 338 *Lancet* 552-553 (1991).

35. Joe Abernathy, "City Health Clinics Unveil Controversial 'Smart Card'," *Houston Chronicle*, October 11, 1992, sec. A, p. 1.

36. See, e.g., M. Shaw, "Conditional Prospective Rights of the Fetus," 5 *J. Legal Med.* 63 (1989).

37. Moreover, it should be noted that this risk (transmission of genetic disease to offspring) is one that society has always lived with, and seems to have flourished despite that risk.

38. For example, in *The New York Times v. United States*, 403 U.S. 713 (1971), the U.S. Supreme Court, in a per curiam opinion held that the government had not met its "heavy burden" of proving that national security required that the Pentagon Papers be suppressed. The logic of the case was explained further in the concurrences; the right of free speech is to be infringed by a prior restraint only when disclosure "will surely result in direct, immediate, and irreparable damage to our Nation or its people." *Id.* at 730 (Stewart, J., concurring). Or when there is "governmental allegation and proof that publication must inevitably, directly, and immediately cause the occurrence of an event kindred to imperiling the safety of a transport already at sea . . ." during wartime. *Id.* at 726-727 (Brennan, J., concurring).

The standard of irreparability for granting an injunction against protected speech is an absolute, not a comparative standard. Even if the speech could cause great harm, that would not be sufficient. As Justice White pointed out in his concurrence in *New York Times*, it is not sufficient that there may be "substantial damage to public interests." *Id.* at 731 (White, J., concurring). Similarly, Justice Stewart said "I am convinced that the Executive is correct with respect to some of the documents involved [i.e., they should not, in the national interest, be published]. But I cannot say that disclosure of any of them will surely result in direct, immediate, and irreparable harm to our Nation or its people. That being so, there can under the First Amendment be but one judicial resolution of the issue before us." *Id.* at 730 (White, J., concurring).

Even if irreparable harm were a possibility, *New York Times* indicates that an injunction should not be issued against the press unless such harm would come about directly and immediately. The term "immediately" is easy enough to understand; it requires a present, not future, harm. The term "directly" relates to the lack of intervening influences during that time period. The irreparable harm would not occur directly if another important influence would or could intervene. Another way of expressing the immediacy and directness that is necessary is by saying the harm is "inevitable"—it will occur within a short period of time during which nothing will or could change it or stop it.

Even when a prior restraint is not at issue, high standards are required for showing a compelling state interest when a fundamental right is at issue. Also in the First Amendment area, speech that is not false should not be the basis for subsequent punishment unless it provided an immediate threat of serious harm. (See, e.g., *Bridges v. California*, 314 U.S. 252, 263 (1941) ("the substantial evil must, be extremely serious and the degree of imminence extremely high before utterances can be punished").)

39. AIDS, of course, is an infectious disease that cannot be cured and that is strongly identified with certain minority groups (e.g., homosexuals). It is interesting to note that for many of the same reasons that are applicable to mandatory genetic screening, mandatory AIDS screening has not been adopted. Instead, anonymous voluntary screening has been the model.

40. C. Damme, "Controlling Genetic Disease Through Law," 15 *U. Cal. Davis L. Rev.* 801, 807 (1982).

41. Such charges were leveled by blacks when mandatory sickle cell carrier screening was put into place.

42. L. Andrews, *Medical Genetics: A Legal Frontier* 233 (1987).

43. A. G. Motulsky, "The Significance of Genetic Disease," 59, 61 in B. Hilton, D. Callahan, M. Harris, P. Condliffe, B. Berkley, eds., *Ethical Issues in Human Genetics: Genetic Counseling and the Use of Genetic Knowledge* (Fogarty International Proceedings No. 13, 1973).

44. Statement of D. Brock in B. Hilton et al., eds., *id.* at 90.

45. The idea of choosing by category was discussed by Alta Charo, J.D., at the committee's June 1992 workshop.

46. e.g., *Cobbs v. Grant*, 8 Cal.3d 829, 104 Cal. Rptr. 505, 502 P.2d 1, 12 (1972). Some states' informed consent statutes explicitly recognize a right to refuse information. Alaska Stat. § 09.55.556(b)(2) (1983); Del. Code Ann. tit. 18, § 6852(b)(2) (Supp. 1984); N.H. Rev. Stat. Ann. § 507-C:2(II)(b)(3) (1983); N.Y. Public Health Law § 2805-d(4)(b) (McKinney 1985); Or. Rev. Stat. § 677.097(2) (1985); Utah Code Ann. § 78-14-5(2)(c) (1977); Vt. Stat. Ann. tit. 12, § 1909(c)(2) (Supp. 1991); Wash. Rev. Code Ann. § 7.70.060(2) (Supp. 1991).

47. *Prince v. Massachusetts*, 321 U.S. 158, 170 (1944).

48. *In re Green*, 448 Pa. 338, 292 A.2d 387, 392 (1972). See also Brown and Truit, "The Right of Minors to Medical Treatment," 28 *DePaul L. Rev.* 289, 299 (1979).

49. *Jehovah's Witnesses v. King County Hospital* 278 F. Supp. 488 (W.D. Wash. 1967), 390 U.S. 598 (1968), denied, 391 U.S. 961 (1968).

50. D.C. Code Ann. § 6-314(3) (1989); Md. Health-Gen. Code Ann. §§ 13-102(10) and 109(e)-(f) (1982).

51. Iowa Admin. Code § 641-4.1 (136A) (1992); Mich. Comp. Laws Ann. § 333.5431(1) (West 1992); Mont. Code Ann. § 50-19-203(1) (1991); W. Va. Code Ann. § 16-22-3 (Supp. 1992).

52. Mo. Ann. Stat. § 191.331(5) (Vernon 1990); S.C. Code § 44-37-30(B) (1991).

53. Council of Regional Networks for Genetic Services (CORN), *Newborn Screening: 1990*, Final Report (February 1992). New York.

54. R. R. Faden, A. J. Chwalow, N. A. Holtzman, and S. Horn, "A Survey to Evaluate Parental Consent As Public Policy for Neonatal Screening," 72 *Am. J. Pub. Health* 1347 (1982).

55. "Consensus Statement Proposed for Routine Newborn Genetic Screening." Based on October 1989 conference in Quebec, Canada. Reported in Bartha Maria Knoppers and Claude M. LaBerge (eds.), "Genetic Screening: From Newborns to Data Typing," *Excerpta Medica* 382 (1990).

56. Currently, Colorado and Wyoming include cystic fibrosis testing as a part of their mandatory newborn screening program; Wisconsin includes cystic fibrosis in newborn screening as part of an experimental research protocol.

57. Neil A. Holtzman, "What Drives Neonatal Screening Programs," 325 *New Engl. J. Med.* 802-809 (Sept. 12, 1991), referring to K.B. Hammond, S.H. Abman, R.J. Sokol, F.J. Accurso, "Efficacy of

Statewide Newborn Screening for Cystic Fibrosis by Assay of Trypsinogen Concentration, 325 *New Engl. J. Med.* 769-74 (1991).

58. *Id.*

59. *Id.*, citing P. Farrell, personal communication.

60. Norm Fost presentation, June 1992 committee workshop.

61. Statement of Claude LaBerge at June 1992 committee meeting.

62. See T. McNeil, B. Harty, T. Thelin, E. Aspergren-Jansson, T. Sveger, "Identifying Children at High Somatic Risk: Long-Term Effects on Mother-Child Interactions," *Acta-Psychiatrica Scandinavica* 74(6):555-562 (December 1986).

63. Ellen Wright Clayton, "Screening and Treatment of Newborns," 29 *Houston L. Rev.* 85 (1992).

64. The federal regulations governing informed consent in the context of human experimentation provide that informed consent is not necessary for research on pathological or diagnostic specimens "if these sources are publicly available or if the information is recorded by the investigator in such a manner that subjects cannot be identified, directly or through identifiers linked to the subjects." 45 C.F.R. § 46.101(b)(4)(1991).

Similarly, some state human experimentation laws do not seem to extend their coverage to research on removed parts. In Virginia, for example, the law does not cover "the conduct of biological studies exclusively utilizing tissue or fluids after their removal or withdrawal from a human subject in the course of standard medical practice." Va. Code Ann. § 37.1-234(1) (1990). Under the New York law, human research is defined to exclude "studies exclusively utilizing tissue or fluids after removal or withdrawal from a human subject in the course of medical practice."

Some researchers argue that blood and urine left over after a patient's tests are done should be available without requiring the patient's informed consent. However, the issue is not as straightforward as it might seem. Research surreptitiously done on a patient's blood might generate information that could be damaging to the patient. If a cystic fibrosis test were being developed with excess blood from a PKU test, and the blood tested positive for cystic fibrosis, it could be argued that, depending on how reliable the test seemed, the infant's parents should be informed. But if the result ultimately turned out to be a false positive, the family may have been harmed by unnecessary worry. With respect to research on leftover blood from adults, if testing is being developed for a potentially stigmatizing disorder (such as AIDS) or a disorder that might influence employment or other opportunities for the person (such as Huntington disease) the risks to the patient if confidentiality were compromised might be so high that it would seem unethical not to solicit the individual's consent before the research is undertaken.

65. ASHG Ad Hoc Committee on Individual Identification by DNA Analysis, "Individual Identification by DNA Analysis: Points to Consider," *Am. J. Hum. Genet.* 46:631-634 (1990).

66. *Id.* at 632.

67. Nancy Wexler, "The Tiresias Complex: Huntington's Disease as a Paradigm of Testing for Late-Onset Disorders," *FASEB Journal* 6:2820-2825 (1990).

68. See, e.g., *Skillings v. Allen*, 143 Minn. 323, 173 N.W. 663 (1919); *Davis v. Rodman*, 147 Ark. 385, 227 S.W. 612 (1921). For a more recent case, regarding a duty to warn third parties of communicable diseases, see *Gammill v. U.S.*, 727 F.2d 950 (10th Cir. 1984).

69. *Tarasoff v. Regents of the University of California*, 131 Cal. Rptr. 14, 17 Cal. App. 3d 425, 551 P.2d 334 (1976).

70. *Id.*

71. *Collins v. Howard*, 156 F. Supp. 322, 325 (S.D. Ga. 1957) (dicta).

72. The individual generally asks that his or her spouse be informed as well. Statement of J. Lejeune in B. Hilton, D. Callahan, M. Harris, P. Condliffe, B. Berkeley, eds., *Ethical Issues in Human Genetics: Genetic Counseling and the Use of Genetic Knowledge*, 70 (Fogarty International Proceedings No. 13, 1973).

In a March of Dimes-sponsored national public opinion survey, 71 percent of respondents said that if a doctor of a woman who plans to have children finds through testing that her children might inherit a serious or fatal genetic disease, the doctor has an obligation to tell her husband. March of Dimes Birth Defects Foundation, *Genetic Testing and Gene Therapy: National Survey Findings* 7 (New York, September 1992). However, in some instances, an individual may or may not want personal genetic information disclosed to his or her spouse.

73. *Berry v. Moensch*, 8 Utah 2d 191, 331 P.2d 814 (1958); *Curry v. Corn*, 52 Misc.2d 1035, 277 N.Y.S.2d 470 (1966) (during marriage, each has the right to know the existence of any disease that may have bearing on the marital relation).

74. See, e.g., *Simonsen v. Swenson* 104 Neb. 224, 177 N.W. 831 (1920).

75. The man whose nonpaternity is shown through prenatal screening might argue that, in addition to its relevance to his future childbearing plans, the information that he is not the father of his wife's child has an immediate financial implication since he might not wish to support the child. However, state paternity statutes preserve that a child born during a marriage is the husband's child and require him to support the child, even if it could conceivably be shown through genetic testing that he was not the biological father of the child. The logic behind such cases is that there is a societal interest in the integrity of the family.

76. *Eisenstadt v. Baird*, 405 U.S. 438 (1972).

77. *Planned Parenthood v. Danforth*, 428 U.S. 52 (1976).

78. *Planned Parenthood v. Casey*, ___ U.S. ___, 112 S.Ct. 2791 (1992).

79. *Id.*

80. If a patient is the carrier of the gene for a serious autosomal recessive disorder, his or her relatives might also argue that they would be harmed by not knowing that they, too, are at risk of having children with that disorder. However, the risk to future offspring may be too remote to warrant breaching confidentiality, as it is in the case of a spouse.

81. The President's Commission for the Study of Ethical Problems in Medicine and Biomedical and Behavioral Research, *Screening and Counseling for Genetic Conditions* 6 (1983).

82. See, e.g. *Simonsen v. Swenson*, 104 Neb. 224, 177 N.W. 831 (1920).

83. In one instance, for example, a woman was denied disability insurance when her father's medical records were released to the insurer.

84. Office of Technology Assessment, U.S. Congress, *Medical Testing and Health Insurance* 73 (1988).

85. S. Rep. 100-360, 100th Cong., 1st Sess. 20 (1988).

86. Report of Committee on Employer-Based Health Benefits, citing Seeman (1993).

87. *McGann v. H. & H. Music Co.*, 946 F.2d 401 (5th Cir. 1991), *cert. denied sub nom.*; *Greenberg v. H. & H. Music Company*, ___ U.S. ___, 112 S.Ct. 1556 (1992).

88. Eric Zicklin, "More Employers Self-Insure Their Medical Plans, Survey Finds," *Business and Health* 74 (April 1992).

89. Mark Rothstein, "The Use of Genetic Information in Health and Life Insurance," in *Molecular Genetic Medicine*, ed., Ted Friedman (New York: Academic Press, 1993).

90. According to *American Healthline*, Briefing on Health Insurance, November 17, 1992, more than half of Americans would not accept a job that did not provide health insurance.

91. "EEOC Said Ready to 'Fast Track' Complaints of Insurance Caps under Title 1 of the ADA," 7 No. 18 *AIDS Policy & Law* 1-2 (October 2, 1992).

92. N. Kass, "Insurance for the Insurors," *Hastings Center Report*, 6-11 (November-December 1992).

93. Institute of Medicine (IOM), National Academy of Sciences, M. Field and D. H. Shapiro (eds.) Employment and Health Benefits: A Connection at Risk. Committee on Employer-Based Health Insurance (Washington, D.C.: National Academy Press, 1993).

94. OTA, 1992a, p. 180.

95. OTA, 1992b.

96. See, e.g., P.R. Billings, M.A. Kohn, M. de Cuevas, J. Beckwith, J.S. Alper, M.R. Natowicz, "Discrimination as a Consequence of Genetic Testing," 50 *Am. J. Hum. Genet.* 476-482 (1992).

97. U.S. Congress, Office of Technology Assessment, *Cystic Fibrosis and DNA Tests: Implications of Carrier Screening* (Washington, D.C.: U.S. Government Printing Office, 1992a).

98. The disorders included adult polycystic kidney disease, Huntington disease, neurofibromatosis, Marfan syndrome, Down syndrome, Fabray disease.

99. The conditions included a balanced translocation.

100. The disorder was cystic fibrosis.

101. Kass, 1992.

102. *Id.* at 10.

103. Report of Institute of Medicine Committee on Employer-Based Health Benefits.

104. See Kass, 1992 for descriptions of these plans.

105. P. Reilly, *Genetics, Law and Social Policy* 62-86 (Cambridge, Mass.: Harvard University Press, 1977).

106. Fla. Stat. Ann. § 626.9706(1) (West 1984); La. Rev. Stat. Ann. § 22:652.1(D) (West Supp. 1992).

107. 22 Fla. Stat. Ann. § 626.9707(1) (West 1984); La. Rev. Stat. Ann. § 22:652.1(D) (West Supp. 1992).

108. Fla. Stat. Ann. § 626.9706(2) (West 1984) (life insurance), § 626.9707(2) (West 1984) (disability insurance); La. Rev. Stat. Ann. § 22:652.1(D) (West Supp. 1992).

109. This same law appears in three places in the Florida statutes: Fla. Stat. Ann. § 448.076 (West 1981); § 228.201 (West Supp. 1989); and § 63.043 (West 1985).

110. Fla. Stat. Ann. § 448.075 (West 1981); N.C. Gen. Stat. § 95-28.1 (1989); La. Rev. Stat. Ann. § 23:1002(A)(1) (West 1985).

111. La. Rev. Stat. Ann. § 23:1002(C)(1) (West 1985).

112. Cal. Ins. Code § 10143 (West Supp. 1992).

113. 1991 Wisc. Act 269, codified as Wisc. Stat. Ann. § 631.89.

114. Council on Ethical and Judicial Affairs, "Use of Genetic Testing by Employers," 266 *JAMA* 1827 (1991).

115. *Id.* at 1828.

116. *Id.* at 1828.

117. N.J. Stat. Ann. § 10:5-12(a) (West Supp. 1992).

118. N.Y. Civ. Rights Law § 48 (McKinney 1992).

119. 1992 Iowa Legis. Serv. 93 (West); Or. Rev. Stat. § 659.227 (1991); 1991 Wis. Laws 117.

120. 104 Stat. 327 (1991). For sections of the Americans With Disabilities Act relating to employment, see 42 U.S.C.A. §§ 12101-12117 (Supp. 1992).

121. L. Gostin and W. Roper. "Update: The Americans with Disabilities Act," *Health Affairs* 11(3):248-258.

122. Alaska Stat. § 18.80.220(a)(1) (1991); Cal. Gov't Code § 12940(d) (West Supp. 1991); Colo. Rev. Stat. § 24-34-402(1)(d) (1988); Kan. Stat. Ann. § 44-1009(a)(3) (Supp. 1991); Mich. Comp. Laws Ann. § 37.1206(2) (West 1985); Minn. Stat. Ann. § 363.02(1)(8)(i) (West Supp. 1991); Mo. Ann. Stat. § 213.055.1(1)(3) (Vernon Supp. 1992); Ohio Rev. Code Ann. § 4112.02(E)(1) (Anderson 1991); 43 Pa. Cons. Stat. Ann. § 955(b)(1) (1991); R.I. Gen. Laws § 28-5-7(4)(A) (Supp. 1991); Utah Code Ann. § 34-35-6(1)(d) (Supp. 1991).

123. Office of Technology Assessment (OTA), U.S. Congress, *Genetic Screening in the Workplace*, OTA-BA-456 (Washington, D.C.: U.S. Government Printing Office, 1990).

124. See, e.g., *Simonsen v. Swenson*, 104 Neb. 224, 177 N.W. 831 (1920); *Tarasoff v. Regents of the University of California*, 131 Cal. Rptr. 14, 17 Cal. App. 3d 425, 551 P.2d 334 (1976).

125. National Society of Genetic Counselors (NSGC), "Guiding Principles," *Perspectives on Genetic Counseling* (October 1991).

126. American Council on Life Insurance, *1992 Life Insurance Fact Book* 19 (1992).

127. Medical underwriting is the evaluation of a person's insurability, usually assessed through a combination of answers to a written questionnaire and physical examination to identify certain condi-

tions determined by medical underwriters (and underwriting manuals) to reduce life expectancy below actuarial norms. Standards for medical underwriting vary substantially by insurance company, and underwriting decisions are considered crucial business decisions by insurers and are thus considered "trade secrets."

128. Paul Billings, "Testimony Before Human Resources and Intergovernmental Relations Subcommittee of the Committee on Government Operations," U.S. House of Representatives, 102nd Congress, July 23, 1992.

129. Canadian Privacy Commission, *Genetic Testing and Privacy* (Ottawa, 1992).

130. Neil A. Holtzman and Mark A. Rothstein, "Invited Editorial: Eugenics and Genetic Discrimination," 50 *Am. J. Hum. Genet.* 457-459 (1992).

9

Research and
Policy Agenda

Existing gaps in data, research, and policy analysis impede informed policy making for the future. The committee found surprisingly few data on the extent of genetic testing and screening today, for example, and no system in place to gather data or to assess practices in relation to the committee's principles and recommendations for the future. Moreover, the lack of continuing policy oversight—at the national, state, and professional levels—impedes the development and implementation of coherent, effective standards for the anticipated explosion in genetic testing, screening, and counseling.

This chapter presents the committee's recommendations for addressing the key policy, research, and data needs in genetic testing and screening. Some of these recommendations are addressed to the Ethical, Legal, and Social Implications Program of the Human Genome Project of the National Institutes of Health (NIH) and the Department of Energy (DOE); other recommendations are addressed to relevant agencies, including other components of the National Institutes of Health, the Agency for Health Care Policy and Research, other agencies of the Public Health Service, the Health Care Financing Administration, the Department of Health and Human Services (DHHS), the National Science Foundation (NSF), and a broad range of private organizations.

POLICY OVERSIGHT FOR GENETIC TESTING AND SCREENING

National Policy Oversight

The need for continuing policy oversight for genetic testing has occupied the attention of the Committee on Assessing Genetic Risks from its inception. With the prospect of widespread genetic testing, the committee believes that effective oversight is essential to ensure that tests are validated before becoming standard medical practice and that such tests are used appropriately, with respect for the potential harms such testing may pose.

The committee believes that a national oversight body is needed to serve this function (see below). Such a body would help to bring order, over the coming years, to the continuing oversight of genetic testing and the evaluation of the readiness of new genetic tests for widespread use in medical practice, and to monitor professional practices. Such a body would collect and evaluate data on genetic testing, and advise state and federal agencies and other interested organizations with regulatory authority on establishing and enforcing standards for genetic tests. Among the organizations to whom this body could provide advice are the Human Genome Project (HGP), Health Care Financing Administration (HCFA), Food and Drug Administration (FDA), Centers for Disease Control and Prevention (CDC), Agency for Health Care Policy and Research (AHCPR), and the Congress, as well as legislatures, health agencies, and genetics advisory commissions at the state level.

Among genetics professionals, the American Society for Human Genetics (ASHG) has served some of the functions that the committee has in mind for the proposed National Advisory Committee on Genetic Testing and a Working Group on Genetic Testing (see below). ASHG has issued policy statements on maternal serum alpha-fetoprotein (MSAFP) screening; on cystic fibrosis (CF) testing and screening; on DNA banking, DNA data banking, and related confidentiality issues; and on freedom of choice related to prenatal diagnosis and to the selective abortion of fetuses diagnosed with, or at significant risk of, serious genetic disorders and birth defects. The National Society of Genetic Counselors (NSGC) has also developed a Code of Ethics and Guiding Principles that includes policy statements on access to care, nondiscrimination, and freedom of choice, as well as confidentiality of test results and informed consent. The Council of Regional Networks for Genetic Services (CORN) has developed policies and practices for laboratory quality assurance standards, proficiency testing programs, and essential data collection for newborn screening, cytogenetics, biochemical genetics, alpha-fetoprotein, and hemoglobinopathy screening; more recently, CORN has helped develop quality standards and proficiency testing for molecular genetics in conjunction with ASHG and the College of American Pathologists (CAP).

Many other professional groups also have an interest in genetic testing. The American Academy of Pediatrics (AAP) has issued a series of policy statements and fact sheets on newborn screening, including statements on screening for phenylketonuria and hypothyroidism, the subsequent use of newborn screening spots for DNA diagnosis, and the limits of consent in children and genetic testing in children. The American College of Obstetricians and Gynecologists (ACOG) has issued policy statements on MSAFP screening, prenatal diagnosis for advanced maternal age, and standards for the training of medical students and residents in obstetrics and gynecology related to genetics. Many disease-specific specialty organizations also have a strong interest in the rapidly developing field of genetic testing related to their disciplines and disorders (e.g., oncology, cardiology, diabetology). The development of an international code of ethics for geneticists has also been proposed (Wertz, 1992).

Genetic testing has moved beyond the domain of genetics specialists alone however. **Beyond the role of professional bodies, therefore, the committee recommends broad public involvement in the development of public policy and professional practice concerning genetic testing and screening.** As discussed throughout this report, genetic testing has broad health and social implications of both immediate and future concern to individuals and families with genetic disorders, genetic support groups, and the public at large. The Alliance of Genetic Support Groups has played an important role in coordinating and informing such support groups and, increasingly, in representing their interests in policy discussions. Most recently, the Alliance, in conjunction with ASHG, held a workshop and developed important guidelines for informed consent in research involving genetic testing (see Chapter 4).

Beyond the role of genetic support groups, there is a need for increased public awareness, understanding, and participation in the development of policy for genetic testing. Increased public education will be required to equip the public to make informed personal and policy decisions in genetic testing (see Chapter 5).

National Advisory Committee and Working Group

The committee deliberated at length about the best way to proceed in this complex professional and public policy climate and considered a variety of mechanisms for accomplishing the goals of technical and policy oversight. Some members felt that the existing Joint Working Group on the Ethical, Legal, and Social Implications (ELSI) of the Human Genome Project could serve as the needed oversight body if it had a more formalized mandate, along with expanded staff and funding. (The ELSI program has already supported consensus conferences to help to develop policy statements on issues such as CF screening, p53 screening for cancers, the implications of presymptomatic identification of late-onset genetic disorders in relation to implementation of the Americans with Disabilities Act, and research guidelines for large family studies in genetics.) In contrast, some members felt that overall policy oversight for genetic testing would be best provided in the context of a broader body overseeing biomedical ethics generally.

The majority of the committee recommends a broadly based, continuing, independent National Advisory Committee on Genetic Testing to provide policy advice and oversight for genetic testing, in conjunction with a Working Group on Genetic Testing to provide a forum for gathering and disseminating data—both scientific and social—to help develop common principles

and standards for evaluating when genetic tests are ready for widespread use in medical practice and overseeing the use of such testing. The National Advisory Committee and its Working Group should be appointed by the Secretary of Health and Human Services to give advice to DHHS and to the Congress, including the Joint NIH-DOE Human Genome Project. Its policy recommendations must be directed wherever appropriate, however, including other NIH components, CDC, FDA, AHCPR, HCFA, DHHS, the Congress, and other public and professional bodies. This National Advisory Committee should consist of scientists and physicians with expertise in genetic tests, as well as consumers aware of the problems of genetic testing, including members of the genetics community (particularly the American College of Medical Genetics (ACMG), ASHG, CORN, CAP, and the Alliance of Genetic Support Groups), other professional societies (e.g., ACOG and AAP), as well as other interested parties from law, business, and ethics.

The majority of the committee urges DHHS to fund the proposed National Advisory Committee on Genetic Testing with its Working Group on Genetic Testing and to fund an adequate staff. The Advisory Committee should be appointed by the Secretary of Health and Human Services and funded independently in order to ensure oversight of the full range of federal agencies involved in genetic testing and to professional societies making "standard of care" decisions. The Working Group should be capable of (1) collecting data on the validity and safety of tests already in use; (2) evaluating new tests by helping to design and evaluate pilot programs; and (3) measuring the performance of specific tests against the principles and criteria described in this report, and others that may be needed. The Advisory Committee would set priorities for which tests or types of tests should be evaluated and what additional data should be acquired by the Working Group. Based on the findings of the Working Group, the National Advisory Committee could make recommendations on altering current genetic testing practices, on when new tests are ready for widespread use, and on modifying or adding to this committee's principles and criteria for testing. The Advisory Committee should make reports as needed, but at least every two years, to the Secretary of Health and Human Services and the Congress. This policy mechanism should allow more comprehensive consensus and policy development, as well as the monitoring and oversight of professional practices related to genetic testing.

There have been discussions of and recommendations for a national commission on genetics to develop essential policy and provide oversight for this rapidly developing field, with its many scientific, ethical, legal, and social implications. The House Committee on Government Operations, Subcommittee on Information, Justice, and Agriculture (1992) issued a report recommending a national commission on genetic privacy at the level of the Secretary of Health and Human Services and the Secretary of Energy (Gellman, 1992; see Chapter 8). Issues in genetic privacy that are especially complex may warrant independent national review, depending *in part* on the outcome of the current round of health insurance reform at the national level. This will require careful monitoring over the next few years. If the committee's recommended National Advisory Committee on Genetic Testing and a Working Group on Genetic Testing are not created and funded—or are not successful—it will be necessary to reconsider the need for creation of a statutory national commission on genetics with a full legislative mandate negotiated through the Congress.

State Oversight: Role of State Commissions

The committee also sees a particular need for broadly representative advisory bodies at the state level. These advisory bodies should guide state health departments and legislatures on such issues as deciding when tests should be added to state-run screening programs and should ensure that the offering, testing, and associated education and counseling are always conducted in accord with principles outlined in this report. **State statutes affecting genetic testing should not be unduly prescriptive or restrictive, and should provide latitude to such advisory bodies to modify state-run genetic testing programs.** The committee believes that a federally supported national advisory body with a Working Group on Genetic Testing would be of great help to states in assessing genetic tests, in deciding which tests to adopt, and in tailoring national policy to meet state needs. Some states may not have the necessary expertise or resources to develop their own advisory structure, and may wish to collaborate with neighboring states, or to obtain their advice from the recommended national advisory group.

Research Policy for Studies Involving Genetic Testing

Much of current genetic testing grew out of and is still conducted within the context of research studies. Research initiatives involving genetic testing are being supported and developed not only within the Human Genome Project, but also within the research programs of various NIH components (including the National Institute of General Medical Sciences; National Institute of Child Health and Human Development; National Cancer Institute; National Heart, Lung, and Blood Institute; National Institute of Diabetes and Digestive and Kidney Diseases; National Institute of Neurological Disorders and Stroke, etc.).

In developing and approving research protocols, the committee recommends that the NIH implement the recommendations of this committee within the context of research studies. In particular, the committee recommends that all projects involving genetic testing consider the relevant psychosocial implications of genetic testing, and the potential for harm from the use and misuse of resulting genetic information. This is especially significant where there is no treatment available for the disorders, as will often be the case for many disorders in the near future. In developing requests for proposals or requests for applications, and in reviewing research, demonstration projects, pilot studies, clinical trials, and family studies in genetics, NIH and other funding agencies should also assess the availability of appropriate genetic counseling and follow-up services in evaluating study designs.

NEED FOR ADDITIONAL STANDARDS FOR GENETIC TESTING

The committee identified several areas in which additional standards are needed to indicate who should be tested, for what disorders, and at what age. These include prenatal diagnosis, predispositional testing, the age and circumstances for testing of minors, and multiplex genetic testing.

Prenatal Diagnosis

One area requiring additional standards is prenatal diagnosis, a form of genetic testing that is already widespread. Before informed policy can be developed for some of these issues, key research questions need to be addressed. These include the special impact of prenatal diagnosis on women, the issues posed by carrier detection during pregnancy rather than prior to conception, the complexities of MSAFP screening, the issues posed by seeking "perfection," including the use of prenatal diagnosis and selective abortion to choose the sex of the fetus.

The committee recommends additional research on the impact of prenatal diagnosis, particularly its immediate and long-term effects on women. Such research should include the psychosocial implications—both at the time of pregnancy and later in the woman's life—of decision making about selective abortion of a fetus diagnosed with a genetic disorder. The committee believes that such research will provide important information for the design, conduct, and evaluation of genetic counseling for prenatal diagnosis in the future.

The nature of MSAFP screening involves a high rate of initial identification of increased risk for a wide variety of conditions in the fetuses where the fetus later turns out not to be affected. This can cause substantial anxiety during the waiting period for follow-up confirmatory test results. These factors highlight the need for intensive follow-up of prenatal genetic testing, both to confirm the predictive value of tests and to ensure counseling for women with abnormal MSAFP screening results. **The committee recognizes that carrier screening sometimes takes place during pregnancy, but it recommends the development of carrier screening before pregnancy.** There is a need for innovative and practical methods for carrier screening of adults before pregnancy, as well as the evaluation of such programs through pilot studies. Better public and provider education may increase preconception carrier testing.

With parents having fewer children, and often having them later in life, there may be increasing emphasis on having children who are not only healthy, but have certain desired characteristics. This possibility raises the issues of "designer children," "designer genes," and "genetic perfectibility." **The committee recommends that prenatal diagnosis only be used to assess genetic disorders and** birth defects; it is concerned about the offering of prenatal diagnosis for trivial reasons. **The committee is particularly concerned about the use of prenatal diagnosis for sex selection.** It is concerned that—with increasing entrepreneurial pressures in prenatal diagnosis—the use of prenatal diagnosis for selection of fetal sex may become more widespread in the future. The committee believes this issue warrants careful scrutiny over the next three to five years as the availability of genetic testing becomes more widespread, and especially as simpler, safer technologies for prenatal diagnosis are developed (see Chapter 2).

ACOG, ASHG, CORN, and NSGC have issued a variety of policy statements about aspects of prenatal diagnosis. However, the committee believes that issues in genetic testing have moved beyond the domain of professional groups alone. While existing standards may have been adequate for the past, new standards will be needed in the future, particularly to respond to rapid developments in genetic testing methods that are now experimental, such as the use of fetal cells isolated from maternal blood, triple-marker screening, and preimplantation diagnosis. Reproductive genetic decisions raise some of the most deeply personal and troubling issues in genetic testing. **The committee recommends that professional groups work together, and develop innovative methods for involving the public, in the development of standards for the use of these technologies.**

Predispositional Genetic Testing and Screening

There is at the present time an important "window of opportunity" now to consider all the ramifications of predispositional genetic testing before such testing becomes widespread. For common disorders, the committee believes that tests for predisposition will vary in predictive value both among tests and among disorders; and that the disorders will vary in treatability, thereby affecting the utility of the information to be gained even from highly predictive tests. Genetic testing for very common, high-profile disorders such as heart disease, diabetes mellitus, and cancers will be subject to entrepreneurial pressure to expand testing once such tests are available; this, in turn, may have substantial potential for harm to individuals and families, at least in terms of insurability and employability.

The committee recommends the development of standards for genetic tests designed to detect predispositions to disorders of late onset. Strict guidelines for efficacy will be necessary to prevent the premature introduction of this technology. The development of such standards would be an appropriate early task for the National Advisory Committee on Genetic Testing with a Working Group on Genetic Testing.

The committee believes that population screening for late-onset monogenic diseases should be considered only for treatable or preventable conditions of relatively high frequency. Under such guidelines, population screening should be offered only after appropriate, reliable, sensitive, and specific tests become available. Such tests do not yet exist. Once appropriate tests become available, pilot studies will be required to demonstrate that the proposed interventions are safe and effective before their wide-scale introduction can be recommended. These tests may have long-term impacts, and extensive pretest counseling is critical to ensure voluntary participation and informed consent. The committee recommends research on education and counseling both before and after predispositional genetic testing to ensure that an individual is fully aware of the potential use and usefulness of test results, as well as possible harms of having the information. Research on issues related to predispositional genetic testing should include the key policy issues identified in Chapters 4, 6, and 8. For example, the potential abuse of such information in employment or insurance practice must be fully understood by the individual undergoing predispositional genetic screening or testing, and the provider should ensure that confidentiality is respected.

Providers who conduct predispositional genetic testing should also be well schooled in the principles of genetics and genetic counseling, including the ethical, legal, and social issues involved in genetic testing. In the future, for example, genetic testing for psychiatric diseases will require all psychiatrists to have more training in genetics and genetic counseling, again including the ethical, legal, and social implications of such testing (see Chapters 4 and 6).

Testing of Minors

The committee believes that special concerns are posed by the prospect of increased genetic testing of minors. The committee believes that its principles for newborn screening are appropriate policy guidance for genetic testing in minors, particularly the principle of benefit to the minor and avoiding the possibility that genetic information will be generated about a child when there is no likely benefit to the child in the immediate future (see Chapters 1, 2, 4, and 8). In general, the committee does not recommend predispositional genetic testing for minors unless delays would result in significant harm to the child. **Research should be undertaken to define factors relating to the appropriate age for testing and screening for genetic disorders in order to maximize the benefits of therapeutic intervention and minimize the potential for harms.** The committee was concerned about the use of genetic information in adoption in ways that might represent harmful and unwarranted intrusions on individual privacy, for example, to determine "suitability" as parents or as a potential adopted child. Alternatively, some genetic information might be helpful to parents in the care of an adopted child. **Further study is needed to determine the appropriate use of genetic— and other medical—information in adoption cases.**

Multiplex Testing

Multiplex testing represents one of the key innovations likely to be introduced in genetic testing; it involves performing multiple genetic tests on a single blood or other tissue sample. This will be a very important issue for the future of genetic testing and genetic counseling (see Chapters 1, 2, 4, and 8).

The committee recommends the development both of standards for multiplex genetic testing and of innovative methods for applying multiplex testing. The latter could involve the grouping of tests by related types of disorders that raise similar issues in terms of their significance, including severity, variability, the availability of effective treatment, how soon treatment needs to be instituted, and other specifics of each disorder), to allow time for appropriate education, informed consent, and genetic counseling.

The committee opposes the multiplexing of all available genetic tests merely because it is technologically possible to do so (see Chapter 2). Research will be required to develop and evaluate innovative methods for the grouping of genetic tests in a way that will make it possible for multiplex testing to embody the committee's fundamental principles of informed consent, as well as its principles for genetic education and counseling (see Chapters 4 and 8).

RESEARCH NEEDS

Assessment of ELSI Research and Policy Studies

One key contribution to our state of knowledge concerning research and policy issues in genetic testing would be a state-of-the-art analysis of what has been learned to date from projects supported under the joint Ethical, Legal, and Social Implications Program of NIH and DOE. Three years of developmental work has gone into this innovative effort to assess a major new area of technology before its full impact has been felt; this is an appropriate time to assess what has been learned.

The committee endorses the concept that the ELSI program support "meta-analyses" of what has been learned in the key areas of its program investment. Such meta-analyses can help inform policy debate and development, as well as aid those working in the field—and those developing projects and concepts—to make use of this important investment in our understanding of all the implications of genetic testing posed by the Human Genome Project.

Pilot Studies

It is critical to conduct adequate pilot studies and related investigations before genetic tests move from research to widespread or routine clinical use (see Chapters 1 and 3). The 1975 committee of the National Academy of Sciences (NAS, 1975) also identified the importance of pilot studies to precede genetic testing and screening. Since that time, not all genetic testing and screening programs have been subject to the discipline of pilot testing and evaluation, and some have undergone pilot studies but not undergone outside evaluation.

The committee recommends that pilot studies be conducted on all genetic testing and screening programs—with outside, peer-reviewed evaluation—before they become widespread in newborn screening or any other types of genetic testing or screening. Effective pilot studies should be implemented as early as possible in genetic testing and screening situations for which there is no prior experience, for example, testing for predisposition to late-onset disorders. Once multiplex testing becomes possible, appropriate pilot studies must be carried out before this kind of simultaneous testing for multiple disorders is implemented (see Chapters 1, 3, and 4). Third-party payers should look to such pilot studies in considering reimbursement for genetic testing. Pilot testing is a legitimate and appropriate area for federal assistance.

Laboratory Quality Assurance

Centralization raises potential issues that, in the past, have been considered restraint of trade for commercial testing laboratories. Nevertheless, centralization of laboratory testing offers opportunities for improving the all-important quality of genetic test results and reaching the goal of close to "zero-error" tolerance in laboratory genetic testing. The committee has stopped short of recommending the kind of centralization of genetic testing laboratories adopted, for example, by California for its newborn, Tay-Sachs, and MSAFP screening programs. Instead, the committee has recommended other means of ensuring quality and proficiency in genetic testing (see Chapter 3). Research is needed to develop and evaluate these methods of laboratory quality assurance for genetic testing, including quality control and proficiency testing. However, centralized laboratory testing is recommended now to ensure the quality of genetic tests for rare disorders (see Chapter 3).

Genetics Knowledge and Attitudes of Health Professionals

Since genetic testing is increasingly likely to be delivered in primary care settings in the future, the adequacy of genetics education and counseling in such settings will have to be evaluated. Research on knowledge and practices related to genetics and genetic testing among the professionals who are to provide this education and counseling, is essential to the development of proper reforms in education, training, and professional standards related to genetic testing (see Chapters 4 and 6).

The committee recommends that genetics education and counseling tasks be analyzed to determine what level of complexity can appropriately be delivered by primary care providers and what degree of complexity requires the training and experience of specialized genetics personnel. The committee believes that the more complex and significant the implications and decisions to be made are—including reproductive decisions and testing for *untreatable* late-onset disorders—the more training will be needed for the people who are providing genetics education and counseling. Research is also needed on the knowledge, attitudes, and behavior of health professionals concerning untreatable disorders or reproductive decisions, particularly related to nondirectiveness.

Genetics Education and Counseling

Research is required on the essential components of genetic counseling services, including education and counseling before and after testing, and on the need for follow-up support services. A number of pressing research issues need to be addressed in genetic education and counseling: Can counseling be streamlined and still be appropriate? Can supplemental support techniques (e.g., introductory videos, computer models, interactive video, workbooks, audiotapes of counseling sessions) provide important education and increase the cost-effectiveness of genetic counseling, whoever provides such services in the future? What is needed for appropriate informed consent? What impact do psychosocial factors related to genetic testing have on the effects and effectiveness of genetic counseling and education? What can be done to increase the cultural appropriateness of genetic counseling and education? What more can be done to inform people effectively about various genetic disorders, including the development of balanced materials?

Informed Consent

For example, most people have less interest in information about the name of the disorder and its mechanisms of action, than in information about the certainty with which the test predicts a disorder, what effects the disorder has on physical and mental functioning, whether treatment exists, and how intrusive any existing treatment protocol would be.

The committee recommends that research be undertaken to determine what people feel they need to know in order to decide whether or not to undergo a genetic test.

Research is also needed on what constitutes informed consent. This includes the level of information needed for various types of disorders (e.g., accepted testing for treatable disorders such as PKU, versus untreatable disorders of late onset such as Huntington disease), as well as how it may be affected by a variety of variables such as ethnic, racial, cultural, and socioeconomic differences. Research is needed to determine the advantages and disadvantages of various means of conveying that information (e.g., through specialized genetic counselors, primary care providers, single-disorder counselors, brochures, videos, audiotapes, computer programs).

Psychosocial Factors in Genetic Testing

Research is needed on the barriers to and the psychosocial impacts of

genetics services, for example, (1) social stigma; (2) insurance and employment discrimination; and (3) the organization, delivery, availability, and financing of genetic testing services. This research should address factors such as geographic distribution, cost, and differences in cultural perceptions and values (see Chapters 2, 4, 6, and 8). It might also include research on the meanings and implications of commonly used health terminology, and the changes in application of that terminology to the field of genetics. Important among these issues of the language of genetics are the use of terms such as "defect" versus "condition"; more attention to the functional status of persons with genetic disorders; and assessment of how people consider the "eradication" of genetic disorders versus the eradication of communicable diseases (see Chapter 4, Box 4-1).

Culturally Appropriate Genetic Testing and Counseling

The committee recommends research to determine how best to provide genetic counseling in ways that are sensitive and appropriate to a variety of cultures and languages. Such research should be planned, conducted, and evaluated with the participation of persons from the cultures being studied. It should attempt to elucidate the effects of cultural differences on the delivery and receipt of genetic counseling with special attention to differing cultural perspectives on the role of persons in authority when the person is offering genetic counseling. Research should also include the analysis of key issues in genetics of particular importance to various cultures.

Once understood, these analyses should be widely disseminated and used in training, not only throughout the professional genetics community, but also among health care professionals in general. Materials developed for culturally sensitive genetics education and counseling, both print and video, should be evaluated and model materials distributed widely.

Development of Balanced Materials on Genetic Disorders

The committee recommends the development and evaluation of balanced descriptions of genetic disorders, in culturally appropriate language, that are respectful of persons with the disorder(s) and avoid the use of pejorative terms or language. Appropriate genetics professional groups should undertake the development and evaluation of such descriptions with the participation of individuals and families affected by the disorder, as well as specialized genetics personnel. These descriptions should carefully balance available information about the sensitivity and specificity of the test, as well as about the severity, variability, and treatability, and what is not known about various disorders. The proposed National Advisory Committee and Working Group would be one mechanism for producing such documents. These materials should be evaluated to determine their effectiveness and possible sources of bias in communicating information both about a particular disorder and about the potential risks and harms of tests for the disorder.

Materials should be developed on particular disorders, perhaps starting with more common ones. Good examples for such balanced materials would include neural tube defects and Down syndrome, for which screening is already widespread. Cystic fibrosis might also be a good subject for this approach because (1) it exemplifies problems of variable expressivity; (2) the tests are complex in terms of sensitivity and specificity; and (3) treatments are estimated to be improving the overall prospects for many persons born with cystic fibrosis.

Measuring the Effectiveness of Genetic Education and Counseling

The committee believes that measuring a client's understanding and recall of numerical risks is too limited an indication of the success of or need for counseling. Beyond mere comprehension of numerical risk, genetic counseling must assist individuals in determining their own acceptable risk. Since risk perceptions vary among individuals and among counselees and counselors, there is no one right way to present or interpret risk information; information must be balanced, and the process must be tailored to each client.

The committee recommends that research on the best ways to provide essential genetics education and counseling—by a variety of providers in a variety of settings—precede efforts to streamline genetic counseling. Specifically, a variety of approaches to counseling and informing of results should be evaluated to determine (1) what the client has learned; (2) how counseling has affected her or him; and (3) his or her satisfaction with the way counseling was provided and information reported (see Chapter 4).

Public Education

New policy and research initiatives should be launched to enhance public knowledge and impart the skills needed to make informed personal and public policy decisions related to genetic testing (see Chapter 5). The Human Genome Project's ELSI program should coordinate a public education initiative in genetics and expand its support for such efforts. To accomplish essential changes in policy, it will be necessary to bring together leaders from education and other professions, other federal agencies, support groups, foundations, and consumers to explore common interests and to formulate appropriate goals and strategies in public education related to genetic testing. CORN has already held one meeting of this kind related to a project to develop an on-line data base on genetic testing for consumers (Proud, 1992). This activity could serve as the basis for further coordination and collaboration on public information on genetic testing.

Components of this public education effort include the following:

• Incorporating the principles, concepts, and skills training that support informed decision making about genetic testing into all levels of schooling—kindergarten through college. These should include concepts of respect for genetic diversity (differences) and kinship, as well as consideration of sensitive issues of reproduction in terms appropriate to the age and stage of development of students.

• Ensuring that appropriate educational messages about genetic tests and their implications reach the public, to enhance informed public decision making about either seeking or accepting genetic tests.

• Establishing systems for designing, implementing, and maintaining community-based interventions for genetics education among population groups at higher risk of particular genetic disorders (e.g., increased risk related to race or ethnicity).

• Encouraging broad public participation in the development of educational approaches that respect the widely varying personal and cultural perspectives on issues of genetics and are tolerant of individuals with genetic disorders of all kinds. Particular effort will be needed to include the perspectives of women, minorities, and persons with disabilities, who may feel especially affected by developing genetics technologies.

• Enlisting the mass media to help decrease public confusion and increase the knowledge and skills that will equip consumers to make appropriate decisions for themselves.

• *Developing a consumer's guide to genetic testing* and other consumer materials that provide reliable, self-explanatory, easily understood, and readily available information about genetic services and the many possible implications of the tests.

• Developing model genetics education initiatives to incorporate both the science and the social issues associated with genetic testing. NSF and other organizations should (1) expand programs that support model educational initiatives in science for precollege and college programs in molecular biology; (2) collaborate with the ELSI program of the Human Genome Project to encourage such programs to focus the attention of students on the health, social, legal, and ethical issues raised by genetic testing and screening; and (3) require evaluation of educational interventions.

Computer Innovation in Genetics Education

Innovative and interactive computer-assisted systems should be developed to provide clients and professionals with the latest information on genetic disorders and on genetic diagnosis, testing, and screening, as one way to improve the quality of genetic testing, education, and counseling services in the future (see Chapters 5 and 6). If designed and used appropriately, computer technologies could assist genetics specialists and primary care practitioners by

presenting patients with basic, self-paced genetics education and even by presenting possible decision options for consideration of patients.

The on-line AIDS bibliography could serve as one example of the use of
computerized techniques to enhance public education for joint action by the ELSI
program and the National Library of Medicine (NLM). NLM's program with the
American College of Physicians (ACP), which provides access to NLM resources
to ACP members, is another possible model. The system should include access to
the recommendations and assessments of the proposed National Advisory Committee on Genetic Testing and its Working Group on Genetic Testing. The ELSI
program should coordinate with professional genetics organizations and NLM to
develop such a genetics education and dissemination program for interested health
professionals (see Chapter 6). However, more research is needed to determine
which tasks in genetics education and counseling can be appropriately accomplished using such techniques and to evaluate these techniques in various settings
and populations.

Cost-Effectiveness Analysis of Genetic Testing

The original Institute of Medicine (IOM) request for funding for this study
included, among the issues the committee might address, the cost-effectiveness
and cost-benefit of genetic testing and screening. This is a murky and often arcane area where, unfortunately, more attention is usually paid to the cost side of
the equation than to benefits or effectiveness—at least in these economically difficult times. It is difficult enough to apply these analytical constructs to technological innovations in medical practice, such as the model of quality of life factors
in assessing medical interventions such as the artificial heart (Hogness and
VanAntwerp, 1991). Genetic testing and screening, with its attendant social, legal, and ethical issues, increases the complexity of the analysis still further. The
President's Commission (1983, p. 84) summed up these issues succinctly:

> Cost-benefit analysis is most useful when the costs and benefits of the
> action under consideration are tangible, can be measured by a common
> unit of measurement, and can be known with certainty. These conditions
> are rarely satisfied in public policy situations and they can be particularly
> elusive in genetic screening and counseling programs. For example, cost-
> benefit calculations can accurately evaluate the worth of a projected prena-
> tal screening program if the only costs measured are the financial outlays
> (that is, administering a screening and counseling program and performing
> abortions when defects are detected) and the benefits measured are the
> dollars that would have been spent on the care of affected children. But
> the calculations become both much more complex and much less accurate
> if an attempt is made to quantify the psychological "costs" and "benefits"
> to screenees, their families, and society.
>
> A more fundamental limitation on cost-benefit analysis is that in its
> simplest form it assumes that the governing moral value is to maximize the

general welfare (utilitarianism). Simply aggregating gains and losses across all the individuals affected omits considerations of equity or fairness. Indeed, cost-benefit methodology itself does not distinguish as to *whose* costs and benefits are to be considered. It is possible, however, to incorporate considerations of equity or fairness and thereby depart from a strictly utilitarian form of cost-benefit analysis either by weighing some costs or benefits or by restricting the class of individuals who will be included in the calculation. In any case, **cost-benefit analysis must be regarded as a technical instrument to be used within an ethical framework (whether utilitarian or otherwise), rather than as a method of avoiding difficult ethical judgments.**

Many issues are involved in applying the difficult measures of cost, burden, benefit, and effectiveness to genetic testing and screening, where risks and costs are distributed disproportionally to benefits among individuals, and even across generations. Increasing the effectiveness of the tests (i.e., specificity, sensitivity, reliability, and validity) *is a necessary but not sufficient* answer to critical questions about the value of genetic testing and screening. The availability or absence of treatment for genetic conditions must also weigh heavily in any assessment of the benefits and costs of genetic testing and screening for individuals, their families, and society.

Additional research is needed in improved analytic thinking and techniques to provide a better foundation for cost-effectiveness analysis for genetic testing and screening. The work of the National Advisory Committee on Genetic Testing and its Working Group on Genetic Testing should provide essential information on the readiness of genetic tests for wide-scale use. However, genetic testing is not an end in itself. The committee, therefore, recommends that this research address such broader policy questions as: Where do genetic services and genetic assessment fit into the broad picture of health care priorities? What is the appropriate relative priority for genetic services compared to alternative investments in prenatal care, childhood immunization, or prevention of child abuse, all of which have better-documented cost-effectiveness than genetic testing and screening now has (e.g., GAO, 1992).

CRITICAL DEFICIENCIES IN DATA ON GENETICS SERVICES

The committee found that basic data on the number and kinds of genetic testing procedures are not available on most genetic testing and counseling services. With support from the Genetic Services Branch of the Maternal and Child Health Bureau, DHHS, CORN has worked to develop data on genetic services. In the only area of genetic services for which basic data exist—newborn screening—the data report and policy recommendations were developed through the efforts of CORN (1992).

One reason for the paucity of data about genetic testing is the wide variety of settings in which such services are delivered, including many research laboratories and physician offices. New data show that slightly more than 2 million MSAFP screening tests were performed in 1991 based on a survey of laboratories performing MSAFP analysis (J. Haddow, Foundation for Blood Research, personal communication, January 1993). CORN has made an effort to collect more comprehensive data on prenatal diagnosis (Meaney, 1992), but it has limited reporting sources and no access to data on obstetrical office procedures. Without basic data on prenatal genetic services, there is no way to monitor current or future professional practices in relation to professional society guidelines or the recommendations of this committee.

The committee recommends the systematic development of basic data on the full range of genetic testing and screening services that is needed to provide a sound basis for policy development for the future. A minimum data set on genetic services should be developed by a joint working group on genetic testing and services. This group should consist, at a minimum, of the National Center for Health Statistics, the Genetic Services Branch, the Human Genome Project, the Centers for Disease Control and Prevention, and Medicaid data experts, as well as CORN and other interested professional groups, and other relevant data experts.

Two critical areas for immediate development of data sets are prenatal diagnosis and predispositional genetic testing. Both areas pose difficulties in the design and collection of basic data. In the case of prenatal diagnosis, most services are provided in private physician offices; although Medicaid can provide reimbursement information on prenatal diagnosis among its population, states vary widely in coverage of prenatal diagnosis and possible abortion of fetuses identified with genetic disorders (see Chapter 7). Predispositional testing is newer and likely to expand in the future (see Chapter 2). Much of such testing is now performed in research settings (see Chapter 3), but like prenatal diagnosis, it is likely to be done in physicians' offices as it moves into widespread use. The development of data and collection methods early in the dissemination of predispositional testing can provide a model for studying the dissemination of genetic testing into medical practice generally, as well as for monitoring professional practices in relation to professional guidelines and the recommendations of this committee.

RESEARCH ON POPULATION GENETICS

There is a need for better information on the frequency and distribution of disease-related mutations in defined populations, an important part of population genetics. The availability of better information is critical in refining the risk estimates given to clients and their families in genetics education and in counseling about various genetic disorders. Such information is also essential in determining changing patterns in genetic disorders, such as the reduction in Tay-Sachs disease in North Americans over the past 20 years.

The committee believes that such intensive population genetics studies are needed, but that the design of such studies requires the utmost care in the protection of study participants. In particular, these studies need to ensure that participants understand that their participation is for research purposes only and that no health or other personal benefit will come from the research. The committee also notes that data and analysis from population studies have in the past been used against some population groups, as in the often bitter debates about the genetic basis of intelligence. **Special care is needed in the design and implementation of all genetics studies to ensure that their unintended consequences do not jeopardize future genetic testing and screening programs that have direct health benefits.**

REFERENCES

Committee on Government Operations. 1992. Designing Genetic Information Policy: The Need for an Independent Policy Review of the Ethical, Legal, and Social Implications of the Human Genome Project, House Report 102-478. U.S. House of Representatives. Washington, D.C.

Council of Regional Networks for Genetic Services (CORN). 1992. Newborn Screening: 1990 (Final Report). New York: CORN.

Gellman, R. 1992. Genetic privacy. Presentation before the Committee on Assessing Genetic Risks. Washington, D.C. September.

General Accounting Office (GAO). 1992. Child Abuse: Prevention Program Needs Greater Emphasis. Washington, D.C.

Hogness, J., and VanAntwerp, M. 1991. The Artificial Heart: Prototypes, Policies, and Patients. Washington, D.C.: National Academy Press.

House Committee on Government Operations, Subcommittee on Information, Justice, and Agriculture. 1992. Designing Genetic Information Policy: The Need for an Independent Policy Review of the Human Genome Project. House Report 102-478. Washington, D.C.: U.S. Government Printing Office.

Kaback, M. 1993. Tay-Sachs disease. In Scriver, C., et al. (eds.) The Metabolic Basis of Inherited Diseases (6th ed.). New York: Liss.

Meaney, J. 1992 (published in 1994). National data on genetic services: Council of Regional Networks for Genetic Services. In Fullarton, J. (ed.) Proceedings of the Committee on Assessing Genetic Risks. Washington, D.C.: National Academy Press.

National Academy of Sciences (NAS). 1975. Genetic Screening: Programs, Principles, and Research. National Research Council. Washington, D.C.: NAS.

National Academy of Sciences (NAS). 1992. DNA Technology in Forensic Science. National Research Council. Washington, D.C.: National Academy Press.

President's Commission for the Study of Ethical Problems in Medicine and Biomedical and Behavioral Research. 1983. Screening and Counseling for Genetic Conditions: The Ethical, Social, and Legal Implications of Genetic Screening, Counseling, and Education Programs. Washington, D.C.: U.S. Government Printing Office.

Proud, V. 1992 (published in 1994). On-line genetics public education. In Fullarton, J. (ed.) Proceedings of the Committee on Assessing Genetic Risks. Washington, D.C.: National Academy Press.

Wertz, D. 1992 (published in 1994). International code of ethics for genetics. In Fullarton, J. (ed.) Proceedings of the Committee on Assessing Genetic Risks. Washington, D.C.: National Academy Press.

APPENDIX A

Workshop Participants

**PARTICIPANTS IN THE FEBRUARY 1992 WORKSHOP
ON LABORATORY ISSUES IN GENETICS**

Arthur Beaudet, M.D.
Institute of Molecular Genetics
Baylor College of Medicine
One Baylor Plaza, T-619
Houston, TX 77030

David Blumenthal, M.D.
Medical Practices Evaluation
    Center
Massachusetts General Hospital
50 Staniford Street
Boston, MA 02114

Jessica Davis, M.D.
President, Council of Regional
    Networks
Cornell University Medical Center
Genetics Box 3
1300 York Avenue
New York, NY 10021

Wayne Grody, M.D., Ph.D.
UCLA School of Medicine
Assistant Professor
Divisions of Medical Genetics and
    Molecular Pathology
Los Angeles, CA 90024-1732

Frits Hommes, Ph.D.
Voluntary National Biochemical
    Genetics Laboratory Proficiency
    Testing Program
Professor, Department of
    Biochemistry and Molecular
    Biology, Medical College of
    Georgia
1120 Fifteenth Street
Augusta, GA 30912

Thaddeus Kelly, M.D., Ph.D.
Vice Chair
American Board of Medical
    Genetics
Division of Human Genetics
University of Virginia Hospital
Charlottesville, VA 22908

Katherine Klinger, Ph.D.
Vice President for Science
Integrated Genetics, Inc.
31 New York Avenue
Framingham, MA 01701

George Knight, Ph.D.
Foundation for Blood Research
P. O. Box 190
Scarborough, ME 04070

Karla Matteson, Ph.D.
Director, Human Development and
    Genetics Center
University of Tennessee Medical
    Center
1924 Alcon Highway
Knoxville, TN 37920

Douglas McQuilken
Vice President for Business
    Development
Roche Molecular Systems, Inc.
340 Kingsland Street
Nutley, NJ 07110

F. John Meaney, Ph.D.
Office of Risk Assessment and
    Investigation
Division of Disease Prevention
    Services
Arizona Department of Health
    Services
3008 N. 3rd Street, Suite 101
Phoenix, AZ 85012

Patricia Murphy, Ph.D.
Director, DNA Diagnostic
    Laboratory
Laboratory of Human Genetics
State of New York Department of
    Health
Wadsworth Center for Laboratories
    and Research
Empire State Plaza
Albany, NY 12201-0509

Deborah Nickerson, Ph.D.
Division of Biology, 139-74
California Institute of Technology
Pasadena, CA 91125

Seymour Perry, M.D.
Chair
Department of Family and
    Community Medicine
Georgetown University School of
    Medicine
215 Kober-Cogan Building
3750 Reservoir Road
Washington, DC 20007

Hope Punnett, Ph.D.
ASHG Committee on Genetic
    Services
St. Christopher's Children's
    Hospital
Front and Erie Streets
Philadelphia, PA 19134

Max Rabinowitz, M.D.
Division of Clinical Laboratory
    Devices
Office of Device Evaluation, Food
    and Drug Administration
1390 Piccard Drive
Rockville, MD 20850

William Seltzer, Ph.D.
Director
DNA Diagnostic Laboratory
Assistant Professor, Pediatrics and
  Biochemistry, Biophysics and
  Genetics
Department of Pediatrics, Box
  C233
University of Colorado Health
  Sciences Center
Denver, CO 80262

Joseph Shulman, M.D.
President, Genetics and IVF
  Institute
3020 Javier Road
Fairfax, VA 22031

Paul Silverman, Ph.D.
Director of Scientific Affairs
Beckman Instruments, Inc.
2500 Harbor Boulevard D-14-E
Fullerton, CA 92634-3100

Michael Watson, Ph.D.
American College of Medical
  Genetics
Director of Clinical Cytogenetics
St. Louis Children's Hospital
400 South Kingshighway Boulevard
St. Louis, MO 63110

Victor W. Weedn, M.D., J.D.
Major, U.S. Army Medical Corps
DNA Identification Laboratory
Armed Forces Institute of
  Pathology
Washington, DC 20306-6000

Ann Willey, Ph.D.
Director
Laboratory of Human Genetics
Wadsworth Center for Laboratories
  Research
New York State Department of
  Health
P. O. Box 509
Albany, NY 12201-0509

PARTICIPANTS IN THE JUNE 1992 WORKSHOP
ON ISSUES IN GENETIC SERVICES

Barbara Adam
Chief
CDC Infant Screening Quality
  Assurance Laboratory
1600 Clifton Road
Atlanta, GA 30333

Paul R. Billings, M.D., Ph.D.
Chief
Division of Genetic Medicine
Department of Medicine
Pacific Presbyterian Medical Center
San Francisco, CA 94120

Alta Charo, J.D.
Assistant Professor, Law and
  Medical Ethics
University of Wisconsin
308 Law Building
Madison, WI 53706

Ellen Wright Clayton, M.D., J.D.
Assistant Professor of Pediatrics
  and Law
Vanderbilt University School of
  Law
Nashville, TN 37240

Barbara Crandall, M.D.
University of California-Los
  Angeles Medical Center Mental
  Retardation Unit
760 Westwood Plaza
Los Angeles, CA 90024

George Cunningham, M.D., M.P.H.
Chief, Genetic Disease Branch
California Department of Health
  Services
2151 Berkeley Way (Annex Four)
Berkeley, CA 94704-1011

Mark Evans, M.D.
Director
Division of Reproductive Genetics
Wayne State University School of
  Medicine
Department of Obstetrics and
  Gynecology
4707 St. Antoine Boulevard
Detroit, MI 48201

Stephen Friend, M.D.
MGH Cancer Center
Building 149, 13th Street
Charlestown, MA 02129

Patricia A. Gabow, M.D.
Deputy Manager
Medical Affairs
Denver General Hospital
777 Bannock Street
Denver, CO 80202-4507

Elena Gates, M.D.
Assistant Clinical Professor
Department of Obstetrics and
  Gynecology
University of California-San
  Francisco
505 Parnassus Avenue—Box 0132
San Francisco, CA 94143

Michael R. Hayden, Ph.D., FRCPC
Associate Professor of Medical
  Genetics and Director, Adult
  Genetics Clinic
University of British Columbia
2211 Westbrook Mall, Room F-185
Vancouver, BC, Canada V6T 2B5

Claude Laberge, Ph.D., FRCPC
President
Quebec Network of Genetic
  Medicine
CHUL Department of Genetic
  Medicine
2705 Laurier Boulevard, Room
  9355
Ste. Foy, Quebec, Canada G1V4G2

Sue Levi-Pearl
Liaison, Medical and Scientific
  Programs
Tourette Syndrome Association,
  Inc.
42-40 Bell Boulevard
Bayside, NY 11361-2861

Abby Lippman, Ph.D.
Associate Professor, Department of
  Epidemiology and Biostatistics
McGill University
Montreal, Quebec, Canada H3A1A2

Edward McCabe, M.D., Ph.D.
Baylor College of Medicine
Institute for Molecular Genetics
Room S-921
Texas Medical Center
Houston, TX 77030

Gloria Petersen, M.D.
Assistant Professor of
    Epidemiology
Johns Hopkins University
School of Public Health and
    Hygiene
615 N. Wolfe Street
Baltimore, MD 21205

Nancy Press, Ph.D.
Assistant Research Anthropologist
Department of Psychiatry/
    Behavioral Sciences
Medical Center, University of
    California-L.A.
760 Westwood Plaza
Los Angeles, CA 90024

Neil J. Risch, Ph.D.
Yale University School of Medicine
Department of Epidemiology/Public
    Health
60 College Street, PO Box 3333
New Haven, CN 06510

Barbara Katz Rothman, Ph.D.
Professor
Department of Sociology
Baruch College, City University of
    New York
17 Lexington Avenue
New York, NY 10010

Janet Rowley, M.D.
Professor
Departments of Medicine and
    Molecular Genetics and Cell
    Biology
The University of Chicago
5841 South Maryland Avenue, Box
    420
Chicago, IL 60637

Margery Shaw, M.D., J.D.
2617 Pine Tree Drive
Evansville, IN 47711

Elizabeth Thomson, R.N., M.S.
Coordinator
Iowa Statewide Genetic Counseling
    Services
Coordinator, Cystic Fibrosis Pilot
    Project Consortium (National
    Center for Human Genome
    Research)
Division of Medical Genetics
Department of Pediatrics
University Hospitals and Clinics
Iowa City, IA 52242

Barbara Faye Waxman
8883 Pico Boulevard
Los Angeles, CA 90035

Dorothy Wertz, Ph.D.
Social Science, Ethics, and Law
    Program
Shriver Center for Mental
    Retardation
200 Trapelo Road
Waltham, MA 02254

PARTICIPANTS IN THE SEPTEMBER 1992 MINI-WORKSHOPS
ON GENETIC COUNSELING; PUBLIC EDUCATION;
PRIVACY AND INSURANCE

Ruby Bishop
President-Elect
Alliance of Genetic Support Groups
7101 W. 12th, Suite 401
Little Rock, AR 72204

Troy Duster, Ph.D.
Director
Institute for the Study of Social
  Change
University of California/Berkeley
2420 Bowditch Street
Berkeley, CA 94720

John Fanning, J.D.
Office of Health Policy and
  Evaluation
Office of the Assistant Secretary
  for Health
Department of Health and Human
  Services
200 Independence Avenue SW,
  Room 740G
Washington, DC 20201

Robert Gellman, J.D.
Chief Counsel
Subcommittee on Government
  Information, Justice, and
  Agriculture
House Committee on Government
  Operations
Washington, DC 20515-6147

Betsy Gettig, M.S.
President-Elect
National Society of Genetic
  Counselors
Director of Genetic Counseling
West Penn Hospital School of Nursing
2nd Floor, Room 205
Pittsburgh, PA 15224

David Micklos
Director
DNA Learning Center
Cold Spring Harbor Laboratory
Cold Spring Harbor, NY 11724

Walter Nance, M.D., Ph.D.
Department of Medical Genetics
Medical College of Virginia
Box 33, MCV Station
Richmond, VA 23298

Madison Powers, J.D.
Kennedy Institute of Bioethics
Georgetown University
209 Poulton Hall
Washington, DC 20057

Virginia Proud, M.D.
Laboratory of Medical Genetics
University of Alabama at Birmingham
Byrd Building 323, UAB Station
Birmingham, AL 35294

Kimberly Quaid, Ph.D.
Department of Medical Genetics
Indiana University School of
  Medicine
975 West Walnut Street
Indianapolis, IN 46202-5251

Elizabeth Thomson, R.N., M.S.
Coordinator
Iowa Statewide Genetic Counseling
 Services
Coordinator, Cystic Fibrosis Pilot
 Project Consortium (National
 Center for Human Genome
 Research)
Division of Medical Genetics
Department of Pediatrics
University Hospitals and Clinics
Iowa City, IA 52242

Michael Yesley, J.D.
Los Alamos National Laboratory
Department of Energy
M5 A187, P.O. Box 1663
Los Alamos, NM 87545

PARTICIPANTS IN THE SEPTEMBER 1992 PUBLIC FORUM ON ASSESSING GENETIC RISKS: ISSUES AND IMPLICATIONS FOR HEALTH

Judith L. Benkendorf, M.S.
Genetic Counselor and Assistant
 Professor
Division of Genetics
Department of Obstetrics and
 Gynecology
Georgetown University Medical
 Center
Washington, D.C. 20007

Ruby Bishop
President-Elect
Alliance of Genetic Support Groups
7101 W. 12th, Suite 401
Little Rock, AR 72204

Hope Charkins, M.S.W.
Executive Director
Treacher Collins Foundation
P.O. Box 683
Norwich, VT 05055

Elizabeth Fain
2765 Stockwood Drive
Gastonia, NC 28056

Penelope Fischer
983 1st Place
Longwood, FL 32750

Helen Bequaert Holmes
Center for Genetics, Ethics and
 Women
24 Berkshire Terrace
Amherst, MA 01002

Edward M. Kloza, M.S.
President
National Society of Genetic
 Counselors, Inc.
233 Canterbury Drive
Wallingford, PA 19086

Sue Levi-Pearl
Liaison for Medical and Scientific
 Programs
Tourette Syndrome Association,
 Inc.
42-40 Bell Boulevard
Bayside, NY 11361

Abbey S. Meyers
Executive Director
National Organization for Rare
    Disorders, Inc.
100 Route 37, P.O. Box 8923
New Fairfield, CT 06812-1783

C. Ben Mitchell, M.Div.
Director of Biomedical and Life
    Issues
The Christian Life Commission of
    the Southern Baptist Convention
901 Commerce Street, Suite 550
P.O. Box 25266
Nashville, TN 37202-5266

Theresa E. Morelli
200 Fernwood Road, Apt. 22
Wintersville, OH 43952

Marsha Saxton, J.D.
Project on Women and Disabilities
1 Ashburton Place, Room 130
Boston, MA 02108

Dorothy C. Wertz, Ph.D.
Social Science, Ethics and Law
The Shriver Center
200 Trapelo Road
Waltham, MA 02254

Nachama Wilker
Executive Director
The Council for Responsible
    Genetics
19 Garden Street
Cambridge, MA 02138-3622

APPENDIX B

Committee Biographies

LORI B. ANDREWS is a Visiting Professor of Law at Chicago-Kent College of Law, on leave from her position as Research Fellow at the American Bar Foundation. For the past six years, she has also been a Senior Scholar at the Center for Clinical Medical Ethics at the University of Chicago. She has been a member of advisory panels to the World Health Organization, the Centers for Disease Control and Prevention, the U.S. Department of Health and Human Services, and the Office of Technology Assessment of the U.S. Congress, and she has taught health law courses at the University of Houston Law Center, the University of Chicago School of Law, and the Graduate School of Business at the University of Chicago. Ms. Andrews is the author of *Medical Genetics: A Legal Frontier* (1987). She has also written three other books and more than fifty scholarly articles, monographs, and book chapters on subjects including medical genetics, informed consent, and alternative modes of reproduction. She received her B.A. *summa cum laude* from Yale College and her J.D. from Yale Law School.

BARBARA BOWLES BIESECKER is Genetic Counselor and Section Head in the Medical Genetics Branch of the National Center for Human Genome Research at the National Institutes of Health, Bethesda, Maryland. She obtained her M.S. degree from the University of Michigan in 1981 and has held six genetic counseling positions at several universities in the midwest. She has been President of the National Society of Genetic Counselors and Associate Director of the Genetic Counseling Graduate Program at the University of Michigan. Her areas of interest include research in genetic counseling, the psychological ramifications of genetic disorders, and the implications of gene testing.

JAMES F. CHILDRESS is the Edwin B. Kyle Professor of Religious Studies and professor of medical education at the University of Virginia, where he is also chairman of the Department of Religious Studies and principal of the Monroe Hill Residential College. He is the author of numerous articles and several books on biomedical ethics, including *Principles of Biomedical Ethics* (with Tom L. Beauchamp), *Priorities in Biomedical Ethics*, and *Who Should Decide? Paternalism in Health Care*. Formerly vice chairman of the National Task Force on Organ Transplantation, he serves on the Board of Directors of the United Network for Organ Sharing and is a member of the Recombinant DNA Advisory Committee, the Human Gene Therapy Subcommittee, and the Biomedical Ethics Advisory Committee. He is a fellow of the American Academy of Arts and Sciences and of the Hastings Center, and he has been the Joseph P. Kennedy, Sr., Professor of Christian Ethics at Georgetown University and a visiting professor at the University of Chicago Divinity School and Princeton University. He received his B.A. from Guilford College, his B.D. from Yale Divinity School, and his M.A. and Ph.D. from Yale University.

BARTON CHILDS is Emeritus Professor of Pediatrics at The Johns Hopkins University School of Medicine. He obtained his M.D. degree at Johns Hopkins and trained there in pediatrics. His education in genetics was obtained at University College, London. Dr. Childs was chairman of the National Research Council committee on Genetic Screening in 1972-1975.

FRANCIS S. COLLINS is Director of the National Center for Human Genome Research at the National Institutes of Health. He was formerly a Howard Hughes Medical Institute investigator and professor in the Departments of Internal Medicine and Human Genetics at the University of Michigan School of Medicine in Ann Arbor. Dr. Collins pioneered the development of positional cloning, which utilizes the inheritance pattern of a disease within families to pinpoint the location of a gene. He and his colleagues have used the technique to isolate the genes for cystic fibrosis, neurofibromatosis type 1, and Huntington disease. Dr. Collins received a Ph.D. degree in physical chemistry from Yale University and an M.D. degree from the University of North Carolina School of Medicine. Dr. Collins is a member of the National Academy of Sciences and the Institute of Medicine. He is also a member of the Board of Directors of the American Society of Human Genetics, the American Federation for Clinical Research, the American Society for Clinical Investigation, the Association of American Physicians, and sits on the executive council of the International Human Genome Organization. He serves as an associate editor for several publications.

P. MICHAEL CONNEALLY is Distinguished Professor of Medical and Molecular Genetics and of Neurology at Indiana University Medical Center, Indianapolis, Indiana. He obtained his Ph.D. degree at the University of Wisconsin in 1962.

He serves on several editorial boards and also on the scientific advisory boards of eight lay organizations for specific genetic disorders. Dr. Conneally has been involved in the genetic mapping of numerous human inherited diseases and has trained a number of human population geneticists.

HELEN R. DONIS-KELLER is Professor of Surgery and Genetics in the Department of Surgery at Washington University School of Medicine in St. Louis, Missouri. She is also Director of the Division of Human Molecular Genetics in the Surgery Department. She obtained her Ph.D. degree in biochemistry and molecular biology at Harvard University in 1979. Her research interests include mapping genes responsible for human diseases, such as cystic fibrosis and multiple endocrine neoplasia type 2. She has also been active in the development of predictive DNA tests for these and other disorders. Prior to joining Washington University, she was Director of the Department of Human Genetics at Collaborative Research Incorporated and a former Assistant Director for Research at Biogen Incorporated.

NORMAN C. FOST is Professor and Vice Chairman of Pediatrics and Director of the Program in Medical Ethics at the University of Wisconsin School of Medicine. He is a graduate of Princeton (A.B., 1960), Yale (M.D., 1964), and Harvard (M.P.H., 1973). He is Past-Chairman of the American Academy of Pediatrics Committee on Bioethics and was a member of the White House Interagency Task Force on Health Reform. At the University of Wisconsin he is Director of the Residency Training Program, Chairman of the Hospital Ethics Committee, Chairman of the Institutional Review Board, and heads the Child Protection Team. His interest in ethical issues in genetics goes back to 1973 when he was a consultant to the National Academy of Sciences Committee on Screening for Inborn Errors of Metabolism, whose report, *Genetic Screening: Programs, Principles and Research*, was published in 1975. He was a member of the National Institutes of Health Workshop on Population Screening for the Cystic Fibrosis Gene, a member of the American Society of Human Genetics (ASHG) Committee on Cf Heterozygote Detection, and Cochair of the ASHG Committee on Insurance. Dr. Fost is the author of numerous publications on ethical and legal issues in genetics, including recent papers with Benjamin Wilfond on the social implications of the discovery of the gene for cystic fibrosis.

NEIL A. HOLTZMAN is Professor of Pediatrics at the Johns Hopkins University School of Medicine and has joint appointments in Health Policy and Management and in Epidemiology at the School of Hygiene and Public Health. Dr. Holtzman conducted biochemical research on genetic diseases before turning to policy studies dealing primarily with genetic screening and technology diffusion. He also organized the Pediatric Genetics Unit at the Johns Hopkins Hospital and was Coordinator for Hereditary Disorders Services for the Maryland Department of

Health and Mental Hygiene. He served as a Senior Analyst at Office of Technology Assessment of the U.S. Congress. In 1989, Dr. Holtzman's book *Proceed with Caution: Predicting Genetic Risks in the Recombinant DNA Era*, was published by the Johns Hopkins University Press. Dr. Holtzman currently has grants from the NIH Ethical, Legal, and Social Implications (ELSI) component of the Human Genome Project to study the diffusion of genetic technologies.

MICHAEL M. KABACK is Professor of Pediatrics and Reproductive Medicine and Chief of the Division of Medical Genetics (Peds) at the University of California at San Diego School of Medicine. He also serves as the Director of the State of California Tay-Sachs Disease Prevention Program, past president of the Western Society for Pediatric Research, past president (1991) of the Society of Human Genetics, and North American Editor of "Prenatal Diagnosis." Dr. Kaback's major research interests include: the application of genetic technologies to the control of human genetic disease, psychosocial issues in genetic screening, and genotype-phenotype correlations in the lysosomal storage disorders.

MARY-CLAIRE KING is Professor of Epidemiology and Human Genetics at the University of California at Berkeley. Her research centers on the genetics and epidemiology of breast cancer and other common chronic diseases, pedigree analysis, and human and primate molecular evolution. Dr. King received her B.A. from Carleton College and her Ph.D. in genetics from the University of California at Berkeley. She is a member of the American Epidemiological Society, the American Society of Human Genetics, and the Society for Epidemiological Research.

PATRICIA A. KING is a Professor of Law at Georgetown University Law Center. She is a graduate of Wheaton College (1963) and Harvard Law School (1969). She specialized in family law and the relationship between biomedical ethics, law, and public policy, particularly related to reproduction. Professor King has served on numerous public bodies concerning biomedicine and public policy. They include the National Commission for Protection of Human Subjects of Biomedical and Behavioral Research, the President's Commission for the Study of Ethical Problems in Medicine and Biomedical and Behavioral Research, and the Human Fetal Tissue Transplantation Research Panel. Professor King is a member of the Institute of Medicine.

ALEXANDER LEAF is Jackson Professor of Medicine, Emeritus, Harvard Medical School and former Chief of Medicine, Massachusetts General Hospital and former Ridley Watts Professor of Preventive Medicine and Chairman, Department of Preventive Medicine and Clinical Epidemiology, Harvard Medical School. He is currently a Distinguished Physician at the West Roxbury VA Medical Center. He is a member of the National Academy of Sciences and of the

Institute of Medicine. Professor Leaf has participated on several NAS and IOM committees. He has authored over 300 scientific and policy articles and books.

PETER LIBASSI is Dean of the Barney School of Business and Public Administration at the University of Hartford. His prior careers have included business, law, nonprofit and government service, including: Senior Vice President, Travelers Insurance Company; General Counsel, U.S. Department of Health, Education, and Welfare; Deputy Staff Director, U.S. Commission on Civil Rights; and Executive Director, National Urban Coalition. He has served on several national and state commissions on health, aging, and public policy, including: the Department of Health and Human Services Secretary's Task Force on Long-Term Care; Governor's Commission on Long-Term-Care Insurance; National Academy of Sciences Committee on an Aging Society; Pew Commission on Health Professionals; and Commonwealth Fund Commissions on Elderly Living Alone and on Health Care Reform. He is a graduate of Colgate University and Yale Law School.

ARNO G. MOTULSKY is Professor of Medicine and Genetics at the University of Washington, Seattle, Washington. He obtained his M.D. degree at the University of Illinois in 1947, and trained in internal medicine and medical genetics. He was President of the American Society of Human Genetics, and editor of the *American Journal of Human Genetics*. He serves on multiple editorial boards. Dr. Motulsky is a member of the National Academy of Sciences and the Institute of Medicine. In the 1970s he participated in the NRC committee on genetic screening and in the 1980s he served on the President's Commission for the Study of Ethical Problems in Medicine and Biomedical and Behavioral Research. He has received a variety of awards for his work. Dr. Motulsky has authored over 300 scientific publications, is coauthor of an influential textbook in his field, and has trained many medical geneticists.

ROBERT F. MURRAY, JR., is Chief of the Division of Medical Genetics in the Department of Pediatrics and Child Health, and Professor of Pediatrics, Medicine, and Oncology at Howard University College of Medicine. He is also Chairman of the Graduate Department of Genetics and Human Genetics in the Graduate School of Arts and Sciences at Howard University. He is a member of the Institute of Medicine and has served on the IOM Council and also on several National Research Council and IOM task forces and working groups. He is a fellow and member of the Board of Directors of the Hastings Center on Bioethics, and a fellow of the American Association for the Advancement of Science. He has served on the Recombinant DNA Advisory Committee (RAC) and the Human Gene Therapy Subcommittee of the RAC and the Working Group on Ethics, Law, and Social Issues (ELSI) of the National Center for Human Genome Research at NIH. He is coauthor with Dr. James Bowman of "Genetic Variation and Disorders in Peoples of African Origin," published in 1990 by Johns Hopkins University Press and has coedited two other books on mental retardation and genetic counseling. Dr. Murray is a graduate of Union College (B.S.) and the University of Rochester School of Medicine (M.D.). He is board certified in both internal medicine and medical genetics.

MARK A. ROTHSTEIN is Law Foundation Professor of Law and Director of the Health Law and Policy Institute of the University of Houston. He is a graduate of the University of Pittsburgh (B.A., 1970) and Georgetown University Law Center (J.D., 1973). Professor Rothstein specializes in the ethical and legal issues raised by the use of medical information in the nonclinical setting, including employment and insurance. He is the author of numerous books and articles on these and related issues. Professor Rothstein also has served as an adviser to the Office of Technology Assessment of the United States Congress, the U.S. Department of Energy, American Medical Association, and other organizations.

CLAUDIA T. WEICKER serves on the boards of the National Mental Health Association, the Stewart B. McKinney Foundation, and the National Abortion Rights Action League. She serves on the advisory boards of the University of Connecticut Children's Cancer Fund and the Department of Psychiatry at the Yale University School of Medicine. She was Staff Director of the Subcommittee on Appropriations and then Staff Director of the Subcommittee on Labor, Health, Human Services and Education of the U.S. Senate. She is a graduate of Hartford College for Women and of Marymount College. Since 1991, when her husband, Lowell P. Weicker, Jr. became Governor of Connecticut, she has been an advocate on health and children's issues, and has served as the honorary chairwoman of the Connecticut Commission on Children's "Kids Count" Campaign, which emphasizes school readiness and preventive health care for the state's children.

NANCY SABIN WEXLER is Professor of Clinical Neuropsychology in the Departments of Neurology and Psychiatry at Columbia University and President of the Hereditary Disease Foundation, Santa Monica, California. She received an A.B. degree *cum laude* from Radcliffe College in 1967, and a Ph.D. in clinical psychology from the University of Michigan in 1974. Beginning in 1968, Dr. Wexler's most important scientific contribution is her work on Huntington disease. For the last 13 years she and her colleagues have studied the disease and collected blood samples from members of the world's largest family with Huntington disease in Venezuela. These samples led to the localization of the Huntington disease gene in 1983 and the discovery of the gene in March 1993. Dr. Wexler is a member of the Program Advisory Committee of the National Center for Human Genome Research at the National Institutes of Health (NIH). She chairs the Joint NIH/DOE Ethical, Legal, and Social Implications Working Group on the Human Genome (ELSI) and co-chairs the Ethics Committee of the Human

Genome Organization (HUGO). Within the last two years, Nancy Wexler was elected to the Board of Directors, American Association for the Advancement of Science, awarded an Honorary Doctor of Humane Letters from New York Medical College, an Honorary Doctor of Science from the University of Michigan, the Distinguished Service Award from the National Association of Biology Teachers, and the Albert Lasker Public Service Award.

Index